Sampling for Health Professionals

PAUL S. LEVY
School of Public Health
University of Illinois

STANLEY LEMESHOW
Division of Public Health
University of Massachusetts

Lifetime Learning Publications
Belmont, California
A Division of Wadsworth, Inc.

To our wives, Lorraine and Elaine and our children

Printed in the United States of America

2   3   4   5   6   7   8   9   10———84   83   82   81

Library of Congress Cataloging in Publication Data

Levy, Paul S
    Sampling for health professionals.

    Includes bibliographies and index.
    1. Health surveys—Statistical methods.   2. Sampling (Statistics)   I. Lemeshow, Stanley, joint author.   II. Title.   [DNLM: 1. Sampling studies.   2. Statistics. WA950   L668s]
RA409.L49   362.1′0723   80-14733
ISBN 0-534-97986-6

Contents

List of Tables

List of Boxes

Preface

Statistical methods are now being used widely at all levels by health agencies and organizations. Correspondingly, there are now many individuals who serve as resident statisticians to these organizations. The primary objective of this book is to meet the needs of these working statisticians.

Since a person does not need a license to serve as a statistician, in contrast to the situation for a physician or a plumber, the backgrounds of health statisticians show tremendous variation. While some have graduate training to the masters or even doctoral level in a statistical science, many others have minimum formal education in statistics but considerable field and bench experience gained from actual work situations. We have endeavored to write this book in such a way that it could be understood by anyone having familiarity with basic statistical concepts yet at the same time not offend or be useful to someone with considerable formal statistical education.

Since this book addresses as primary audience the working health statistician, it should serve to fulfill his or her professional needs with respect to sample survey methodology. With this in mind, we list the following skills that the reader should acquire from studying this material.

1. Ability to recognize the type of inputs that are needed in planning a sample survey and to gather, with the aid of consultants, if needed, sufficient information to write a detailed survey plan.

2. Ability to handle the statistical aspects of a sample survey from the initial sampling plan to the writing of the final statistical report, provided that the

complexity of the survey is not greater than that treated in this book and the scope of the survey is relatively small. This objective would include data management (quality control, preparation, processing, analysis) as well as sampling.

3. Ability to furnish advice concerning costs, feasibility, statistical problems, and measurement problems in connection with a proposed sample survey.

We do not feel that the reader of this book will emerge as an expert in sample survey methodology. We do feel, however, that this book will enable the reader to handle the statistical aspects of the type of surveys likely to be encountered in practice.

Although this book is designed primarily for the working statistician, we feel that it can serve, in addition, as a primary text for a course in sample survey methods that emphasizes applications rather than theory. Portions of this book have been used by the authors as notes for a one-semester course in sample survey methodology at the University of Massachusetts and for a one-quarter course given at the University of Illinois. The book might also be useful as supplementary reading for more formal theoretical sampling courses, since it can help furnish a bridge linking theory and practical use.

Over the past fifteen years there has been a proliferation of books on statistical methods. Only a handful of these, however, are concerned with sample survey methodology. Statisticians with primary interests in sample survey methodology are generally found not at academic institutions but at organizations that are responsible for planning and conducting sample surveys. Typically these statisticians do not put a high priority on writing textbooks. Since the relatively small number of existing books on sample survey methods have objectives different from ours, we feel that our book will satisfy a need not presently met.

There are several books on sampling methodology that could serve as supplementary reading to this text. For example, W. G. Cochran's book, *Sampling Techniques* (New York: Wiley, 1977), now in its third edition, is written at a higher mathematical level than this book. The two-volume classic text by Hansen, Hurwitz, and Madow, *Sample Survey Methods and Theory* (Vols. 1 and 2; New York: Wiley, 1953), is of most use to the professional survey statistician as a reference book, as are the books by Kish, *Survey Sampling* (New York: Wiley, 1965), and Jessen, *Statistical Survey Techniques* (New York: Wiley, 1978). A recent book by Scheaffer, Mendenhall, and Ott, *Elementary Survey Sampling* (2d ed.; N. Scituate, MA: Duxbury Press, 1979), is at approximately the same mathematical level as this book and has many examples and exercises. Another recent book, *A Sampler on Sampling* (New York: Wiley, 1978), by B. Williams, makes use of examples and an intuitive approach. Finally, the excellent monograph series on health survey methods published by the National Center for Health Statistics treats topics of importance in health surveys. The publications mentioned above are all excellent companion readings to this book.

We anticipate that this book will be read by several types of practitioners as well as by students taking formal courses in sample survey methodology. We list below the parts of this book that would be most important for each type of reader.

USER	CHAPTERS OR SECTIONS TO BE READ
Practitioner requiring knowledge of major issues involved in survey sampling (e.g., administrator of an agency that makes decisions on the basis of surveys conducted by contractors).	1–7, 9, 10.1, 11.1, 12.1, 13.1, 13.2, 13.4, 14, 15.1, 15.2
Practitioner serving as project officer on a contract involving a sample survey conducted by a contractor; statistician being trained to work in a survey research organization.	All
Student taking a one-semester course in sample survey methods (42 lecture hours).	1–7, 9–15
Student taking a one-quarter course in sample survey methods (30 lecture hours).	1–7, 9, 10.1, 11.1, 12.1, 13.1, 13.2, 14, 15

Acknowledgments

We are grateful to our public health students, both at the University of Massachusetts and the University of Illinois, who have used earlier versions of this book and have given us the benefits of their comments. In particular, Jill Spitz, Harriet Peterson, and Jim Melius have spent many hours jotting down problems occurring in earlier versions and working out numerical examples. In addition, we are indebted to Suzanne Harris for her excellent typing of the final versions of this book, to Connie Grant for her typing of earlier versions, to Carol Beal for her substantive comments and fine editing of the manuscript, and to Alex Kugushev for his continuous encouragement and support. Finally, we would like to thank the dean of the School of Health Sciences, University of Massachusetts, William Darity, and the chairman of the Biostatistics/Epidemiology Program Area, Stuart Hartz, for providing us with the resources to pursue this project to its final conclusion, and Christine Forman for organizing and coordinating these resources.

1

Uses of Sample Surveys in Health Professions

1.1 WHY SAMPLE SURVEYS ARE USED

Suppose the Massachusetts State Health Department is interested in determining the proportion of the state's elementary schoolchildren who have been immunized against polio and measles. For administrative reasons only one month is available to gather the necessary information.

At first glance this task would seem to be most formidable, involving the careful coordination of a large staff attempting to collect information, either from parents or medical records, on each and every elementary schoolchild in the state. Clearly the necessary budget for such an undertaking would be enormous because of the time, travel expenses, and numbers of children involved. Even with a sizable staff, it would be difficult to meet the relatively tight time constraint.

To handle problems like the one outlined above, this text will present a variety of methods for selecting a subset—a **sample**—from the original set of all measurements—the **population**—of interest to the researchers. It is the members of this sample who will be interviewed, studied, or measured. For example, in the problem above the net effect of such methods will be that precise estimates of the proportions of children who have been immunized will be obtained at a great reduction of time, expense, and effort.

The use of a sample reduces costs and time

More formally, a **sample survey** may be defined as a study involving a subset (or sample) of individuals selected from a larger population. Variables or characteristics of interest are observed or measured on each of the sampled individuals. These measurements are then aggregated over all individuals in the

Sample surveys produce summary statistics

1

Summary statistics produce estimates of population values

sample to obtain **summary statistics** (e.g., means, proportions, totals) for the sample. It is from these summary statistics that extrapolations can be made concerning the entire population. The validity and reliability of these extrapolations depend on how well the sample was chosen and how well the measurements were made. These issues constitute the subject matter of this text.

A census measures all members of a population

When all the individuals in the population are selected for measurement, the study is called a **census.** The summary statistics obtained from a census are not extrapolations, since all members of the population are measured. The validity of the resulting statistics, however, still depends on how well the measurements are made. The main advantages of sample surveys over censuses lie in the reduced cost and greater speed made possible by taking measurements on a subset rather than on an entire population. In addition, studies involving complex issues requiring elaborate measurement procedures are often feasible only if a sample of the population is selected for measurement, since limited resources can be allocated to getting detailed measurements if the number of individuals to be measured is not too great.

In the health professions sample surveys are widely used to obtain information for both research and administrative purposes. In fact, the National Center for Health Statistics (NCHS), a bureau within the Department of Health, Education, and Welfare, is mandated by Public Law 91-515 to develop and conduct a program of periodic and ongoing sample surveys designed to obtain information about illness, disability, and utilization of health care services in the United States (5).* The surveys developed by NCHS usually have very complex designs and require very large, highly skilled staffs (and hence large budgets) for their execution. While such elaborate and expensive procedures are justifiable for the type of general purpose health survey conducted by NCHS, in which typically a very large amount of data is obtained from each individual selected, the costs inherent in such complex surveys are generally not justified in the types of surveys needed by most health professionals. Very often, health professionals require answers to a limited set of questions that can be obtained in a single one-shot survey. Thus in this text we will discuss only those survey methods that we feel will meet the needs of most health professionals.

Sample surveys along with cohort studies and case-control studies are three types of observational studies used in the health sciences

Sample surveys belong to a larger class of nonexperimental studies generally given the name "observational studies," which include cohort studies as well as retrospective case-control studies. An example of a cohort study in the health sciences is the famous Framingham cardiovascular disease study in which a sample of individuals 30 years and over was chosen and observed throughout the years with the objective of determining those factors related to development of cardiovascular disease (2). Retrospective case-control studies are those in which a group of persons with a condition or disease is selected

---

* Numbers in parentheses in the text refer to a source cited in the Bibliography found at the end of each chapter. Each bibliography contains an annotated listing of publications that you may find useful in studying or applying the material of that chapter.

and a *control group* of persons without the condition or disease is chosen; both groups are measured with respect to variables thought to be associated with the condition or disease. Examples of such retrospective studies are abundant in epidemiologic literature (1, 3). Studies such as those mentioned above are generally designed with the objective of testing some statement—or **hypothesis** (e.g., association between heart disease and elevated serum lipids)—concerning a set of dependent variables and another set of independent variables.

While these studies are very important in the health sciences, they do not comprise the subject matter of this text. The type of study of concern here is often known as a **descriptive survey.** Its main objective is that of **estimating** the level of a set of variables in a population. For example, in the hypothetical problem presented at the outset of this chapter, the major objective is to estimate, through the use of a sample, the proportion of all elementary school-children who have been immunized for polio and measles. In descriptive surveys much attention is given to the selection of the sample since extrapolation is made from the sample to the population. Although hypotheses can be tested based on data collected from descriptive surveys, this is generally a secondary objective in surveys. Estimation is almost always the primary objective.

Estimation of population values is the primary objective of sample surveys

1.2 DESIGNING SAMPLE SURVEYS

In this section we will discuss the four major components involved in designing sample surveys. These are sample design, survey measurements, survey operations, and statistical analysis and report writing.

Sample Design

In a sample survey the major statistical components are often referred to as the **sample design** and include both the sampling plan and the estimation procedures. The **sampling plan** is the methodology used for choosing the sample from the population. The **estimation procedures** are the algorithms or formulas used for obtaining estimates of population values from the sample data and for estimating the reliability of these population estimates.

The choice of a particular sample design should be a collaborative effort involving input from the statistician who will design the survey, the persons involved in executing the survey, and those who will use the data from the survey. The data users should specify what variables will be measured, what estimates are required, what levels of reliability and validity are needed for the estimates, and what restrictions are placed on the survey with respect to time and budget. Those individuals involved in executing the survey should furnish input about costs for personnel, time, and materials as well as input about the feasibility of alternative sampling and measurement procedures. Having received such input, the statistician can then propose a sample design that will meet the required specifications of the users at the lowest possible cost.

The statistician provides the sample design

Survey Measurements

Just as sampling and estimation are the statistician's responsibilities in the design of a sample survey, the choice of measurements to be taken and the procedures for taking these measurements are the responsibilities of those individuals who are experts in the subject matter of the survey and also of those individuals who are experts in taking measurements. Those individuals who are experts in the substantive issues of the study (often called "subject matter persons") give most input into specifying what measurements are needed to meet the objectives of the survey. Once these measurements are specified, the measurement experts—who are often sociologists or psychologists with special skills in survey research—begin designing the questionnaires or forms to be used in eliciting the data from the sample individuals. The design of a questionnaire or other survey instrument, which must produce valid and reliable data, is often a very complex task; it requires considerable care and sometimes a preliminary study, especially if some of the variables to be measured have never been measured before by survey.

Subject matter experts and measurement experts plan the survey measurements

Once the survey instruments have been drafted, the statistician provides input with respect to measures to be taken to evaluate and assure the quality of the data. In addition, the statistician ensures that the data can be easily coded and processed for statistical analysis.

Survey Operations

Once the sample has been chosen and the measuring instruments or questionnaires drafted, pretested, and modified, the field work of the survey—including data collection—can then begin. But before the data collection starts, there should be a dry run or a pilot survey on a small sample, with the objective of testing the measuring instruments and eliminating the imperfections in the survey procedures.

The first step in survey operations is data collection

In order for the estimates resulting from the sample survey to be valid and reliable, it is important that the data be collected in accordance with the survey design, and it is the task of those individuals responsible for survey operations to oversee this procedure. The nature of the survey operations staff depends on the size and scope of the sample survey, the complexity of the measurements, and the nature of the survey (i.e., a one-shot study or an ongoing study). For example, the Health and Nutrition Examination Survey (HANES), a complex nationwide sample survey conducted through NCHS by means of physical examinations and interviews, has a large operations staff and an operations budget of over $1 million annually (4). On the other hand, a sample survey having only a limited set of objectives can be executed with a small operations staff.

Whether the survey is large or small, complicated or relatively simple, the survey operations should be very carefully planned so that the data can be collected according to design in an orderly manner and with enough flexibility to enable occasional crises to be handled.

In addition to data collection, survey operations also include preparation and processing of data. Data preparation generally involves those operations performed after the data are collected that result in the production of an edited (or clean) data set. Modern data preparation operations include coding the data, putting data in machine-readable form by keypunching or some other method, and editing the data by use of computer programs. To ensure the quality of the final data set, it is important that these operations be carefully planned and that quality control procedures be instituted as part of the data preparation activities. Data processing generally involves production of the desired statistics or estimates from the edited data set and production of estimates of the reliability (e.g., variances, standard errors) of these estimates. Often data processing involves the use of standard statistical computer programs such as the *Statistical Package for the Social Sciences* (SPSS) (7), the *Biomedical Computer Programs* (BMD) (6), or other so-called packaged programs. Such general purpose statistical programs have the advantages of being well developed and tested for accuracy, readily available on most computer systems, and easy to use. They have the disadvantage inherent in all general systems—namely, that they are not specific to any single data set. Sometimes, however, they can be used in conjunction with programs written specifically for the data set being processed.

The second step is data preparation and processing

Statistical Analysis and Report Writing

After the data have been collected, coded, edited, and processed, the data can be analyzed statistically and the findings incorporated into a final report. As in all components of a sample survey, considerable care should be taken in the interpretation of the findings of the survey. These findings are in the form of estimated characteristics of the population from which the sample was taken. These estimates, however, are subject to both sampling and measurement errors, and any interpretation of the findings should take these errors into consideration. In many projects involving sample surveys, ample time and resources are allocated to the design of the sample, the development of the measuring instruments or questionnaires, and the survey operations, but very little time and resources are allocated to the final statistical analysis and report writing. This situation is unfortunate, because the impact of the findings is often lost through lack of effort at this last stage. In this text an entire chapter (chapter 15) is devoted to the analysis of data arising from sample surveys and to the writing of statistical reports about the findings of sample surveys.

Sampling and measurement errors must be considered in this final stage

1.3 PRELIMINARY PLANNING OF A SAMPLE SURVEY

In the previous section we discussed the major components involved in a sample survey. From that discussion it should be evident that a sample survey can be a considerable undertaking, requiring much in the way of time and resources, both material and human. It should also be evident that serious consideration should be given to deciding whether or not to conduct a sample survey. And once the decision to go ahead is made, serious thought should be given to formulating the survey objectives and specifications before work on the survey design begins.

First, consider objectives, alternatives, and uses of data

In the preliminary-planning stage those individuals contemplating a sample survey should formulate the objectives of the proposed survey. The objectives should include specification of the information to be gathered and of the population to which the findings of the survey will be extrapolated. Alternatives to a survey should be discussed, such as secondary analysis of data already collected. Careful consideration should be given to the use of the data collected from the proposed survey, especially the decisions that will be made on the basis of the findings of the survey. This step will determine whether it is worthwhile to conduct the survey at all and, if so, how accurate the resulting estimates should be.

Second, consider subdomains of population and resources available

In the preliminary-planning stage thought should be given to the various subdomains of the population (e.g., age groups, sex groups, race groups) for which estimates are required and to the level of accuracy required for these estimates. Additional thought should be given to the resources that are available in terms of budget and personnel and the time frame in which the data are needed. The resolution of these issues helps to determine whether it is feasible to plan and conduct a sample survey and, if so, to determine the required configuration of the survey in terms of its components.

BIBLIOGRAPHY

The following publications give good examples of the use of sample surveys in the health professions.

1. HERBST, A. L.; ULFEDLER, H.; and POSKANZER, D. C. Association of maternal stilbestrol therapy with tumor appearance in young women. *New England Journal of Medicine* (1971) 284:878.
2. KANNEL, W. B. An epidemiologic study of cerebrovascular disease. In *Fifth conference on cerebral vascular diseases*, ed. R. G. Siekert, and J. P. Whisnat. New York and London: Grune and Stratton, 1966.
3. SARTWELL, P. E. Oral contraceptives and thromboembolism: A further report. *American Journal of Epidemiology* (1971) 94:102.

The following publications contain data that are useful for sample surveys in the health professions.

4. National Center for Health Statistics. *Plan and operation of the health and nutrition examination survey, United States, 1971–1973.* Vital and Health Statistics, Series 1, No. 10a, DHEW Publication No. (HRA) 76-1310. Washington, DC: U.S. Government Printing Office, 1973.
5. National Center for Health Statistics. *Current listing and topical index to the vital and health statistics,* Series 1962–1972, DHEW Publication No. (HSM) 73-1301 (revised). Washington, DC: U.S. Government Printing Office, 1973.

The following packaged programs are useful for performing many statistical calculations involved in sample surveys.

6. DIXON, W. J., and BROWN, M. B., eds. *BMDP-77: Biomedical computer programs,* P-Series. Berkeley: University of California Press, 1977.
7. NIE, N. H.; HULL, C. H.; JENKINS, J. G.; STEINBRENNER, K.; and BENT, D. H. *SPSS: Statistical package for the social sciences.* 2d ed. New York: McGraw-Hill, 1973.

2

The Population and the Sample

In the previous chapter we discussed sample surveys as studies that estimate characteristics of a population by means of a subset taken from the population. Sample selection is performed according to some method that allows reliable and valid inferences to be drawn from the sample to the population. In this chapter we develop the foundations of sampling methodology by first defining the components of a population in terms that are meaningful with respect to taking a sample from it. Once these properties of the population have been defined and discussed, we then begin the development of sampling methodology.

2.1 THE POPULATION

The **population** (or **universe** or **target population**) is the entire set of individuals to which the findings of the survey are to be extrapolated. In this text we use the terms "universe," "target population," and "population" interchangeably.

The individual members of the population whose characteristics are to be measured are called the **elementary units** or **elements** of the population. For example, if we are conducting a sample survey for purposes of estimating the number of persons living in Illinois who have never visited a dentist, the universe includes all persons living in Illinois, and each person living in Illinois is an elementary unit. If we are conducting a sample survey of in-hospital records for purposes of estimating the number of discharges during a given year with specified diagnoses, each discharge occurring during the year is an element, and the totality of such discharges constitutes the population.

In the conduct of sample surveys it is often not convenient to sample the elementary units directly because lists of elementary units from which the sample can be taken are not readily available and cannot be constructed without great difficulty or expense. Often, however, elementary units can be associated with other kinds of units for which lists can be constructed for purposes of sampling. These other kinds of units are known as **enumeration units** or **listing units.** An enumeration unit or listing unit may contain one or more elementary unit and can be identified prior to the drawing of the sample. For example, suppose that a sample survey is being planned in western Massachusetts for purposes of determining the number of persons in Hampshire County who have been immunized for measles. The population in this instance consists of all persons living in this county, and the elementary units are the individual persons in the county. It is very unlikely that an accurate and up-to-date list of all persons living in this county will be available or easily obtainable. If it were, a sample could be drawn from this list. However, it is conceivable that a list of all households in the county is available or at least could be obtained without great difficulty or expense. If such a list is available, a sample of households can be drawn, and those persons residing in the sample households are taken as the sample elementary units. The households are the enumeration units.

Enumeration units contain one or more elementary units and can be identified more easily than elementary units

If a sample is to be drawn from a list of enumeration units, it is necessary to specify by some algorithm the elementary units that are to be associated with each enumeration unit. Such an algorithm is called a **counting rule** or **enumeration rule.** In the household survey mentioned above for estimating the number of persons in Hampshire County who are immunized for measles, the elementary units are the persons living in the county, and the households are the enumeration units. The counting rule in this example might specify that all individuals living in a particular household be associated with that household.

The counting rule links the elementary units to the enumeration units

In the Hamsphire County example the counting rule is obvious and straightforward. Sometimes, however, the counting rule that associates elementary units with enumeration units is not so obvious. For example, suppose we wish to estimate the number of persons in California who have a relatively rare and severe disease such as multiple sclerosis. It would make sense in this instance to take a sample survey of health care providers (e.g., physicians and hospitals) and to obtain from them information about the individuals under their care for the particular disease. Since an individual with the disease may be receiving or may have received care from several sources, there is more than one reasonable way of linking cases (elementary units) to sources (enumeration units). For example, one counting rule might allow a case to be linked to the health care provider (source) that is responsible for primary treatment of the individual. A second counting rule might allow a case to be linked to all sources that have treated the individual. A third might link the case to the source that first diagnosed the case. A recent development in sampling theory has been the realization that the choice of an appropriate counting rule can improve considerably the reliability of the estimates in a sample survey (1).

Sometimes there may be more than one way of specifying a counting rule

The primary purpose of almost every sample survey is to estimate certain values relating to the distributions of specified characteristics of a population (universe). These values are most often in the form of means, totals or aggregates, and proportions or ratios. They might also be percentiles, standard deviations, or other features of a distribution. For example, in a household survey in which a sample of Chicago residents is taken, we might wish to estimate the average number of acute illness episodes per person (a population mean), the total days of work or school lost among all members of the population because of acute illnesses (a population total or aggregate), and the proportion of persons having two or more acute illnesses within the past year (a population proportion). We also might wish to estimate the median annual household expenditure for health care and the standard deviation of the distribution of days lost from work each year due to acute illnesses. In the following discussion we develop formal notation for discussing the concepts mentioned above.

Elementary Units

The **number of elementary units** in the population is denoted by N, and each elementary unit will be identified by a label in the form of a number from 1 to N. A **characteristic** (or **random variable**) will be denoted by a letter such as $\mathcal{X}$ or $\mathcal{Y}$. The **value of a characteristic** $\mathcal{X}$ in the ith elementary unit will be denoted by X_i. For example, in a survey of hospital discharges occurring in a hospital over a particular year, the population might be the set of all hospital discharges occurring during the time period, and each discharge would be an elementary unit. If 2000 discharges occurred during the year, then N would be equal to 2000, and each discharge would be given (for the purposes of the survey) an identifying label in the form of a number from 1 to 2000. Let us suppose that we are interested in the distribution of number of days hospitalized (length of stay) among the discharges. Then X_1 would represent the length of stay with respect to the hospital discharge labeled "1"; X_2, the length of stay with respect to the discharge labeled "2"; and so on.

Here is the population notation we will use

Population Parameters

We mentioned above that the objectives of a survey include estimation of certain *values* of the distribution of a specified variable or characteristic in a population. These values for a population are called **parameters,** and for a given population a parameter is constant. Definitions of the parameters most often of interest in terms of estimation are given in the following discussion.

POPULATION TOTAL. The **population total** of a characteristic $\mathcal{X}$ is generally denoted by X and is the sum of the values of the characteristic over all elements in the population. The population total is given by

$$X = \sum_{i=1}^{N} X_i$$

POPULATION MEAN.   The **population mean** with respect to a characteristic $\mathscr{X}$ is denoted by $\bar{X}$ and is given by

$$\bar{X} = \frac{\sum\limits_{i=1}^{N} X_i}{N}$$

POPULATION PROPORTION.   When the characteristic being measured represents the presence or absence of some *dichotomous* attribute, it is often desired to estimate the proportion of elementary units in the population having the attribute. If the attribute is denoted by $\mathscr{X}$, and if X is the total number of elementary units in the population having the attribute, then P_x denotes the **population proportion** of elements having the attribute and is given by

Proportions are used only when the attribute is dichotomous

$$P_x = \frac{X}{N}$$

It should be noted that a population proportion is a population mean for the special situation in which the variable $\mathscr{X}$ is given by

$$X_i = \begin{cases} 1 & \text{if the attribute } \mathscr{X} \text{ is present in element } i \\ 0 & \text{if the attribute } \mathscr{X} \text{ is not present in element } i \end{cases}$$

Thus $X = \sum_{i=1}^{n} X_i$ would represent the total number of elements having the attribute.

POPULATION VARIANCE AND STANDARD DEVIATION.   The variance and the standard deviation of the distribution of a characteristic in a population are of interest, because they measure the *spread* of the distribution. The **population variance** of a characteristic $\mathscr{X}$ is denoted by σ_x^2 and is given by

$$\sigma_x^2 = \frac{\sum\limits_{i=1}^{N} (X_i - \bar{X})^2}{N}$$

The **population standard deviation,** denoted by σ_x, is simply the square root of the variance and is given by

$$\sigma_x = \left[\frac{\sum\limits_{i=1}^{N} (X_i - \bar{X})^2}{N} \right]^{1/2}$$

For computational purposes the following two formulas, which are algebraically equivalent to the expression given above for σ_x^2, are sometimes used:

These are computational formulas for variance

$$\sigma_x^2 = \frac{\sum\limits_{i=1}^{N} X_i^2 - \left(\sum\limits_{i=1}^{N} X_i \right)^2 \Big/ N}{N} \qquad \text{or} \qquad \sigma_x^2 = \frac{\sum\limits_{i=1}^{N} X_i^2 - N\bar{X}^2}{N}$$

When the characteristic being considered is a dichotomous attribute, it can be shown that the population variance as defined above reduces to the expression

For a dichotomous attribute

$$\sigma_x^2 = P_x(1 - P_x)$$

For convenience in later reference, the formulas given above are summarized in the following box.

Box 2.1 Population Parameters

Total

$$X = \sum_{i=1}^{N} X_i \tag{2.1}$$

Mean

$$\bar{X} = \frac{\sum_{i=1}^{N} X_i}{N} = \frac{X}{N} \tag{2.2}$$

Proportion

$$P_x = \frac{X}{N} \tag{2.3}$$

Variance

$$\sigma_x^2 = \frac{\sum_{i=1}^{N} (X_i - \bar{X})^2}{N} \tag{2.4}$$

Standard Deviation

$$\sigma_x = \left[\frac{\sum_{i=1}^{N} (X_i - \bar{X})^2}{N} \right]^{1/2} \tag{2.5}$$

Variance, Dichotomous Attribute

$$\sigma_x^2 = P_x(1 - P_x) \tag{2.6}$$

In these definitions N is the number of elementary units in the population and X_i is the value of the ith elementary unit.

Now let's see how these formulas might be used in practice.

ILLUSTRATIVE EXAMPLE

Suppose we are interested in the distribution of household visits made by physicians in a community over a specified year. The 25 physicians in the community are labeled from 1 to 25, and the number of visits made by each physician is shown in table 2.1.

Table 2.1   Number of Household Visits Made During a Specified Year

Physician	No. of Visits	Physician	No. of Visits
1	5	14	4
2	0	15	8
3	1	16	0
4	4	17	7
5	7	18	0
6	0	19	37
7	12	20	0
8	0	21	8
9	0	22	0
10	22	23	0
11	0	24	1
12	5	25	0
13	6		

In this instance the elementary units are physicians and there are 25 of them. In other words, $N = 25$. If we let X_i = the number of household visits made by physician i, the population mean, total, variance, and standard deviation are (see formulas in box 2.1)

$$\bar{X} = 5.08 \text{ visits} \qquad \sigma_x^2 = 67.91 \text{ (visits)}^2$$
$$X = 127 \text{ visits} \qquad \sigma_x = 8.24 \text{ visits}$$

If we let $\mathcal{Y}$ represent the attribute of having performed one or more household visits during the specified time period, we have

$$P_y = \frac{14}{25} = .56$$

where P_y is the proportion of physicians in the population who performed one or more household visits during the period. We also have

$$\sigma_y^2 = (.56)(1 - .56) = .246 \qquad \text{and} \qquad \sigma_y = \sqrt{.246} = .496$$

Another parameter of a population—which is of importance in sampling theory yet is rarely used in other areas of statistics—is the **coefficient of variation,** denoted by V_x, of a distribution, which is the ratio of the standard deviation to the mean of the distribution:

$$V_x = \frac{\sigma_x}{\overline{X}} \tag{2.7}$$

The coefficient of variation measures the spread of a distribution relative to the mean of the distribution. For the distribution of household visits in the illustrative example above, the coefficient of variation is

$$V_x = \frac{8.24}{5.08} = 1.62$$

For a dichotomous attribute $\mathscr{Y}$ it can be shown that the coefficient of variation V_y is given by

For a dichotomous attribute

$$V_y = \left(\frac{1 - P_y}{P_y}\right)^{1/2} \tag{2.8}$$

For the distribution of physicians with respect to the attribute of having performed one or more household visits during the specified time period (see the illustrative example), the coefficient of variation is

$$V_y = \left(\frac{.44}{.56}\right)^{1/2} = .886$$

The square of the coefficient of variation, V_x^2, is known as the **relative variance** or **rel-variance** and is a parameter that is widely used in sampling methodology.

ILLUSTRATIVE EXAMPLE

The coefficient of variation can be used to compare two characteristics measured in different units

As an illustration of the use of the coefficient of variation as a descriptive statistic, let us suppose that we wish to obtain some insight into whether cholesterol levels in a population are more variable than systolic blood pressure levels in the same population. Let us suppose that the mean systolic blood pressure level in the population is 130 mmHg (millimeters of mercury) and the standard deviation is 15 mmHg. Let us suppose further that the mean cholesterol level is 200 mg/100 mL (milligrams per 100 milliliters) and that the standard deviation is 40 mg/100 mL. Examination of the respective standard deviations does not tell us which characteristic has more variability in the population, because they are measured in different units (millimeters of mercury versus milligrams per 100 milliliters in this instance). Comparison of the two variables, however, can be made by examination of the respective coefficients of variation: 15/130, or .115, for systolic blood pressure versus 40/200, or .200, for cholesterol. The coefficients of variation can be compared because they are dimensionless numbers. Thus since the coefficient of variation for cholesterol level is greater than that for systolic blood pressure, we can conclude that cholesterol has more variability than systolic blood pressure in the population.

In the example given above the standard deviations could not be used to compare the variability of two variables because the variables were not measured in the same units of measurement. Let us now consider two variables that are measured in the same measurement units, for example, systolic blood pressure and diastolic blood pressure. Suppose that the mean diastolic blood pressure in the population is 60 mmHg with a standard deviation equal to 8 mmHg and that systolic blood pressure has a mean and a standard deviation as given in the previous example (i.e., $\bar{X} = 130$ mmHg and $\sigma_x = 15$ mmHg). Then in *absolute* terms systolic blood pressure is more variable than diastolic blood pressure ($\sigma_x = 15$ mmHg for systolic versus 8 mmHg for diastolic). However, in *relative terms*, as measured by the coefficient of variation, diastolic blood pressure has the greater variability. The coefficients of variation are $\frac{8}{60} = .133$ for diastolic and $15/130 = .115$ for systolic. In the design of sample surveys, relative variation is often of more concern than absolute variation—hence the importance of the coefficient of variation.

The coefficient of variation can also be used to compare the variance of two distributions whose means differ widely even when they are measured in the same units

2.2 THE SAMPLE

In section 2.1 we introduced concepts relating to the universe or target population. We emphasize that the parameters of the population discussed in section 2.1—such as the mean level of a characteristic, the total amount of a characteristic in the population, or the proportion of elements in the population having some specified attribute—are almost always unknown. Thus the primary objectives of a sample survey are to take a sample from the population and to estimate population parameters from the sample. In this section we introduce certain concepts relating to samples and discuss how estimates of population parameters are made from the sample.

We need samples because population parameters are almost always unknown

Probability and Nonprobability Sampling

Sample surveys can be categorized into two very broad classes on the basis of how the sample was selected, namely, probability samples and nonprobability samples. A **probability sample** has the characteristic that every element in the population has a known, nonzero probability of being included in the sample. A **nonprobability sample** is one based on a sampling plan that does not have that feature. In probability sampling, because every element has a known chance of being selected, the reliability of the resulting population estimates can be evaluated, and those individuals using the survey estimates can have some insight into how much value can be placed on the estimates. In nonprobability sampling, no such insight can be obtained mathematically.

In probability sampling every element of the population must have some known chance of being selected for the sample

Selection probabilities cannot be associated with nonprobability samples

Nonprobability samples are used quite frequently, especially in market research and public opinion surveys. They are used because probability sampling is often a time-consuming and expensive procedure and, in fact, may not be feasible. An example of a nonprobability survey is the so-called *quota survey* in which interviewers are told to contact and interview a certain number of individuals from specified demographic subgroups. For example, an interviewer might be told to interview five black males, five black females, ten white males, and ten white females, with the selection of the individuals left in the hands of the interviewer. It is highly likely that such a method of selecting a sample can lead to estimates that are very biased. For example, for reasons of convenience the interviewer might choose the five black males and five black females from only upper-socioeconomic black neighborhoods, which may not be representative of the black community as a whole.

A quota survey is a nonprobability sample

A judgmental sample is also a nonprobability sample

Another type of nonprobability sampling that is sometimes used is called *purposive* or *judgmental sampling*. In this type of sampling, individuals are selected who are considered to be most representative of the population as a whole. For example, we might attempt to estimate the total number of venipunctures performed during a given year in an outpatient clinic by choosing a few typical days and reviewing the clinic records for those sampled days. If we had the resources to sample only a few days, this approach might lead to more valid and reliable estimates than the approach of using a random sample of days, because the judgmental procedure would avoid the possibility of including unusual days (e.g., days in which the patient load was atypically high or low or unusual in some other way). The disadvantage of judgmental procedures is that no insight can be obtained mathematically concerning the reliability of the resulting estimates.

We will use only probability samples

In this text we will only consider probability samples, since we feel very strongly that sample designs in the health sciences should yield estimates that can be evaluated mathematically with respect to their reliability.

Sampling Frames, Sampling Units, and Enumeration Units

In probability sampling the probability of any element appearing in the sample must be known. For this to be accomplished, some list should be available from which the sample can be selected. Such a list is called a **sampling frame** and should have the property that every element in the population has some chance of being included in the sample by whatever method is used to select elements from the sampling frame. A sampling frame does not have to list explicitly all elements in the population. For example, if a city directory is used as a sampling frame for a sample survey in which the elements are residents of the city, then clearly the elements would not be listed in the sampling frame, which in this instance is a listing of households. However, every element has some chance of being selected in the sample if the sampling frame, in reality, contains all households in the city.

Often a particular sampling design specifies that the sampling be performed in two or more stages; this design is called a **multistage sampling design.** For example, a household interview survey conducted in Illinois might have a sampling design that specifies that a sample of counties be drawn; that within each sample county a sample of minor civil divisions (townships) be drawn; and that within each minor civil division a sample of households be drawn. In multistage surveys a different sampling frame is used at each stage of sampling. The units listed in the frame are generally called **sampling units.** In the example mentioned here the sampling frame for the first stage is the list of counties in Illinois, and each county is a sampling unit for this stage. The list of townships within each county selected at the first stage is the sampling frame for the second stage, and each township is a sampling unit for this stage. Finally, the list of households within each selected township is the sampling frame for the third and final stage, and each household is a sampling unit for this stage. The sampling units for the first stage are called **primary sampling units** (PSUs). The sampling units for the final stage of a multistage sampling design are called **enumeration units** or **listing units;** these have been discussed earlier.

Multistage samples have more than one sampling frame

Sample Measurements and Summary Statistics

Let us suppose that in some way we have taken a sample of n elements from a population containing N elements and that we measure each sample element with respect to some variable $\mathscr{X}$. For convenience we label the sample elements from 1 to n (no matter what their original labels were in the population): we let x_1 denote the value of $\mathscr{X}$ for the sample element labeled "1"; we let x_2 denote the value of $\mathscr{X}$ for the sample element labeled "2"; and so on. Having taken the sample, we can then compute for the sample such quantities as totals, means, proportions, and standard deviations, just as we did for the population. However, when these quantities are calculated for a sample, they are not parameters in the true sense of the word, since they are subject to sampling variability (a true parameter is a constant). Instead these sample values are generally referred to as **statistics,** as **summary statistics,** or as **descriptive statistics.** Definitions of some statistics that are used in many sample designs, either for descriptive purposes or in formulas for population estimates, are given in the following discussion; others will be introduced as needed.

Here is the sample notation we will use

SAMPLE TOTAL.   The **sample total** of a characteristic $\mathscr{X}$ is generally denoted by x and is the sum of the values of the characteristic over all elements in the sample:

$$x = \sum_{i=1}^{n} x_i$$

SAMPLE MEAN.   The **sample mean** with respect to a characteristic $\mathscr{X}$ is generally denoted by $\bar{x}$ and is given by

$$\bar{x} = \frac{\sum\limits_{i=1}^{n} x_i}{n}$$

SAMPLE PROPORTION.   When the characteristic $\mathscr{X}$ being measured represents presence or absence of some dichotomous attribute, the **sample proportion** is generally denoted by p_x and is given by

$$p_x = \frac{x}{n}$$

where x is the number of sample elements having the attribute.

SAMPLE VARIANCE AND STANDARD DEVIATION.   For any characteristic $\mathscr{X}$ the **sample variance** s_x^2 is given by

$$s_x^2 = \frac{\sum\limits_{i=1}^{n} (x_i - \bar{x})^2}{n-1}$$

For computational purposes we often use these algebraically equivalent forms:

These are computational forms

$$s_x^2 = \frac{\left(\sum\limits_{i=1}^{n} x_i^2 - n\bar{x}^2\right)}{n-1} \quad \text{or} \quad s_x^2 = \frac{\sum\limits_{i=1}^{n} x_i^2 - (x^2/n)}{n-1}$$

When the characteristic $\mathscr{X}$ is a dichotomous attribute, the sample variance s_x^2 as defined above reduces to

For a dichotomous attribute

$$s_x^2 = \frac{np_x(1 - p_x)}{n-1}$$

If the sample size n is large (say greater than 20), we can use the following approximation:

$$s_x^2 \approx p_x(1 - p_x)$$

The **sample standard deviation** s_x is simply the square root of the sample variance:

$$s_x = \left[\frac{\sum\limits_{i=1}^{n} (x_i - \bar{x})^2}{n-1}\right]^{1/2}$$

For convenience in later reference, these formulas are summarized in the following box.

Box 2.2 Sample Statistics

Total

$$x = \sum_{i=1}^{n} x_i \qquad (2.9)$$

Mean

$$\bar{x} = \frac{\sum_{i=1}^{n} x_i}{n} = \frac{x}{n} \qquad (2.10)$$

Proportion

$$p_x = \frac{x}{n} \qquad (2.11)$$

where x is the number of sample elements having the dichotomous attribute.

Variance

$$s_x^2 = \frac{\sum_{i=1}^{n} (x_i - \bar{x})^2}{n - 1} \qquad (2.12)$$

Variance, Dichotomous Attribute

$$s_x^2 = \frac{n p_x (1 - p_x)}{n - 1} \qquad (2.13)$$

Standard Deviation

$$s_x = \left[\frac{\sum_{i=1}^{n} (x_i - \bar{x})^2}{n - 1} \right]^{1/2} \qquad (2.14)$$

In these definitions n is the number of elements in the sample and x_i is the value of the ith element.

Estimates of Population Characteristics

Estimates of population means and proportions can be obtained directly from the sample means and proportions.

An **estimate of the population total** X obtained from the sample total x is given by

$$x' = \left(\frac{N}{n}\right)(x) \tag{2.15}$$

In other words, if we multiply the sample total x by the ratio of the number of elements in the population to the number in the sample, we can use the resulting statistic x' as an estimate of the population total X.

An **estimate** $\hat{\sigma}_x^2$ **of the population variance** σ_x^2 is given by

The symbol $\frown$ over a letter denotes an estimate of that quantity

$$\hat{\sigma}_x^2 = \left(\frac{N-1}{N}\right)(s_x^2) \tag{2.16}$$

If the number of elements N in the population is moderately large,* we can use the approximation

$$\hat{\sigma}_x^2 \approx s_x^2$$

We emphasize here that the sample statistics and population estimates presented above would not be used for every sample design. They are discussed here as illustrations of the ways in which the sample measurements might be aggregated to form summary statistics and estimates of population characteristics. As we discuss specific sample designs in later chapters, we will present the methods of estimating population characteristics that are specific to the particular design being discussed.

ILLUSTRATIVE EXAMPLE

Let us illustrate these concepts by using the data on physician household visits given in table 2.1. Suppose that in some way we take a sample of nine physicians in the population and suppose that our sample includes the nine physicians listed in table 2.2.

The sample total, mean, and variance for these data are (see the formulas in box 2.2)

$$x = 80 \qquad \bar{x} = 8.89 \qquad s_x^2 = 125.11$$

The sample proportion with one or more household visits is

$$p_y = .78$$

---

* When N is reasonably large, $(N-1)/N$ can be approximated by $N/N = 1$.

Table 2.2   Sample Data for Number of Household Visits

Physician	No. of Visits	Physician	No. of Visits
1	5	17	7
6	0	19	37
7	12	21	8
12	5	25	0
13	6		

The sample variance with respect to having made one or more household visits is

$$s_y^2 = .1944$$

If we wish to estimate from this sample the total X of all household visits made by physicians in the population during the specified time period, we first obtain the sample total x of household visits among the nine sample physicians. Then we obtain x' by multiplying x by N/n, where in this case $N = 25$ and $n = 9$. A summary of population parameters and sample estimates (based on the formulas above and in boxes 2.1 and 2.2) follows.

POPULATION PARAMETER	ESTIMATE FROM SAMPLE	
$X = 127$	$x' = (\frac{25}{9})(80) = 222.22$	***Summary of***
$\bar{X} = 5.08$	$\bar{x} = 8.89$	***calculations***
$\sigma_x^2 = 67.91$	$\hat{\sigma}_x^2 = (\frac{24}{25})(125.11) = 120.11$	
$P_y = .56$	$p_y = \frac{7}{9} = .78$	
$\sigma_y^2 = .246$	$\hat{\sigma}_y^2 = (\frac{24}{25})(.1944) = .1866$	

We see from the summary of calculations in the example above that the estimates of population parameters obtained from the particular sample taken not only are not equal to the population parameters being estimated, but they are not even very close to the true values of these parameters. If we had taken a different sample, we would have obtained different estimates of these parameters, which may have been either closer or further away from the true parameter values. Since we never know in reality the true values of the population parameters that we are estimating from a sample, we never know how bad or how good our sample estimates really are. If, however, our sampling plan uses a probability sample, then we can get some mathematical insight into how far away from the unknown true values our sample estimates are likely to be. In order to do this, we must know something about the distribution of our population estimates over all possible samples that can arise from the particular sampling plan being used. In the next section we develop methodology for obtaining such information from probability samples.

2.3 SAMPLING DISTRIBUTION

In the previous section we discussed estimation of population parameters from a sample. In this section we consider the distribution of these estimated population parameters over all possible samples that can be generated by using a particular sampling plan.

d can be any
population
parameter and
d̂ is its estimate

Let us suppose that a particular sampling plan and estimation procedure could result in T possible samples from a given population and that a particular sample results in an estimate $\hat{d}$ of a population parameter d. The relative frequency distribution of $\hat{d}$ over the T possible samples is called the **sampling distribution** of $\hat{d}$ with respect to the specified sampling plan and estimation procedure.

To illustrate a sampling distribution, let us look at an example.

ILLUSTRATIVE EXAMPLE

Suppose that a hypothetical community has six schools. This population of six schools is given in table 2.3. Now suppose that we wish to take a sample of two of these schools for purposes of estimating the total number of students not immunized for measles among the six schools in the community.

Table 2.3   Data for Number of Students Not Immunized for Measles Among Six Schools in a Community

School	No. of Students	STUDENTS NOT IMMUNIZED FOR MEASLES	
		Total	Proportion
1	59	4	.068
2	28	5	.179
3	90	3	.033
4	44	3	.068
5	36	7	.194
6	57	8	.140
Total	314	30	.096

Let us specify a sampling plan in which six identical sealed envelopes, each containing a card numbered from 1 to 6, are placed in a hat and are thoroughly shuffled. Two envelopes are then drawn from the hat and the two schools corresponding to the two numbers on the cards in the selected envelopes are included in the sample. Suppose that information concerning immunization status for measles is elicited from each child in the sample schools. The total number of students in the population not immunized for measles is obtained by inflating the sample totals over the two schools by the ratio N/n, where $N = 6$ and $n = 2$. This procedure yields 15 possible samples, each having the same chance of being selected. In terms of the notation described in the definition of a sampling distribution, we have $T = 15$, $d = X = 30$, and each $\hat{d} = x'$, where X and x' are the population total and estimated population total, respectively. The 15 possible samples obtained from this sampling plan, along with values of x', are listed in table 2.4.

Table 2.4   Possible Samples and Values of x'

Sample	Sample Schools	x'	Sample	Sample Schools	x'	Sample	Sample Schools	x'
1	1, 2	27	6	2, 3	24	11	3, 5	30
2	1, 3	21	7	2, 4	24	12	3, 6	33
3	1, 4	21	8	2, 5	36	13	4, 5	30
4	1, 5	33	9	2, 6	39	14	4, 6	33
5	1, 6	36	10	3, 4	18	15	5, 6	45

Since each of the 15 samples listed in table 2.4 has the same chance ($\frac{1}{15}$) of being selected, we can obtain the frequency distribution of x' by grouping similar values of x'. Table 2.5 represents the sampling distribution of the estimated total x'.

Table 2.5   Sampling Distribution for Data
of Table 2.4

x'	Frequency	Relative Frequency
18	1	$\frac{1}{15}$
21	2	$\frac{2}{15}$
24	2	$\frac{2}{15}$
27	1	$\frac{1}{15}$
30	2	$\frac{2}{15}$
33	3	$\frac{3}{15}$
36	2	$\frac{2}{15}$
39	1	$\frac{1}{15}$
45	1	$\frac{1}{15}$

This is the sampling distribution of x'

The relative frequencies given in the last column of table 2.5 show the fraction of all possible samples that take on the corresponding values of x'. Using these relative frequencies, we can draw a picture of the sampling distribution of x', as shown in figure 2.1.

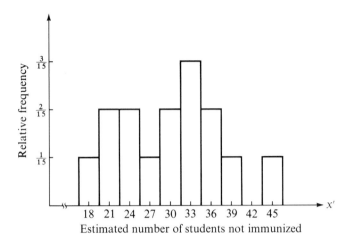

Figure 2.1   Relative Frequency Histogram of Sampling Distribution of x'

Sampling distributions have certain characteristics associated with them. For our purposes the two most important of these are the mean and the variance (or its square root, the standard deviation). These are defined next.

The **mean of the sampling distribution** of an estimated parameter $\hat{d}$ with respect to a particular sampling plan that yields T possible samples resulting in C possible values of $\hat{d}$ is also known as the **expected value** of $\hat{d}$, denoted by $E(\hat{d})$, and is defined as

$$E(\hat{d}) = \sum_{i=1}^{C} \hat{d}_i \pi_i \tag{2.17}$$

where $\hat{d}_i$ is a particular value of $\hat{d}$ and π_i is the probability of obtaining that particular value of $\hat{d}$. (Note that $\pi_i = f_i/T$, where f_i is the number of samples in which a particular value of $\hat{d}_i$ occurs.)

The **variance** $\text{Var}(\hat{d})$ **of the sampling distribution** of an estimated parameter $\hat{d}$ with respect to a particular sampling plan is given by

$$\text{Var}(\hat{d}) = \sum_{i=1}^{C} [\hat{d}_i - E(\hat{d})]^2 \pi_i \tag{2.18}$$

The algebraic equivalent of this equation, which can be used for computations is

$$\text{Var}(\hat{d}) = \sum_{i=1}^{C} \hat{d}_i^2 \pi_i - E^2(\hat{d}) \tag{2.19}$$

The **standard deviation** $\text{SE}(\hat{d})$ **of the sampling distribution** of an estimated parameter $\hat{d}$ is more commonly known as the **standard error** of $\hat{d}$ and is simply the square root of the variance $\text{Var}(\hat{d})$ of the sampling distribution of $\hat{d}$:

$$\text{SE}(\hat{d}) = [\text{Var}(\hat{d})]^{1/2} \qquad (2.20)$$

Using these general equations, we can derive expressions for the mean and variance (and hence the standard error) of the sampling distribution for totals, means, and proportions. For convenience in later reference, these expressions are summarized in the next two boxes.

Box 2.3 Mean and Variance of Sampling Distribution When Each Sample Has Same Probability $(1/T)$ of Selection

For Totals

$$E(x') = \frac{\sum\limits_{i=1}^{T} x_i'}{T} \qquad \text{Var}(x') = \frac{\sum\limits_{i=1}^{T} [x_i' - E(x')]^2}{T} \qquad (2.21)$$

where x_i' is the sample total computed from the ith possible sample selected from a population. Note that some of the values of x_i' may be the same from sample to sample, but each realization appears in the sum even if there is duplication.

For Means

$$E(\bar{x}) = \frac{\sum\limits_{i=1}^{T} \bar{x}_i}{T} \qquad \text{Var}(\bar{x}) = \frac{\sum\limits_{i=1}^{T} [\bar{x}_i - E(\bar{x})]^2}{T} \qquad (2.22)$$

For Proportions

$$E(p_y) = \frac{\sum\limits_{i=1}^{T} p_{y_i}}{T} \qquad \text{Var}(p_y) = \frac{\sum\limits_{i=1}^{T} [p_{y_i} - E(p_y)]^2}{T} \qquad (2.23)$$

In these expressions T is the number of possible samples.

When each sample does not have the same probability of selection, or if we wish to compute means and variances of sampling distributions directly from a sampling distribution such as the one given in table 2.5, then we must use the expressions given in the next box.

Box 2.4 Mean and Variance of Sampling Distribution When Each Sample Does Not Have Same Probability of Selection*

For Totals

$$E(x') = \sum_{i=1}^{C} x_i' \pi_i \qquad \mathrm{Var}(x') = \sum_{i=1}^{C} [x_i' - E(x')]^2 \pi_i \qquad (2.24)$$

For Means

$$E(\bar{x}) = \sum_{i=1}^{C} \bar{x}_i \pi_i \qquad \mathrm{Var}(\bar{x}) = \sum_{i=1}^{C} [\bar{x}_i - E(\bar{x})]^2 \pi_i \qquad (2.25)$$

For Proportions

$$E(p_y) = \sum_{i=1}^{C} p_{y_i} \pi_i \qquad \mathrm{Var}(p_y) = \sum_{i=1}^{C} [p_{y_i} - E(p_y)]^2 \pi_i \qquad (2.26)$$

In these expressions C is the number of possible unique values of a statistic and $\pi_i = f_i/T$ is the proportion of the sample in the sampling distribution yielding the ith unique value, where f_i is the frequency of occurrence in the sampling distribution of the ith realization and T is the number of possible samples.

* Or when the possible values of the totals, means, or proportions do not occur with the same relative frequency over all possible samples.

Now let us see how some of these formulas can be used in practice. We will use the data given in the previous example.

ILLUSTRATIVE EXAMPLE

For the previous example we have $\hat{d} = x'$, $T = 15$, and $C = 9$, and the π_i are the relative frequencies associated with any particular value of x'. The mean $E(x')$ of the sampling distribution of x' for that example is (using the expressions in box 2.4)

$$E(x') = \sum_{i=1}^{9} x_i'(f_i/15)$$

$$= 18(\tfrac{1}{15}) + 21(\tfrac{2}{15}) + 24(\tfrac{2}{15}) + 27(\tfrac{1}{15}) + 30(\tfrac{2}{15})$$

$$+ 33(\tfrac{3}{15}) + 36(\tfrac{2}{15}) + 39(\tfrac{1}{15}) + 45(\tfrac{1}{15})$$

$$= 30$$

Notice that
E(x') = X = 30

The variance $\text{Var}(x')$ of the sampling distribution of x' is

$$\text{Var}(x') = (18 - 30)^2(\tfrac{1}{15}) + (21 - 30)^2(\tfrac{2}{15}) + (24 - 30)^2(\tfrac{2}{15})$$

$$+ (27 - 30)^2(\tfrac{1}{15}) + (30 - 30)^2(\tfrac{2}{15}) + (33 - 30)^2(\tfrac{3}{15})$$

$$+ (36 - 30)^2(\tfrac{2}{15}) + (39 - 30)^2(\tfrac{1}{15}) + (45 - 30)^2(\tfrac{1}{15})$$

$$= 52.8$$

The standard error of x' is

$$\text{SE}(x') = (52.8)^{1/2} = 7.27$$

2.4 CHARACTERISTICS OF ESTIMATES OF POPULATION PARAMETERS

In the previous section we introduced the concept of the sampling distribution of an estimate of a population parameter with respect to a particular sampling plan. Also, we introduced the concepts of the mean of the sampling distribution of a population estimate and the standard error of the estimate. We can now discuss certain properties of population estimates in terms of these concepts. It would seem intuitively clear that a desirable property of a sampling plan and estimation procedure is that it should yield estimates of population parameters for which the mean of the sampling distribution is equal to, or at least close to, the true unknown population parameter and for which the standard error is very small. In fact, the accuracy of an estimated population parameter is evaluated in terms of these two characteristics. In this section we introduce the concepts that are used to evaluate sample designs.

The characteristics of estimates discussed in this section are used to evaluate sample designs

Bias

The **bias** $B(\hat{d})$ of an estimate $\hat{d}$ of a population parameter d is defined as the difference between the mean $E(\hat{d})$ of the sampling distribution of $\hat{d}$ and the true value of the unknown parameter d. In other words,

$$B(\hat{d}) = E(\hat{d}) - d \qquad (2.27)$$

An estimate $\hat{d}$ is said to be **unbiased** if $B(\hat{d}) = 0$, or, in other words, if the mean of the sampling distribution of $\hat{d}$ is equal to d.

In the example considered in the previous section, the estimate x' of the total number of children not immunized for measles is an unbiased estimate of the true population total X, since it was demonstrated that $E(x') = 30 = X$.

We emphasize that the same estimation procedure that is unbiased for one sampling plan can be biased for another sampling plan. The next example illustrates this idea.

ILLUSTRATIVE EXAMPLE

Let us consider the same population of six schools used in the previous example (p. 22), but now let us use the following sampling plan: Place cards with numbers from 1 to 10 in ten sealed envelopes, and place the sealed envelopes in a hat. Take one envelope from the hat and choose two schools in the sample according to the procedure shown in table 2.6. This procedure is a probability sample since each school has a known, nonzero chance of being selected in the sample.

Table 2.6   Sampling Procedure for Population of Six Schools

Number Picked	Schools Chosen in Sample	Number Picked	Schools Chosen in Sample
1	1 and 2	6	2 and 3
2	1 and 3	7	2 and 4
3	1 and 4	8	2 and 5
4	1 and 5	9	2 and 6
5	1 and 6	10	3 and 4

The distribution of estimated totals if this procedure is used is shown in table 2.7.

Table 2.7   Possible Samples and Values of x'

Sample	Sample Schools	x'	Sample	Sample Schools	x'
1	1, 2	27	6	2, 3	24
2	1, 3	21	7	2, 4	24
3	1, 4	21	8	2, 5	36
4	1, 5	33	9	2, 6	39
5	1, 6	36	10	3, 4	18

Since each of the 10 possible samples is equally likely, we have the distribution of x' that is shown in table 2.8.

Table 2.8   Sampling Distribution of x'

x'	π
18	$\frac{1}{10}$
21	$\frac{2}{10}$
24	$\frac{2}{10}$
27	$\frac{1}{10}$
33	$\frac{1}{10}$
36	$\frac{2}{10}$
39	$\frac{1}{10}$
Total	1

From the distribution in table 2.8 we see that the mean $E(x')$ of the sampling distribution of x' under this sampling plan is

$$E(x') = 18(\tfrac{1}{10}) + 21(\tfrac{2}{10}) + 24(\tfrac{2}{10}) + 27(\tfrac{1}{10}) + 33(\tfrac{1}{10}) + 36(\tfrac{2}{10}) + 39(\tfrac{1}{10})$$
$$= 27.9$$

Compare this **E(x′)** *with the* **E(x′) = 30** *on page 27*

Therefore, under this sampling plan the estimated population total x' is *not* an unbiased estimate of the true population total X.

Mean Square Error

The **mean square error** of a population estimate $\hat{d}$, denoted by $\text{MSE}(\hat{d})$, is defined as the mean of the squared differences between the values of the estimate and the true value d of the unknown parameter over all possible samples. In terms of the notation developed in the last section, the mean square error of $\hat{d}$ is defined by the relation

$$\text{MSE}(\hat{d}) = \sum_{i=1}^{C} (\hat{d}_i - d)^2 \pi_i \qquad (2.28)$$

Notice the difference between the mean square error and the variance of an estimate. The mean square error of an estimate is the mean value of squared deviations about the true value of the parameter being estimated; the variance of an estimate is the mean value of squared deviations about the mean of the sampling distribution of the estimate. If the estimate is unbiased—or, in other words, if the mean of the sampling distribution of the estimate is equal to the true value of the parameter—then the mean square error of the estimate is equal to the variance of the estimate, since the deviations are taken about the same entity. In general, the mean square error of an estimate is related to its bias and variance by the following relation:

Here MSE is related to variance and bias

$$\text{MSE}(\hat{d}) \doteq \text{Var}(\hat{d}) + B^2(\hat{d}) \tag{2.29}$$

In other words, the mean square error of a population estimate is equal to the variance of the estimate plus the square of its bias.

ILLUSTRATIVE EXAMPLE

In the example considered earlier (p. 26) in which the sampling plan yields an unbiased estimate of the population total, the mean square error is

$$\text{MSE}(x') = 52.8 + 0^2 = 52.8$$

In other words, the MSE is equal to the variance of the estimate.

In the example (p. 28) for which the sampling plan yielded a biased estimate x' of X, the variance of x' is [from equation (2.28)]

$$\text{Var}(x') = (18 - 27.9)^2(\tfrac{1}{10}) + (21 - 27.9)^2(\tfrac{2}{10}) + (24 - 27.9)^2(\tfrac{2}{10})$$
$$+ (27 - 27.9)^2(\tfrac{1}{10}) + (33 - 27.9)^2(\tfrac{1}{10}) + (36 - 27.9)^2(\tfrac{2}{10}) + (39 - 27.9)^2(\tfrac{1}{10})$$
$$= 50.49$$

Thus the MSE for x' is

$$\text{MSE}(x') = 50.49 + (30 - 27.9)^2 = 54.9$$

Note that the second sampling plan yields an estimator x' that has smaller variance but larger overall mean square error than the equivalent estimate yielded by the first sampling plan.

ILLUSTRATIVE EXAMPLE

Let's look at another example of the use of the mean square error. Suppose a survey is being planned to evaluate the seriousness of burn injuries that occur in the United States. In connection with the survey three students are being trained at survey headquarters in the assessment of the percentage of a patient's body suffering third-degree burns. (This is called "full-thickness burn area.")

To assess the students' progress, a senior burn surgeon uses sets of photographs taken of ten patients, each of whom suffered full-thickness burn areas of 37%. These ten patients, whose total burn injuries were equal in total percentage of the body involved rather than in specific body parts involved, were selected from among many seen by the surgeon.

Let us call the three students Dave, Anne, and Stu. Table 2.9 shows the means and variances of the ten burn area estimates made by each student. Now let us evaluate each of the estimates.

Table 2.9 Data for the Burn Area Estimates

Student	Mean (%)	Variance (%^{2})
Dave	37	64
Anne	42	9
Stu	50	9

The average burn assessment made by Dave happens to equal the true average of the photographs under consideration (i.e., bias = 37 − 37 = 0). However, the variability in his measurements is large and, as a result, his mean square error is large (i.e., MSE = 0^2 + 64 = 64).

Anne tended to overestimate the actual full-thickness burn area (i.e., bias = 42 − 37 = 5) but she did so rather consistently. As a result, the mean square error for her readings (MSE = 5^2 + 9 = 34) is smaller than Dave's. Stated differently, the mean of the squared deviations of each of Anne's assessments of burn area about the true burn area is smaller than is Dave's.

Stu's assessment of burn area tended to grossly overestimate the true values (i.e., bias = 50 − 37 = 13), but there is little variability in these assessments. The resulting mean square error (MSE = 13^2 + 9 = 178) is the largest of the three students.

Pictorially, the relationship among bias, variability, and mean square error is seen in figure 2.2, where it is assumed that the measurements are normally distributed with the stated means and variances. Notice that while the mean of Dave's distribution is equal to the true value, it would not be unusual for any one of his assessments to miss the true value by a wide margin (as indicated by the wide spread of his distribution). For instance, suppose we let $Pr(\mathcal{X} > c)$ represent the probability that a particular realization of the random variable $\mathcal{X}$ exceeds the value c. Then the probability that Dave misses the true burn area by more than 10 percentage points is

$$Pr(\mathcal{X} > 47) + Pr(\mathcal{X} < 27) = Pr\left(z > \frac{47 - 37}{8} = 1.25\right) + Pr(z < -1.25) = .21$$

Anne's burn measurements are usually high, but it is not often that she would be more than 10 percentage points away from the true value, since, for Anne,

$$Pr(\mathcal{X} > 47) = Pr\left(z > \frac{47 - 42}{3} = 1.67\right) = .05$$

Finally, as reflected by his large MSE, the probability that Stu misses the target burn area by more than 10 percentage points is quite high:

$$Pr(\mathcal{X} > 47) = Pr\left(z > \frac{47 - 50}{3} = -1\right) = .84$$

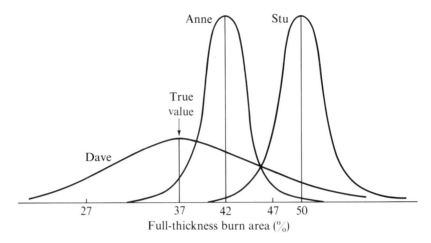

Figure 2.2   Relationship Among Bias, Variability, and MSE for the Data of Table 2.9

Hence, as we have seen in this example, when evaluating potential estimators, it is important to examine both bias and variance. Both these values play important roles in the mean square error.

Validity, Reliability, and Accuracy

In earlier sections we have spoken of the desirability of using sample designs that yield reliable and valid estimates. However, we have never defined just what the terms "reliability" and "validity" mean in terms of characteristics of estimates. We now have developed enough concepts and notation concerning estimates to be able to define these two terms, as well as a third term, the "accuracy" of an estimate, which is derived from the validity and reliability.

Reliability is measured in terms of standard error

The **reliability** of an estimated population characteristic refers to how reproducible the estimate is over repetitions of the process yielding the estimate. If we assume that there is no measurement error in the survey, then the reliability of an estimate can be stated in terms of its sampling variance or, equivalently, its standard error. The smaller the standard error of an estimate, the greater is its reliability.

Validity is measured in terms of bias

The **validity** of an estimated population characteristic refers to how the mean of the estimate, over repetitions of the process yielding the estimate, differs from the true value of the parameter being estimated. Again, if we assume that there is no measurement error, the validity of an estimate can be evaluated by examining the bias of the estimate. The smaller the bias, the greater is the validity.

The **accuracy** of an estimate refers to how far away a particular value of the estimate is, on the average, from the true value of the parameter being measured. The accuracy of an estimate is generally evaluated on the basis of its MSE, or, equivalently, on the basis of the square root of its MSE (denoted by RMSE and called "root mean square error"). The smaller the MSE of an estimate, the greater is its accuracy.

Accuracy is measured in terms of mean square error

2.5 CRITERIA FOR A GOOD SAMPLE DESIGN

Throughout the remainder of this book we will be discussing various sample designs and showing how manipulation of the sampling plan, estimation procedure, or counting rule can affect the reliability and validity of the resulting estimates. We will limit our discussion to probability samples, because these are the only sampling plans that allow the reliability of the estimates to be evaluated from the data collected in the survey. Since the accuracy of an estimate involves both its reliability and its validity, and since accuracy is measured by the mean square error, one of our criteria for choosing a sample design will be the size of the mean square errors anticipated for the resulting estimates.

The criteria are these:
1. size of the MSEs (accuracy)

In addition to the mean square error criterion, the cost involved in conducting a survey according to a specified sample design will be used as a criterion for evaluating the particular sample design. The criteria of cost and accuracy can be combined into a composite criterion by first deciding on the total cost to be allocated to the survey and then choosing that sample design that will yield estimates having the lowest MSE at that particular cost. Conversely, we might make specifications on the MSEs of the estimates and choose the sample design that yields estimates meeting these specified MSEs at the lowest possible cost.

2. cost

Finally, in addition to accuracy and cost, a third criterion we will use is feasibility in executing a particular sample design. No matter how cost-efficient a design is, it is of no use if it is not feasible to execute the design.

3. feasibility

SUMMARY

In this chapter we discussed and developed concepts concerning populations, samples, and estimates.

We defined what we mean by a population, and we discussed how the elements of a population are often grouped for purposes of sampling into enumeration units or listing units. We showed how the elementary units and enumeration units are often linked by a counting rule. We defined certain parameters that characterize the distribution of variables in the population. The parameters discussed include the population mean, total or aggregate, proportion, variance, standard deviation, coefficient of variation, and relative variance or rel-variance.

We discussed the concept of taking a sample from a population, and we distinguished between probability samples and nonprobability samples. We discussed the use of sampling frames in selecting samples from a population and the use of multistage selection of a sample. Summary statistics for samples such as the sample mean, sample total, sample proportion, and sample variance were introduced, and their use in obtaining estimates of population characteristics or variables was discussed.

Concepts relating to the sampling distribution of estimates were developed, including the mean of the sampling distribution of an estimate, its variance and standard error, its bias, and its mean square error. The concepts of validity, reliability, and accuracy of an estimated population characteristic were then defined in relation to the concepts of variance, bias, and mean square error.

EXERCISES

1. The accompanying table presents a population of five hospitals denoted by *A, B, C, D,* and *E.* The total number of beds is given for each hospital.

Hospital	Number of Beds
A	160
B	220
C	850
D	510
E	110

(a) Compute the mean number of beds $\bar{X}$ and the standard deviation σ_x of the distribution of number of beds in the population of 5 hospitals.

(b) How many samples of 2 hospitals can be drawn from this population of 5 hospitals?

(c) List each of the possible samples of 2 hospitals and compute the mean number of beds per hospital for each sample.

(d) Assuming each of the samples listed in part (c) is equally likely, compute the mean $E(\bar{x})$ and variance $\mathrm{Var}(\bar{x})$ of the distribution of sample means $\bar{x}$. How does $E(\bar{x})$ compare with the population mean $\bar{X}$?

(e) Calculate the standard error of $\bar{x}$. How does $\mathrm{SE}(\bar{x})$ compare with the population standard deviation σ_x?

(f) How many different samples of 4 hospitals can be drawn from this population? List each of these samples along with the sample mean $\bar{x}$ for each sample.

(g) Calculate $E(\bar{x})$ and $\mathrm{Var}(\bar{x})$ for the sample means listed in part (f). How do these compare with the values of $E(\bar{x})$ and $\mathrm{Var}(\hat{x})$ obtained in part (d)?

2. For each of the following problems indicate how you would carry out a sample and specify these:
   (1) the population
   (2) the variable
   (3) the elementary unit
   (4) the frame
   (5) the enumeration unit
   (a) Suppose we wish to estimate the average cost of an appendectomy in a certain state. There are 27 hospitals in this state.
   (b) Suppose we wish to do a nutritional survey in order to estimate the average amount of sugar consumed by individuals in a certain city. Suppose there is no list of families available for the city but there is a map of the city showing each block in detail.
   (c) Suppose we are interested in the proportion of calves who die prior to the first year of life at all dairy farms in a particular state.

3. Suppose a survey is being planned for the purpose of estimating the average number of hours spent exercising daily by adults (18 years of age or older) living in a certain community. A list of all the individuals living in the town is not available; however, a list of all households is available at the office of the town clerk. For simplicity, suppose this list consists of six households and that the information you would collect, were you to visit each household, is as shown in the accompanying table.

Household	No. of Adults (18 years or over)	No. of Hours Spent Exercising by All Adults
1	2	1
2	3	3
3	2	1.5
4	4	1.5
5	3	1
6	3	1

   (a) Define these:
       (1) population
       (2) elementary unit
       (3) enumeration unit
       (4) frame
       (5) variable
   (b) Devise a sampling plan to estimate the average daily time expenditure on exercising by adults living in this community.

(c) Select all possible samples of two households from this frame and compute the average exercising time for each sample.

(d) Compute the expected value of your estimate and compare this to the actual population parameters.

(e) Calculate the standard error of your estimate.

BIBLIOGRAPHY

The following reference deals with the concept of counting rules.

1. SIRKEN, M. G. Household surveys with multiplicity. *Journal of the American Statistical Association* (1970) 65: 257–266.

The following publications discuss the concepts of populations and samples.

2. COCHRAN, W. G. *Sampling techniques.* 3d ed. New York: Wiley, 1977.

3. DIXON, W. J., and MASSEY, F. J. *Introduction to statistical analysis.* 3d ed. New York: McGraw-Hill, 1969.

4. HANSEN, M. H.; HURWITZ, W. N.; and MADOW, W. G. *Sample survey methods and theory.* Vols. 1 and 2. New York: Wiley, 1953.

5. KISH, L. *Survey sampling.* New York: Wiley, 1965.

6. SCHEAFFER, R. L.; MENDENHALL, W.; and OTT, L. *Elementary survey sampling.* 2d ed. N. Scituate, MA: Duxbury Press, 1979.

7. WILLIAMS, B. *A sampler on sampling.* New York: Wiley, 1978.

3

Simple Random Sampling

In chapter 2 we laid a foundation for our discussion of sampling by setting forth general concepts concerning the universe or target population, the sample, sampling distributions, and desirable properties of population estimates. Beginning in this chapter we build upon that foundation by relating these concepts to specific sampling plans and estimation procedures that are widely used in sample surveys. We begin this process by discussing those sampling plans in which the elementary units themselves serve as the sampling units. Such sampling procedures are known as **element sampling.** In this chapter we discuss a method of element sampling—namely, simple random sampling—that is important not because it is widely used in actual sample surveys but because it provides the base upon which the statistical theory of sampling is constructed. Thus in practice you may never decide to select a simple random sampling (we discuss why this is so in section 3.7). However, we devote this chapter to its discussion because simple random sampling techniques form the foundation of sampling theory.

In this chapter the general statistical concepts of chapter 2 are related to simple random sampling

3.1 WHAT IS A SIMPLE RANDOM SAMPLE?

Let us suppose that we have a population of N elements and we wish to take a sample of n of these elements. It can be shown from the mathematical theory of permutations and combinations that the number T of possible samples of *n* elements from a population of *N* elements is denoted by $\binom{N}{n}$ and is given by

T *is the number of possible samples*

$$T = \binom{N}{n} = \frac{N!}{n!(N - n)!} \qquad (3.1)$$

where $n! = n(n - 1)(n - 2) \cdots (1)$, and $0! = 1$. For example, if a population contains 25 elements and we wish to take a sample of five elements, then from relation (3.1) with $N = 25$ and $n = 5$, we see that there are

$$T = \frac{25!}{(5!)(25 - 5)!} = 53,130$$

possible samples of five elements from a population of 25 elements.

With this relation in mind, we have the following definition of simple random sampling: A **simple random sample** of *n* elements from a population of *N* elements is one in which each of the $\binom{N}{n}$ possible samples of *n* elements has the same selection probability, namely, $1/\binom{N}{n}$.

It should be mentioned that the type of sampling discussed above—and throughout this volume—is known as **sampling without replacement.** In sampling without replacement a particular element can appear only once in a given sample, whereas if sampling is done with replacement, a given element can appear more than once in a particular sample. In practice, almost all sampling is done without replacement. Sampling with replacement is of interest primarily for theoretical reasons, since the mathematical theory of this type of sampling is less unwieldy than the theory of sampling without replacement. Under certain conditions, results derived under assumptions of sampling with replacement are approximately true even if the sampling is done without replacement. For discussions of sampling with replacement you may wish to consult a more mathematical sampling text such as Cochran (1) or Hansen et al. (2) or Kish (3).

In this text we always use sampling without replacement

How to Take a Simple Random Sample

First, give each population element a number from 1 to N

The first step in taking a simple random sample is to assign a number from 1 to *N* to each element in the population. The next step is to pick a sample of *n* of these numbers by some random process such as using a table of random numbers, a computer, or a calculator with a random number generator. Whatever procedure is used must ensure that the numbers selected are all different and that none are greater than *N*. Once the *n* numbers are chosen, the population elements corresponding to these numbers are taken as the sample.

*Next, select **n** of these numbers by a random process*

For example, if we want to take a random sample of six physicians from the list of physicians in table 2.1, we could use the random number table in the Appendix (table A1). Using two-digit numbers, and beginning at some arbitrary point [e.g., row 7, first two digits in column (1)], we proceed down the column until six different numbers between 01 and 25 are chosen. All numbers equal to 00 or greater than 25 are discarded. For this example the numbers we get are 09, 10, 07, 02, 01, and 13. These random numbers identify those individuals who will be studied in the sample. (If you work through this example by referring to table A1, you will note that we encounter the numbers 07 and 02 twice. Since we are sampling without replacement, they are discarded the second time we encounter them. Also, note that when we come to the bottom line of a particular page, we proceed to the top line of the very next column on that same page. We do not proceed to the next page of random numbers until we run out of columns on the current page.)

Finally, take those population elements that correspond to the numbers selected

Probability of an Element Being Selected

In simple random sampling there are $\binom{N}{n}$ possible samples of n elements from a population of N elements, and each sample has a probability of $1/\binom{N}{n}$ of being selected. Also, in simple random sampling the probability of any element being selected is equal to n/N, the ratio of the sample size to the population size. This can be demonstrated very simply by the following argument: The number of samples of n elements not containing a particular element is equal to $\binom{N-1}{n}$, the number of possible ways in which the $N-1$ other elements can combine in groups of size n. The probability of any element not being included is therefore equal to $\binom{N-1}{n}/\binom{N}{n}$, which is equal to $(N-n)/N$. The probability of a of a particular element being included is equal to $1 - [(N-n)/N]$, or n/N.

The probability of any element's selection is n/N

3.2 SAMPLING DISTRIBUTIONS OF ESTIMATED POPULATION CHARACTERISTICS

The estimates resulting from a simple random sample are unbiased estimates of the corresponding population parameters. Let us illustrate this idea through an example.

ILLUSTRATIVE EXAMPLE

As a simple example, let us consider the population of six schools shown in table 2.3, and let us suppose that we wish to estimate from a simple random sample of three schools the total number X of children in the six schools not immunized for measles. Using the estimated total, $x' = (N/n)x = \frac{6}{3}x$, we have the estimates shown in table 3.1 for the $\binom{6}{3}$ or 20 samples of three schools from a population of six schools.

Table 3.1   Possible Samples of
Three Schools and Values of x'

Schools in Sample	x'	Schools in Sample	x'
1, 2, 3	24	2, 3, 4	22
1, 2, 4	24	2, 3, 5	30
1, 2, 5	32	2, 3, 6	32
1, 2, 6	34	2, 4, 5	30
1, 3, 4	20	2, 4, 6	32
1, 3, 5	28	2, 5, 6	40
1, 3, 6	30	3, 4, 5	26
1, 4, 5	28	3, 4, 6	28
1, 4, 6	30	3, 5, 6	36
1, 5, 6	38	4, 5, 6	36

Note that each school appears in 10 of the 20 possible samples. Thus the probability of any particular school being in the sample is $\frac{10}{20}$, which is also $n/N = \frac{3}{6}$.

The sampling distribution of the estimated total x' ($n = 3$) for the data in table 3.1 is shown in table 3.2.

Table 3.2   Sampling Distribution
of the x' in Table 3.1

x'	f	$\pi = f/T$
20	1	.05
22	1	.05
24	2	.10
26	1	.05
28	3	.15
30	4	.20
32	3	.15
34	1	.05
36	2	.10
38	1	.05
40	1	.05
Total	20	1.00

From table 3.2 we see that the 20 equally likely samples yield 11 different values of x'. The mean, the variance, and the standard deviation of the sampling distribution of x' are as follows:

$$E(x') = \sum_{i=1}^{11} x'_i \pi_i = 20(.05) + 22(.05) + \cdots + 40(.05) = 30$$

$$Var(x') = \sum_{i=1}^{11} [x'_i - E(x')]^2 \pi_i = (20 - 30)^2(.05) + (22 - 30)^2(.05)$$

$$+ \cdots + (40 - 30)^2(.05) = 26.4$$

$$SE(x') = [Var(x')]^{1/2} = (26.4)^{1/2} = 5.138$$

We note that, for the six schools given in table 2.3, the population parameters X, σ_x^2, and σ_x are

$$X = 30 \qquad \sigma_x^2 = 3.67 \qquad \sigma_x = 1.915$$

We further note that, for the sampling distribution of x' shown in table 3.2,

$$E(x') = X = 30$$

That is, the estimated total in simple random sampling appears to be an unbiased estimate of the true population total.

It can be demonstrated that the variance $Var(x')$ and standard deviation $SE(x')$ of the sampling distribution of x' are given by

$$Var(x') = \left(\frac{N^2}{n}\right)(\sigma_x^2)\left(\frac{N - n}{N - 1}\right)$$

and

$$SE(x') = \left(\frac{N}{\sqrt{n}}\right)(\sigma_x)\left(\frac{N - n}{N - 1}\right)^{1/2}$$

For the example above

$$Var(x') = \left(\frac{6^2}{3}\right)(3.67)\left(\frac{6 - 3}{6 - 1}\right) = 26.4$$

which is the same result that we got through direct computation.

Thus we see that for simple random sampling the estimated population total x' is an unbiased estimate of the population total X. The standard error of x' given by the equation above is directly proportional to σ_x, the standard

The fpc influences
SE(x′)

*For **n** much less*
that N the fpc has
little effect on
SE(x′)

*As **n** approaches*
N, the fpc reduces
the value of SE(x′)

deviation of the distribution of $\mathscr{X}$ in the population, and inversely proportional to the sample size n. The standard error also depends on the square root of the factor $(N - n)/(n - 1)$, which is known as the **finite population correction,** fpc.

We can obtain some insight into the role played by the fpc by examining its value for a hypothetical population containing $N = 10,000$ elements for sample sizes as given in table 3.3. From the table we see that if the sample size n is very much less than the population size N, then the fpc is very close to 1.00 and thus will have little influence on the numerical value of the standard error $SE(x')$ of the estimated total x'. On the other hand, as n gets closer to N, the fpc decreases in magnitude and thus will cause a reduction in the value of $SE(x')$. If we write the fpc in the form $\sqrt{fpc}$, we have

$$\sqrt{fpc} = \left(\frac{N - n}{N - 1}\right)^{1/2} = \left(\frac{N}{N - 1}\right)^{1/2}\left(1 - \frac{n}{N}\right)^{1/2}$$

In this form we see that its value depends primarily on the ratio of n to N rather than on their absolute magnitudes. That the fpc is a factor in the value of $SE(x')$ makes sense intuitively since n close to N implies that most of the elements in the population are in the sample and that the elements not sampled would have very little effect on the distribution of x'.

Table 3.3   Values of fpc $(N = 10,000)$

Sample Size, n	$fpc = \left(\dfrac{N - n}{N - 1}\right)^{1/2}$
1	1.0000
10	.9995
100	.9950
500	.9747
1,000	.9487
5,000	.7071
9,000	.3162

Under simple
random sampling,
these estimates
are unbiased

A presentation similar to the one given above for the properties of a sample total under simple random sampling could be given for properties of the sampling distribution of sample means $\bar{x}$ and sample proportions p_y having an attribute $\mathscr{Y}$. We will not discuss each sampling distribution separately, but we summarize their properties in box 3.1.

We see from box 3.1 that, under simple random sampling, sample totals, means, and proportions are unbiased estimates of the corresponding population parameters.

Box 3.1 Population Estimates and Means and Standard Errors of Population Estimates Under Simple Random Sampling

Total, $\mathbf{x'}$

$$x' = \frac{N \sum\limits_{i=1}^{n} x_i}{n} = \left(\frac{N}{n}\right)(x) \qquad E(x') = X$$

$$SE(x') = \left(\frac{N}{\sqrt{n}}\right)(\sigma_x)\left(\frac{N-n}{N-1}\right)^{1/2}$$

(3.2)

Mean, $\mathbf{\bar{x}}$

$$\bar{x} = \frac{\sum\limits_{i=1}^{n} x_i}{n} = \frac{x}{n} \qquad E(\bar{x}) = \bar{X}$$

$$SE(\bar{x}) = \left(\frac{\sigma_x}{\sqrt{n}}\right)\left(\frac{N-n}{N-1}\right)^{1/2}$$

(3.3)

Proportion, $\mathbf{p_y}$

$$p_y = \frac{\sum\limits_{i=1}^{n} y_i}{n} = \frac{y}{n} \qquad E(p_y) = P_y$$

$$SE(p_y) = \left(\frac{P_y(1-P_y)}{n}\right)^{1/2}\left(\frac{N-n}{N-1}\right)^{1/2}$$

(3.4)

The notation used in these formulas is defined in boxes 2.1 and 2.2; *n* is the number of elements in the sample taken from a population of *N* elements.

3.3 COEFFICIENTS OF VARIATION OF ESTIMATED POPULATION PARAMETERS

In the previous chapter we defined the coefficient of variation V_x of the distribution of a variable $\mathscr{X}$ in a population as the standard deviation of the distribution of $\mathscr{X}$ divided by the mean value of $\mathscr{X}$ in the population. Similarly, we define the **coefficient of variation** $V(\hat{d})$ **of an estimate** $\hat{d}$ of a population parameter d as its standard error $\text{SE}(\hat{d})$ divided by the true value d of the parameter being estimated. In other words,

$$V(\hat{d}) = \frac{\text{SE}(\hat{d})}{d} \tag{3.5}$$

The square $V^2(\hat{d})$ of the coefficient of variation of an estimated parameter is known as the **relative variance** (or rel-variance) **of the estimated parameter.**

V(d̂) measures sampling variability and is used to assess reliability

The coefficient of variation of an estimated parameter measures the sampling variability of the estimate relative to the parameter being estimated and is used in assessing the reliability of the estimate. As we will see later on, it appears as a factor in many important results in sampling theory.

Box 3.2 presents the coefficients of variation of estimated totals, means, and proportions for a simple random sample.

Box 3.2 Coefficients of Variation of Population Estimates Under Simple Random Sampling

Total, x′

$$V(x') = \left(\frac{V_x}{\sqrt{n}}\right)\left(\frac{N-n}{N-1}\right)^{1/2} \tag{3.6}$$

Mean, x̄

$$V(\bar{x}) = \left(\frac{V_x}{\sqrt{n}}\right)\left(\frac{N-n}{N-1}\right)^{1/2} \tag{3.7}$$

Proportion, p_y

$$V(p_y) = \left(\frac{1-P_y}{nP_y}\right)^{1/2}\left(\frac{N-n}{N-1}\right)^{1/2} \tag{3.8}$$

In these formulas V_x is the coefficient of variation for the variable $\mathscr{X}$, P_y is the population proportion, n is the number of elements in the sample, and N is the number of elements in the population.

Derivation of **V(x′)**

The results shown in box 3.2 are obtained by substituting the values of the standard errors shown in box 3.1 into the formula for the coefficient of variation of an estimate [equation (3.5)]. For example, the coefficient of variation of an estimated total x' is, according to box 3.1 and equation (3.5),

$$V(x') = \frac{\left(\dfrac{N}{\sqrt{n}}\right)(\sigma_x)\left(\dfrac{N-n}{N-1}\right)^{1/2}}{X}$$

But $X = N\bar{X}$, and so

$$V(x') = \left(\frac{1}{\sqrt{n}}\right)\left(\frac{\sigma_x}{\bar{X}}\right)\left(\frac{N-n}{N-1}\right)^{1/2}$$

Since $\sigma_x/\bar{X}$ is by definition the coefficient of variation of the distribution of $\mathscr{X}$ in the population, we have

$$V(x') = \left(\frac{V_x}{\sqrt{n}}\right)\left(\frac{N-n}{N-1}\right)^{1/2}$$

The other results displayed in box 3.2 can be derived in a similar way. Note that under simple random sampling the coefficient of variation of an estimated mean $\bar{x}$ is the same as that for an estimated total x'.

3.4 RELIABILITY OF ESTIMATES

The standard error of an estimate is a measure of the sampling variability of the estimate over all possible samples. Under the assumption that measurement error is nonexistent or negligible, the **reliability of an estimate** can be judged by the size of its standard error: the larger the standard error, the lower is the reliability of the estimate. (See section 2.4.)

If we make the assumption that the estimates discussed in the previous sections have, for reasonably large values of n (say greater than 20), distributions that are close to the normal or Gaussian distribution, then we can use normal theory to obtain approximate confidence intervals for the unknown population parameters being estimated. For example, approximate $100(1 - \alpha)\%$ **confidence intervals** for the population total are given by

$$x' \pm z_{1-\alpha/2}\left(\frac{N}{\sqrt{n}}\right)(\sigma_x)\left(\frac{N-n}{N-1}\right)^{1/2}$$

Confidence interval formula for X

where $z_{1-\alpha/2}$ is the $100(1 - \alpha/2)$th percentile of the standard normal distribution. For example, for a 95% confidence interval, $\alpha = .05$ and $z_{1-\alpha/2} = z_{.975} = 1.96$.

Since σ_x is an unknown population parameter, it must be estimated from the sample. If we replace σ_x in the formula above by

$$\hat{\sigma}_x = \left[\left(\frac{N-1}{N}\right)(s_x^2)\right]^{1/2}$$

we obtain the following approximate confidence intervals for the population total X:

$$x' \pm z_{1-\alpha/2}(N)\left(\frac{N-n}{N}\right)^{1/2}\left(\frac{s_x}{\sqrt{n}}\right)$$

ILLUSTRATIVE EXAMPLE

Suppose that a simple random sample of nine of the 25 physicians listed in table 2.1 is taken for purposes of estimating the total X of household visits made by physicians in the population. Let us suppose that the physicians chosen are 13, 3, 17, 1, 14, 12, 7, 18, 4. The sample data are given in table 3.4

Table 3.4   Sample Data for Number of Household Visits

Physician	No. of Visits	Physician	No. of Visits
1	5	13	6
3	1	14	4
4	4	17	7
7	12	18	0
12	5		

The sample statistics are (from formulas in boxes 2.2 and 3.1)

$$x = 44 \qquad s_x = 3.48 \qquad x' = (\tfrac{25}{9})(44) = 122.22$$

From the previous formula we obtain the upper limit of the 95% confidence interval for X, with $z_{1-\alpha/2} = z_{.975} = 1.96$:

$$122.22 + 1.96(25)\left(\frac{25-9}{25}\right)^{1/2}\left(\frac{3.48}{\sqrt{9}}\right)$$

or

$$122.22 + 45.47 = 167.69$$

Likewise, the lower limit of the 95% confidence interval for X is

$$122.22 - 45.47 = 76.75$$

Note that the true population total, $X = 127$ (see p. 13), is covered by this confidence interval.

These 95% confidence intervals have the usual interpretation: that is, in repeated sampling if other samples of n elements were selected according to the same sampling plan and if, for each sample, confidence intervals were calculated, 95% of such confidence intervals would include the true unknown population parameter.

Box 3.3 summarizes the estimated variances of the sampling distribution for the total, mean, and proportion and gives the form of the corresponding confidence interval.

Box 3.3 Estimated Variances and $100(1 - \alpha)\%$ Confidence Intervals Under Simple Random Sampling

Total, x′

$$\widehat{\mathrm{Var}}(x') = N^2 \left(\frac{N - n}{N}\right)\left(\frac{s_x^2}{n}\right)$$

and

$$x' \pm z_{1-\alpha/2}(N)\left(\frac{N - n}{N}\right)^{1/2}\left(\frac{s_x}{\sqrt{n}}\right) \qquad (3.9)$$

Mean, x̄

$$\widehat{\mathrm{Var}}(\bar{x}) = \left(\frac{N - n}{N}\right)\left(\frac{s_x^2}{n}\right)$$

and

$$\bar{x} + z_{1-\alpha/2}\left(\frac{N - n}{N}\right)^{1/2}\left(\frac{s_x}{\sqrt{n}}\right) \qquad (3.10)$$

Proportion, p_y

$$\widehat{\mathrm{Var}}(p_y) = \left(\frac{N - n}{N}\right)\left[\frac{p_y(1 - p_y)}{n - 1}\right]$$

and

$$p_y \pm z_{1-\alpha/2}\left(\frac{N - n}{N}\right)^{1/2}\left[\frac{p_y(1 - p_y)}{n - 1}\right]^{1/2} \qquad (3.11)$$

In these equations n is the number of elements in the sample, N is the number of elements in the population, s_x^2 is the sample variance, and $z_{1-\alpha/2}$ is the $100(1 - \alpha/2)$th percentile of the standard normal distribution.

Note that we may substitute the relation involving $\hat{\sigma}_x^2$ for s_x^2 [see equation (2.16)] in the expressions for $\widehat{\mathrm{Var}}(x')$ and $\widehat{\mathrm{Var}}(\bar{x})$. Also note that, since $\widehat{\mathrm{SE}}(\hat{d}) = [\widehat{\mathrm{Var}}(\hat{d})]^{1/2}$, the confidence interval may be written in terms of the estimated standard error. That is, we may write the confidence intervals as

$$x' \pm z_{1-\alpha/2}[\widehat{\mathrm{SE}}(x')] \qquad \bar{x} \pm z_{1-\alpha/2}[\widehat{\mathrm{SE}}(\bar{x})] \qquad p_y \pm z_{1-\alpha/2}[\widehat{\mathrm{SE}}(p_y)]$$

Confidence intervals of box 3.3 are based on the assumption of normality for the sample estimate

It should be emphasized that the confidence intervals obtained by using the equations in box 3.3 are based on the assumption that the estimate (e.g., x') is normally distributed. The extent to which this assumption is violated depends on such considerations as the nature of the distribution of the variable in the population and the size of the sample. If the variable has a nearly symmetric distribution and the sample size is not small, then the confidence coefficients expressed in the confidence intervals will be approximately correct. If the data are badly skewed, however, and the sample size is small, the confidence coefficients may be misleading. (Exercise 1 in this chapter illustrates this situation using the data in table 2.1.) For linear estimates such as those discussed in this chapter, the **central limit theorem** of statistics gives a theoretical anchor to the assumption of normality. This theorem states, in effect, that if statistics such as means, totals, and proportions are based on large enough sample sizes, their sampling distributions tend to be normal, irrespective of the underlying nature of the original observations.

Confidence intervals can be obtained for population means and proportions from the appropriate sample estimates in a manner analogous to that demonstrated in the example above for totals.

3.5 ESTIMATION OF PARAMETERS FOR SUBDOMAINS

In this section we consider subdomains identified after the simple random sample is drawn

Often the objectives of sample surveys include estimates of parameters not only for the population as a whole but also for certain **subdomains** (subgroups or subsets) of the population. For example, a nationwide health survey of households might require estimates for the nation as a whole and also for groups defined by age, race, sex, geographical area, or combinations of these. Often the subdomains are identified before the sample is taken, and the sample is drawn separately within each subdomain. This type of sampling plan will be considered in our discussion of stratified sampling in chapters 5 and 6. Sometimes, however, a simple random sample is drawn from the population as a whole, and estimates are expressed separately for each subdomain of interest. It is this type of sampling plan that is considered in this section. We will illustrate the procedure by using an example.

ILLUSTRATIVE EXAMPLE

Let us consider the population of six families living on one city block shown in table 3.5. Using these data, we find that the average out-of-pocket medical expense per family is $296.67 for the total population, $316.67 for white families, and $276.67 for black families.

Let us suppose that we wish to take a simple random sample of four households from the population of six households for purposes of estimating the average per-household,

Table 3.5   Race and Out-of-Pocket Medical Expenses for Six Families (1977)

Family	Race	*Out-of-Pocket Medical Expenses (dollars)*	Family	Race	*Out-of-Pocket Medical Expenses (dollars)*
1	W	500	4	W	280
2	B	350	5	W	170
3	B	430	6	B	50

out-of-pocket medical expenditure for the population as a whole and for each race separately. The procedure for obtaining such an estimate for the population as a whole has been discussed earlier. So in this example we will only consider estimates for the desired subdomains.

We can construct estimates for a particular subdomain (e.g., the black population) in the following way: Let

$$Y_i = \begin{cases} 1 \text{ if the } i\text{th family is black} \\ 0 \text{ if otherwise} \end{cases}$$

Let

$$X_i = \text{the out-of-pocket medical expenses of the } i\text{th family}$$
$$Z_i = X_i Y_i$$

For the six families in the population we have the values of X_i, Y_i, and Z_i shown in table 3.6.

Table 3.6   Data for a Subdomain Based on the Families Listed Table 3.5

Family	Race	X_i	Y_i	Z_i
1	W	500	0	0
2	B	350	1	350
3	B	430	1	430
4	W	280	0	0
5	W	170	0	0
6	B	50	1	50

Letting Y and Z denote population totals and y and z denote sample totals in the usual way, we see that $Z = \$830$ and $Y = 3$ and that the average out-of-pocket medical expense per family for black families is equal to the ratio

$$\frac{Z}{Y} = \frac{\$830}{3} = \$276.67$$

Let us estimate Z/Y from the sample by the ratio z/y, constructed from the sample elements. For samples of $n = 4$ elements the distribution of z/y is given in table 3.7.

Table 3.7   Sampling Distribution of z/y

Sample Elements	z	y	z/y
1, 2, 3, 4	780	2	390
1, 2, 3, 5	780	2	390
1, 2, 3, 6	830	3	276.67
1, 2, 4, 5	350	1	350
1, 2, 4, 6	400	2	200
1, 2, 5, 6	400	2	200
1, 3, 4, 5	430	1	430
1, 3, 4, 6	480	2	240
1, 3, 5, 6	480	2	240
1, 4, 5, 6	50	1	50
2, 3, 4, 5	780	2	390
2, 3, 4, 6	830	3	276.67
2, 3, 5, 6	830	3	276.67
2, 4, 5, 6	400	2	200
3, 4, 5, 6	480	2	240

If we calculate the mean $E(z/y)$ of the sampling distribution of z/y and the standard error $SE(z/y)$, we have*

$$E(z/y) = \$276.67 = \frac{Z}{Y} \quad \text{and} \quad SE(z/y) = \$96.77$$

Thus we see that the sample mean z/y is an unbiased estimate of the population mean.

The sample mean for a subdomain is an unbiased estimate

What we have shown above empirically is true in general for simple random sampling—namely, that the sample mean of a variable among members of a subgroup is an unbiased estimate of the population mean for that subgroup.

A precise expression for the **standard error of an estimated mean for a subgroup** is not available. However, the following approximation is valid if the

---

* The ratio z/y is a special case of a ratio estimate, which will be described in detail in chapter 7. In general, ratio estimates are not unbiased, although the magnitude of their bias is generally small. However, when the denominator is a count of the elementary units, an unbiased estimate is obtained with simple random sampling.

expected number $E(y)$ of elements from the subdomain falling in the sample is greater than or equal to 20:

$$SE(z/y) = \left[\frac{\sigma_z}{\sqrt{E(y)}}\right]\left[\frac{Y - E(y)}{Y - 1}\right]^{1/2} \qquad (3.12)$$

An approximation if the subdomain elements in the sample number 20 or more

where z/y is the mean of the y elements in the sample belonging to the subdomain and σ_z is the standard deviation of the distribution of the variable $\mathscr{Z}$ among members of the subgroup in the population and is given by

$$\sigma_z = \left[\frac{\sum\limits_{i=1}^{Y}(Z_i - \bar{Z})^2}{Y}\right]^{1/2}$$

Since Y, $E(y)$, and σ_z are not usually known, they are generally estimated by y' [which is equal to $(N/n)y$], y, and

$$\hat{\sigma}_z = \left(\frac{y' - 1}{y'}\right)^{1/2}\left[\frac{\sum\limits_{i=1}^{y}(z_i - \bar{z})^2}{y - 1}\right]^{1/2}$$

where z_i represents the value of the variable $\mathscr{Z}$ for the ith sample element and $\bar{z}$ is the sample mean of the z_i. Substituting the estimates y, y', and $\hat{\sigma}_z$ into equation (3.12), we then have the **estimate of the standard error** $\widehat{SE}(z/y)$ of an estimated mean for a subgroup:

$$\widehat{SE}(z/y) = \left(\frac{\hat{\sigma}_z}{\sqrt{y}}\right)\left(\frac{y' - y}{y' - 1}\right)^{1/2} \qquad (3.13)$$

Note that the approximation given by equation (3.12) cannot be used for the data in table 3.5, since the average number of elements in the subgroup falling into the sample is equal to 2 $[E(y) = (n/N)Y$ over all possible samples], which is considerably less than 20.

Now let us illustrate how we would estimate a subgroup mean and its standard error by using the preceding equations.

ILLUSTRATIVE EXAMPLE

Let us consider the data in table 3.8, obtained from a simple random sample of 40 workers taken from a plant employing 1200 workers.

If we are interested in estimating the mean forced vital capacity (fvc) among workers having high exposure to pulmonary stressors, we have the following calculations:

$$y = 28 \qquad n = 40 \qquad N = 1200$$

$$y' = \left(\frac{N}{n}\right)(y) = \left(\frac{1200}{40}\right)(28) = 840$$

Table 3.8   Cumulative Exposure to Pulmonary Stressors and
Forced Vital Capacity (fvc) Among Workers in a Sample
Taken at a Plant Employing 1200 Workers

Worker	Exposure	fvc[a]	Worker	Exposure	fvc[a]
1	high	81	21	medium	70
2	high	64	22	low	64
3	medium	85	23	high	72
4	medium	91	24	medium	72
5	high	60	25	high	95
6	low	97	26	high	96
7	low	82	27	high	62
8	low	99	28	high	67
9	high	96	29	high	95
10	high	91	30	low	87
11	low	71	31	high	84
12	high	88	32	high	89
13	medium	84	33	high	89
14	high	85	34	high	65
15	high	77	35	high	67
16	high	76	36	high	69
17	high	62	37	high	80
18	high	67	38	high	98
19	high	91	39	high	65
20	medium	99	40	high	84

[a] Percentage of value expected on basis of age, sex, and height.

$$z = \sum_{i=1}^{n} z_i = 81 + 64 + \cdots + 84 = 2215$$

$$\frac{z}{y} = \frac{2215}{28} = 79.11$$

$$\hat{\sigma}_z = \left(\frac{y'-1}{y'}\right)^{1/2} \left[\frac{\sum_{i=1}^{y}(z_i - \bar{z})^2}{y-1}\right]^{1/2}$$

$$= \left(\frac{840-1}{840}\right)^{1/2} \left[\frac{(81-79.11)^2 + (64-79.11)^2 + \cdots + (84-79.11)^2}{28-1}\right]^{1/2}$$

$$= 12.55$$

$$\widehat{SE}(z/y) = \left(\frac{\hat{\sigma}_z}{\sqrt{y}}\right)\left(\frac{y'-y}{y'-1}\right)^{1/2} = \left(\frac{12.55}{\sqrt{28}}\right)\left(\frac{840-28}{840-1}\right)^{1/2} = 2.33$$

Thus we would estimate from this sample that there are a total of 840 workers having high exposure to pulmonary stressors, that their average fvc is 79.11%, and that a 95% confidence interval for this estimated mean is

$$\frac{z}{y} - (1.96)[\widehat{SE}(z/y)] \leq \frac{Z}{Y} \leq \frac{z}{y} + (1.96)[\widehat{SE}(z/y)]$$

$$79.11 - (1.96)(2.33) \leq \frac{Z}{Y} \leq 79.11 + (1.96)(2.33)$$

$$74.54 \leq \frac{Z}{Y} \leq 83.68$$

3.6 HOW LARGE A SAMPLE DO WE NEED?

One of the most important problems in sample design is that of determining how large a sample is needed for the estimates obtained from the sample survey to be reliable enough to meet the objectives of the survey. In this section we will formulate this problem in very general terms and then show how it may be solved for a particular sample design, for example, for simple random sampling of elementary units.

In determining sample size the first step is to specify the level of reliability needed for the resulting estimates (see section 2.4). In general, the larger the sample, the greater will be the reliability of the resulting estimates. Validity, on the other hand, is a function of the measurement process rather than the sample size and will not, in general, be improved with an increase in sample size. An improvement in validity requires an improvement in the measuring process.

The reliability needed is the first consideration in determining sample size

In determining the levels of reliability needed for estimates, the statisticians and subject matter persons should examine the objectives of the survey. For example, suppose that, from a hospital admitting 20,000 patients annually a survey of hospital patients is to be taken for purposes of determining the proportion of the 20,000 patients that received optimal care as defined by specified standards. The quality care review committee planning the survey might feel that some remedial action should be taken if fewer than 80% of the patients are receiving optimal care. In this instance the committee would be concerned about overestimates of the true proportion but would probably not be too concerned if the estimated proportion were 80% when the true population proportion were 75%. The statistician might formulate this by saying that the user would like to be "virtually certain" that the estimated proportion differs from the true proportion by no more than $100[(80 - 75)/75]\%$, or 6.67%, of the true proportion.

"Virtual certainty"
as a level of
reliability might
be associated with
an interval of ± 3
standard errors
Now let us see what is meant here by "virtual certainty." In terms of reliability, if we assume that the sample estimates are normally distributed with a mean equal to the unknown population estimate, we know that for approximately 997 of every 1000 samples, the true population parameter will lie within three standard errors of the estimate (see figure 3.1). In terms of the example mentioned above, if p_y is the estimated proportion, P_y is the true unknown population proportion, and $SE(p_y)$ is the standard error of p_y, we can be virtually certain that P_y is greater than $p_y - 3SE(p_y)$ and less than $p_y + 3SE(p_y)$. The statistician's problem, then, is to choose a sample large enough so that $3SE(p_y) \leq .0667P_y$ when P_y is approximately equal to .80 (see the next example).

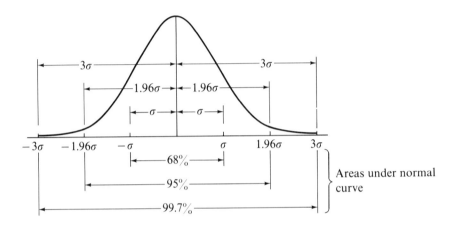

Figure 3.1   Areas Under Normal Curve Within ±1, ±1.96, and ±3 Standard Errors of the Mean

As it is used here, "virtual certainty" is but one of many potential levels of confidence that may be used in the construction of confidence intervals and the determination of necessary sample sizes. This particular level of confidence need not always be used. However, it is commonly used in the determination of sample sizes for sample surveys.

ILLUSTRATIVE EXAMPLE

Let us suppose that our design uses a simple random sample of hospital records from a hospital admitting 20,000 patients annually. From box 3.1 we see that $3SE(p_y)$ is given by

$$3SE(p_y) = 3 \left[\frac{P_y(1 - P_y)}{n} \right]^{1/2} \left(\frac{N - n}{N - 1} \right)^{1/2}$$

We want our sample large enough (see the discussion above) so that

$$3SE(p_y) \leq .0667P_y$$

or

$$3\left[\frac{P_y(1 - P_y)}{n}\right]^{1/2}\left(\frac{N - n}{N - 1}\right)^{1/2} \leq .0667P_y$$

Solving this relation for n, we obtain

$$n \geq \frac{9NP_y(1 - P_y)}{(N - 1)(.0667)^2P_y^2 + 9P_y(1 - P_y)}$$

Setting $P_y = .80$ and $N = 20,000$, we obtain $n \geq 494$. (It should be noted that in all sample size calculations the resulting value of n is rounded up to the nearest integer.) Thus we need a sample of 494 patients or more to be virtually certain of obtaining estimates having the reliability required for meeting the objectives of the survey.

The example above can be generalized to the estimation of any population proportion P_y under simple random sampling. If we wish to be virtually certain that the sample estimate p_y differs in absolute value from the true unknown proportion P_y by no more than εP_y, then the **sample size** n must satisfy the relation given by

$$n \geq \frac{9NP_y(1 - P_y)}{(N - 1)\varepsilon^2P_y^2 + 9P_y(1 - P_y)}$$

Formula for n for the reliability level of virtual certainty

The value of ε is set by the investigator to reflect the objectives of the survey.

If the population size N is very much greater than the required sample size n, the relation above can be approximated by the formula

$$n \geq \frac{9(1 - P_y)}{\varepsilon^2 P_y}$$

This formula is an approximation for the one above

This relation shows that the required sample size depends on three factors: 9, ε^2, and $(1 - P_y)/P_y$. The factor 9 is the virtual certainty factor; the ε^2 factor represents the specifications set on our estimate in terms of the maximum relative difference allowed between it and the unknown true population proportion P_y. The third factor $(1 - P_y)P_y$ is the square of the coefficient of variation (or the relative variance) of the dichotomous variable (in this instance, receiving or not receiving optimal care) upon which the proportion P_y is based. From the approximation formula for n we see that as we make ε more stringent (i.e., smaller), the greater will be the required sample size n.

The sample sizes required under simple random sampling for the estimation of population totals and means can be derived in a similar way and have similar forms to those shown above for proportions. The required sample sizes for totals, means, and proportions are summarized in box 3.4. In this summary z is the **reliability coefficient,** which is based upon the assumption that the sampling distribution of the particular estimate under consideration is normal. That is, for virtual certainty, $z = 3$. If 95% confidence is desired, z is 1.96.

Box 3.4 Exact and Approximate Sample Sizes Required Under Simple Random Sampling

	EXACT	APPROXIMATE

Total, x′

$$n \geq \frac{z^2 N V_x^2}{z^2 V_x^2 + (N - 1)\varepsilon^2} \qquad\qquad n \geq \frac{z^2 V_x^2}{\varepsilon^2} \qquad (3.14)$$

Mean, x̄

$$n \geq \frac{z^2 N V_x^2}{z^2 V_x^2 + (N - 1)\varepsilon^2} \qquad\qquad n \geq \frac{z^2 V_x^2}{\varepsilon^2} \qquad (3.15)$$

Proportion, p_y

$$n \geq \frac{z^2 N P_y(1 - P_y)}{z^2 P_y(1 - P_y) + (N - 1)\varepsilon^2 P_y^2} \qquad n \geq \frac{z^2(1 - P_y)}{\varepsilon^2 P_y} \qquad (3.16)$$

In these equations z is the reliability coefficient (e.g., $z = 3$ for virtual certainty and $z = 1.96$ for a 95% confidence level), N is the population size, V_x^2 is the relative variance for the variable $\mathscr{X}$, ε is a value set by the investigator (e.g., the sample estimate $\hat{d}$ should not differ in absolute value from the true unknown population parameter d by more that εd), and P_y is the population proportion.

With regard to the equations in box 3.4, we note that parameters such as V_x^2, the rel-variance with respect to the distribution of a variable $\mathscr{X}$, in a population are generally not known. Thus in order to calculate required sample sizes, statisticians must usually make educated guesses.

ILLUSTRATIVE EXAMPLE

As another illustration of how sample size might be determined, let us suppose that a sample survey of retail pharmacies is to be conducted in a state that contains 2500 pharmacies. The purpose of the survey is to estimate the average retail price of 20 tablets of a commonly used tranquilizer. An estimate is needed that is within 10% of the true value of the average retail price in the state. A list of all the pharmacies is available, and a simple random sample will be taken from this list. A phone survey of 20 of the $N = 1000$ pharmacies in another state showed an average price of $3.50 for the 20 tablets, with a standard deviation of $0.70.

We can use the information from this small phone survey for purposes of estimating sample size for the proposed study. We estimate V_x^2 as*

$$\hat{V}_x^2 = \frac{\hat{\sigma}_x^2}{\bar{x}^2} = \frac{[(N - 1)/N](s_x^2)}{\bar{x}^2} = \frac{(999/1000)(.70)^2}{(3.50)^2} = .04$$

With $\varepsilon = .1$ and $N = 2500$, we obtain, from the exact formula (3.15),

$$n = \frac{9(2500)(.04)}{9(.04) + 2499(.1)^2} = 35.5 \approx 36$$

Thus a sample of 36 pharmacies is needed for purposes of this study. Note that the approximation $9V_x^2/\varepsilon^2$ in this instance would yield the same value of n.

In actual practice, one variable is rarely singled out as the basis for calculation of sample size. Usually several of the most important variables are chosen and sample sizes are calculated for each of these variables. The final sample size chosen might then be the largest of these calculated sample sizes. If funds are not available to take the largest of these calculated sample sizes, then, as a compromise measure, the median or the mean of the calculated n's might be taken.

In practice, sample size determination is made on the basis of these calculations applied to several variables

We also emphasize that the sample size selected to meet specifications for the reliability of an estimated characteristic in a population as a whole would not be large enough to estimate the characteristic in a subdomain of the

---

* The estimate of V_x^2 is derived as follows: $V_{\bar{x}}^2 = \sigma_{\bar{x}}^2/\bar{X}^2$ from equation (2.7). Hence $\hat{V}_{\bar{x}}^2 = \hat{\sigma}_x^2/\hat{\bar{X}}^2$. But $\hat{\sigma}_x^2 = [(N - 1)/N](s_x^2)$ from equation (2.16) and the estimate of $\bar{X}$ is $\bar{x}$. Thus it follows that

$$\hat{V}_x^2 = \frac{\hat{\sigma}_x^2}{\hat{\bar{X}}^2} = \frac{[(N - 1)/N](s_x^2)}{\bar{x}^2}$$

The sample size needed for reliable population estimates may not yield reliable estimates of subdomain parameters

population. For example, 500 individuals may be an adequate sample size to be virtually certain of estimating the prevalence of hypertension within 10% of the true prevalence. But the estimated prevalence of hypertension in males of that sample is not likely to be as reliable an estimate, since it would be based on a sample size that is considerably smaller than 500. Thus in calculating sample sizes, one should specify the particular subdomains or subgroups for which estimates are needed and the levels of reliability that are desired for the estimates in each subdomain.

3.7 WHY SIMPLE RANDOM SAMPLING IS RARELY USED

It is important as the basis for sampling theory

Simple random sampling is very important as a basis for development of the theory of sampling. Under simple random sampling any particular sample of n elements from a population of N elements can be chosen and, in addition, is as likely to be chosen as any other sample. In this sense it is conceptually the simplest possible method, and hence it is one against which all other methods can be compared.

It may not be feasible

Although simple random sampling is conceptually simple, it can be expensive and simply not feasible in practice since it requires that all elements be identified and labeled *prior* to the sampling. Often this prior identification is not possible, and hence a simple random sampling of elements cannot be drawn.

It may be too costly

Also, since simple random sampling gives each element in the population an equal chance of being chosen for the sample, it may result in samples that are spread out over a large geographic area. And if household interviews are required, this technique can be inordinately expensive.

It may not be an efficient design for the survey's objectives

The fact that every element has an equal chance of selection is likely to result in samples in which subdomains have representation in the sample according to their distribution in the population. While this might be good for some types of surveys, it would not be good for those surveys in which interest is focused on subgroups that comprise a small proportion of the population. For example, a simple random sample of all households in Detroit is not likely to be an efficient design for estimating morbidity in households having income below the poverty level.

In other words, even though it might be possible for a simple random sample of elements to be taken, there are other methods that produce estimates having the same accuracy but at lower total expense. In the remainder of this book we will discuss these other methods.

SUMMARY

In this chapter we introduced the concept of a simple random sample, and we noted its importance as the foundation of sampling theory. We derived general expressions for the mean, variance, standard error, coefficient of variation, and relative variance of estimated means, proportions, and totals under simple random sampling. We discussed the use of confidence intervals for purposes of evaluating the reliability of estimates for sample designs in general, and we illustrated their use for simple random sampling in particular. We showed how to estimate characteristics in subdomains when a simple random sample of the population as a whole has been drawn. We presented methodology for calculating the sample size required under simple random sampling for estimating population characteristics with specified reliability. Finally, mention was made of the disadvantages inherent in simple random sampling.

EXERCISES

1. From the data in table 2.1 (p. 13), and using simple random sampling, take ten different samples of six physicians. For each sample compute approximate 95% confidence intervals for the average number of household visits per physician. For how many of these calculated 95% confidence intervals is the true population mean $\bar{X}$ within the boundaries of the intervals? If this number is much higher or lower than expected, how do you explain it? (Start with the first random number in the upper left-hand corner of table A1 in the Appendix and read down the columns.)

2. How many simple random samples of 15 elements can be taken from a population containing 65 elements?

3. From the data in table 3.8 estimate the proportion of all workers in the plant having a forced vital capacity (fvc) less than 70% of that expected on the basis of age, sex, and height. Give 95% confidence intervals for this estimated proportion.

4. From the data in table 3.8 of the workers having low or medium cumulative exposure to pulmonary stressors, estimate the proportion having an fvc below 90% of that expected on the basis of age, sex, and height. Give 95% confidence intervals for this estimated proportion.

5. From the data in table 3.8 estimate the proportion of workers in the plant having low or medium cumulative exposure to pulmonary stressors. Give 95% confidence intervals for this estimated proportion.

6. A survey of workers is to be taken in a large plant that makes products similar to those made in the plant from which the data of table 3.8 were drawn. The purposes of the survey are to estimate (a) the proportion of all workers having an fvc below 70% and (b) the mean fvc among all workers. Estimates are needed within 5% of the true value of the parameter being estimated. How large a sample of workers is needed? The plant employs 5000 workers.

7. A community within a city contains 3,000 households and 10,000 persons. For purposes of planning a community satellite to the local health department, it is desired to estimate the total number of physician visits made during a calendar year by members of the community. For this information to be useful, it should be accurate to within 10% of the true value. A small pilot survey of 10 households, conducted for purposes of gathering preliminary information, yielded the accompanying data on physician visits made during the previous calendar year. Using these data as preliminary information, determine the sample size needed to meet the specifications of the survey.

Household	No. of Persons in Household	No. of Physician Visits Per Person During Previous Year
1	3	4.0
2	6	4.5
3	2	8.0
4	5	3.4
5	2	0.5
6	3	7.0
7	4	8.5
8	2	6.0
9	6	4.0
10	4	7.5

8. A section of a random number table is reproduced here.

06	97	37	77
08	00	39	81
14	08	58	01
22	17	24	19
75	73	12	79
69	59	32	53
54	03	48	44

(a) Starting with the first random number in the upper left-hand corner of this table and reading down the columns, select a random sample of 6 of the 25 physicians listed in table 2.1 (p. 13).

(b) Estimate the mean number $\bar{X}$ of household visits made by the physicians in the population (use a 90% confidence interval).

(c) Estimate the total number X of household visits made by the physicians in the population (use a 95% confidence interval). How does this confidence interval compare to the one given in the example in the text on page 46?

(d) Estimate, with virtual certainty, the proportion of physicians in the population making two or more household visits per year.

BIBLIOGRAPHY

For a more theoretically oriented discussion of simple random sampling, the following textbooks should be consulted.

1. COCHRAN, W. G. *Sampling techniques*, 3d ed. New York: Wiley, 1977.

2. HANSEN, M. H.; HURWITZ, W. N.; and MADOW, W. G. *Sample survey methods and theory*. Vols. 1 and 2, New York: Wiley, 1953.

3. KISH, L. *Survey sampling*. New York: Wiley, 1965.

4

Systematic Sampling

*Systematic
sampling is
probably the most
widely used
sampling technique*

In the previous chapter we introduced the concept of simple random sampling of elements and discussed its importance as being "conceptually" the simplest kind of sampling since every possible combination of *n* elements from a population of *N* elements has the same chance of being selected. We also discussed some of the problems associated with simple random sampling, including difficulties that may preclude drawing a sample by that method. In this chapter we discuss a type of sampling known as systematic sampling. Systematic sampling is widely used in practice because it is extremely easy to apply and can be easily taught to individuals who have little training in survey methodology. In fact, systematic sampling may be the most widely used method of sampling.

4.1 HOW TO TAKE A SYSTEMATIC SAMPLE

Perhaps the best way to describe the procedure involved in taking a systematic sample is through an example. So let us look first at one specific case.

ILLUSTRATIVE EXAMPLE

Let us suppose that as part of a cost-containment-and-quality-of-care review program, a sample of hospital records is selected on an ongoing basis for a detailed audit. The total

62

number of records in the population is not likely to be known in advance of the sampling since the records are to be sampled on an ongoing basis, and so it would not be possible to use simple random sampling to choose the records. However, it may be possible to guess the approximate number of records that would be available for selection per time period and to select a sample of one in every k records as they become available, where k is an integer having a particular value chosen to meet the requirements of the study.

For example, suppose it is anticipated that ten new discharge records will be available per day and that a total sample of 300 records per year is desired. Then the total number of available records per year is estimated to be 10×365, or 3650. To obtain somewhere in the neighborhood of 300 records per year in the sample, k should be the largest integer in the quotient 3650/300. Since the value of the quotient is 12.17, k would be equal to 12. This value of k is known as the **sampling interval.** Thus we would take a sample of one from every 12 records.

One way to implement this sampling procedure is to identify each record as it is created with a consecutive number, beginning with 1. (There are stamping devices that the quotient 3650/300. Since the value of the quotient is 12.17, k would be equal to 12. chosen as the starting point. Then that record and every twelfth record beyond it would be chosen. For example, if the random number is 4, the records chosen in the sample would be 4, 16, 28, 40, and so on.

To generalize, a systematic sample is taken by first determining the desired sampling interval k, choosing a random number j between 1 and k, and selecting the elements labeled $j, j + k, j + 2k, j + 3k, \ldots$ Note that the **sampling fraction** for such a survey is $1/k$.

Determine k, choose random number j, then select elements j, j + k, j + 2k, and so on

A slight modification of this method based on the decimal system is especially useful if the elements to be sampled are already numbered consecutively and if the actual drawing of the sample is to be done by unskilled personnel. If a sample of one in k units is specified (where k is, for example, a two-digit number), we might select a random two-digit number between 01 and k. If the number selected is j, then the two-digit numbers $j, j + k, j + 2k$, and so on are selected until a three-digit number is reached. All elements ending in the two-digit numbers selected are then included in the sample. For example, if $k = 12$, random two-digit number between 01 and 12 is chosen (e.g., 07). The two-digit sample numbers are then determined (e.g., 07, 19, 31, 43, 55, 67, 79, 91), and all records ending with those two digits would be included in the sample (e.g., 07, 19, 31, 43, 55, 67, 79, 91, 107, 119, 131, 143, 155, 167, 179, 191, 207, 219, 231, etc.). This procedure is sometimes easier to use than the first procedure mentioned, especially if the individuals drawing the sample are unskilled, since they could be instructed to pull only those records ending with the specified digits. Our discussion of the properties of estimates from systematic random samples will be based, however, on the first method described.

A modification if elements are already numbered

In this book we will use the first procedure described

4.2 ESTIMATION OF POPULATION CHARACTERISTICS

x, x̄, and p$_y$ are calculated the same way they were in simple random sampling

If a systematic sample of one in k elements yields a sample of n elements, then the **sample total** x, the **sample mean** $\bar{x}$, and the **sample proportion** p_y are calculated from the sample in the same manner as they were calculated for simple random sampling (see box 3.1). The **estimated population total** x' for systematic sampling is given by

$$x' = \left(\frac{N}{n}\right)(x) \qquad (4.1)$$

and when $k = N/n$ is an integer, $x' = kx$.

It is not necessary that N be known prior to the initiation of sampling. When N is not known prior to sampling (as when taking every kth person to enter an emergency room), N can be determined by counting the number of individuals remaining after the last one is chosen and adding that remainder to nk.

Let us illustrate these ideas with an example.

ILLUSTRATIVE EXAMPLE

Let us take a systematic sample of one in six physicians from the list given in table 2.1 (p. 13). We first take a random number between 1 and 6; for example, we choose 5. The physicians selected in the sample, then, are 5, 11, 17, and 23. The corresponding values of $\mathscr{X}$, the number of household visits, are shown in table 4.1.

Table 4.1   Systematic Sample of One in Six Physicians (from Table 2.1)

Sample Number, i	Physician Number	No. of Visits, x_i
1	5	7
2	11	0
3	17	7
4	23	0
Total		14

The estimated mean number $\bar{x}$ of household visits per physician is

$$\bar{x} = \frac{x}{n} = \frac{14}{4} = 3.5$$

The estimated total number x' of visits made by all physicians in the population is

$$x' = \left(\frac{N}{n}\right)(x) = \left(\frac{25}{4}\right)(14) = 87.5$$

The estimated proportion p_y of physicians making one or more household visits is

$$p_y = \frac{y}{n} = \frac{2}{4} = .50$$

4.3 SAMPLING DISTRIBUTION OF ESTIMATES

In a simple random sample of n elements from a population containing N elements, every one of the $\binom{N}{n}$ total samples not only has a chance of being selected but also has the *same* chance of being selected. In a systematic sample of one in k elements there are only k possible samples, and the particular sample selected depends on the random number initially selected.

Let us compare these two sampling methods in a specific example.

ILLUSTRATIVE EXAMPLE

Suppose that, from the listing in table 2.1, a sample of one in five physicians is desired. The five possible samples are listed in table 4.2 along with estimates $\bar{x}$, x', and p_y of the population parameters $\bar{X}$, X, and P_y.

Table 4.2   Five Possible Samples of One in Five Physicians (from Table 2.1)

Random Number Chosen	Physicians in Sample	Estimated Mean, $\bar{x}$	Estimated Total, x'	Estimated Proportion (Physicians Making One or More Visits), p_y
1	1, 6, 11, 16, 21	2.6	65	.4
2	2, 7, 12, 17, 22	4.8	120	.6
3	3, 8, 13, 18, 23	1.4	35	.4
4	4, 9, 14, 19, 24	9.2	230	.8
5	5, 10, 15, 20, 25	7.4	185	.6

Since each of the five possible samples listed in table 4.2 has the same chance, namely, $\frac{1}{5}$, of being selected, the mean $E(\bar{x})$, of the sampling distribution of the estimated mean is (see box 2.3)

$$E(\bar{x}) = \tfrac{1}{5}(2.6 + 4.8 + 1.4 + 9.2 + 7.4) = 5.08 = \bar{X}$$

In other words, $\bar{x}$ is an unbiased estimate of $\bar{X}$. Similarly,

$$E(x') = \tfrac{1}{5}(65 + 120 + 35 + 230 + 185) = 127 = X$$
$$E(p_y) = \tfrac{1}{5}(.4 + .6 + .4 + .8 + .6) = .56 = P_y$$

Thus we see that in this instance the estimated mean, total, and proportion are unbiased estimates of the corresponding population parameters.

The standard errors of $\bar{x}$, x', and p_y are given next (see box 2.3).

$$SE(\bar{x}) = \{\tfrac{1}{5}\sum[\bar{x} - E(\bar{x})]^2\}^{1/2} = \{\tfrac{1}{5}[(2.6 - 5.08)^2 + (4.8 - 5.08)^2$$
$$+ (1.4 - 5.08)^2 + (9.2 - 5.08)^2 + (7.4 - 5.08)^2]\}^{1/2} = 2.90$$

$$SE(x') = \{\tfrac{1}{5}[(65 - 127)^2 + (120 - 127)^2 + (35 - 127)^2$$
$$+ (230 - 127)^2 + (185 - 127)^2]\}^{1/2} = 72.57$$

$$SE(p_y) = \{\tfrac{1}{5}[(.4 - .56)^2 + (.6 - .56)^2 + (.4 - .56)^2 + (8 - .56)^2$$
$$+ (.6 - .56)^2]\}^{1/2} = .15$$

The means and standard errors of $\bar{x}$, x', and p_y in this example are compared in table 4.3 to the means and standard errors that would have been obtained under simple random sampling. Examining the table, we see that for both sampling schemes the estimates are unbiased. However, the standard errors of the estimates are not the same. In fact, in this example the systematic sampling errors are smaller than those for simple random sampling.

Table 4.3 Comparison of Means and Standard Errors for Simple Random Sampling and for Systematic Sampling ($n = 5$ in All Instances)

| | MEAN | | STANDARD ERROR | |
| | Simple Random | Systematic | Simple Random | Systematic |
Estimate	Sampling	Sampling	Sampling	Sampling
$\bar{x}$	5.08	5.08	3.36	2.90
x'	127	127	84.11	72.57
p_y	.56	.56	.20	.15

The estimated mean, total, and proportion are unbiased if N/k is an integer

In general, the estimated mean, total, and proportion under systematic sampling as described above are unbiased estimates of the corresponding population parameters only if the ratio N/k is an integer. In the previous example $N = 25$, $k = 5$, and hence $N/k = \tfrac{25}{5}$, which is an integer. Thus as was shown above, $\bar{x}$, x', and p_y are unbiased estimates.

If, on the other hand, N/k is not an integer, then the systematic sample estimates may be biased. Let us explore this situation in an example.

ILLUSTRATIVE EXAMPLE

Suppose we specify a one in six systematic sample of physicians from the list in table 2.1. Then we would have the possible samples shown in table 4.4.

Table 4.4   Six Possible Samples of One in Six Physicians (from Table 2.1)

		SAMPLE ESTIMATES		
Random Number Chosen	*Physicians in Sample*	$\bar{x}$	x'	p_y
1	1, 7, 13, 19, 25	12	300	.80
2	2, 8, 14, 20	1	25	.25
3	3, 9, 15, 21	4.25	106.25	.75
4	4, 10, 16, 22	6.5	162.5	.50
5	5, 11, 17, 23	3.5	87.5	.50
6	6, 12, 18, 24	1.5	37.5	.50

Since each of the six possible samples is equally likely, the mean of the sampling distributions of $\bar{x}$, x', and p_y are

$$E(\bar{x}) = \tfrac{1}{6}(12 + 1 + 4.25 + 6.5 + 3.5 + 1.5) = 4.79 \neq \bar{X}$$

$$E(x') = \tfrac{1}{6}(300 + 25 + 106.25 + 162.5 + 87.5 + 37.5) = 119.79 \neq X$$

$$E(p_y) = \tfrac{1}{6}(.80 + .25 + .75 + .50 + .50 + .50) = .55 \neq P_y$$

Thus we see that in this instance systematic sampling does not lead to unbiased estimates.

The reason the estimates in the preceding example are not unbiased is that although each element has the same chance (e.g., $1/k$) of being selected, the impact made on the estimates is not the same for each element. Physician 1, for example, has less impact than physician 2, since physician 1 appears with four other physicians in the sample, whereas physician 2 appears in the sample with three other physicians. Thus physician 1's measurements are diluted more than those of physician 2 in obtaining an estimate. In the previous instance when N/k was an integer, each physician appeared with the same number of other physicians in the sample, and all physicians had the same impact on the estimates.

If N/k is not an integer, the estimates may be biased

If the number of elements N in the population is large, the biases in the estimates from systematic samples will, in general, be quite small and will be of little concern. A slight modification of the method of choosing the initial

When N is large, the biases of the estimates will be very small

random number, however, will result in estimates that are unbiased. This modification will be discussed later in this chapter (section 4.5).

4.4 VARIANCE OF ESTIMATES

Let us now consider the variances of estimates from systematic sampling. As discussed earlier, the variance of an estimate is important since it is a measure of its reliability.

Assumption: N/k
is an integer

In this discussion of variances of estimates from systematic sampling, let us assume for simplicity that N/k is an integer denoted by n. Systematic sampling of one in k elements would then yield a total of k possible samples, each containing N/k elements. The possible samples are shown in table 4.5.

Table 4.5   Possible Samples of One in k Elements (N/k Is an Integer)

Random Number Chosen	Elements in Sample	Value of Variable $\mathscr{X}$
1	$1, 1 + k, 1 + 2k, \ldots, 1 + (n-1)k$	$X_1, X_{1+k}, X_{1+2k}, \ldots, X_{1+(n-1)k}$
2	$2, 2 + k, 2 + 2k, \ldots, 2 + (n-1)k$	$X_2, X_{2+k}, X_{2+2k}, \ldots, X_{2+(n-1)k}$
$\vdots$		
j	$j, j + k, j + 2k, \ldots, j + (n-1)k$	$X_j, X_{j+k}, X_{j+2k}, \ldots, X_{j+(n-1)k}$
$\vdots$		
k	$k, 2k, 3k, \ldots, nk$	$X_k, X_{2k}, X_{3k}, \ldots, X_{nk}$

In examining the systematic samples shown in table 4.5, we see that each sample is a "cluster" of n (equal to N/k) elements, with each element being k "units" apart. Thus systematic sampling is operationally equivalent to grouping the N elements into k clusters, each containing N/k elements that are k units apart on the list, and then taking a simple random sample of one of these clusters. To illustrate this idea, let us look at an example.

ILLUSTRATIVE EXAMPLE

Let us suppose that a systematic sample of one in five workers from table 3.8 (p. 52) is taken. For purposes of illustration the 40 workers in table 3.8 will be considered to be a population rather than a sample from a larger population. Then $N = 40$, $k = 5$, and $N/k = n = \frac{40}{5} = 8$. The five clusters defined by the sampling design are shown in table 4.6. These clusters represent the five possible samples of one in five workers chosen from the list in table 3.8.

Table 4.6   Cluster Samples Based on Data of Table 3.8

Cluster	Workers in Cluster	Forced Vital Capacity of Workers in Cluster
1	1, 6, 11, 16, 21, 26, 31, 36	81, 97, 71, 76, 70, 96, 84, 69
2	2, 7, 12, 17, 22, 27, 32, 37	64, 82, 88, 62, 64, 62, 89, 80
3	3, 8, 13, 18, 23, 28, 33, 38	85, 99, 84, 67, 72, 67, 89, 98
4	4, 9, 14, 19, 24, 29, 34, 39	91, 96, 85, 91, 72, 95, 65, 65
5	5, 10, 15, 20, 25, 30, 35, 40	60, 91, 77, 99, 95, 87, 67, 84

The variance of estimates from systematic samples can be understood more easily if we relabel the elements with double subscripts to denote the particular cluster. For example, the elements in the first cluster, elements 1, $1 + k$, $1 + 2k, \ldots, 1 + (n - 1)k$, would be relabeled with double subscripts as follows:

For convenience we relabel the subscripts shown in table 4.5

ORIGINAL LABEL	NEW LABEL	VALUE OF VARIABLES $\mathscr{X}$
1	1, 1	X_{11}
$1 + k$	1, 2	X_{12}
$1 + 2k$	1, 3	X_{13}
$1 + (n - 1)k$	1, n	X_{1n}

The elements in the jth cluster would be relabeled similarly:

ORIGINAL LABEL	NEW LABEL	VALUE OF VARIABLES $\mathscr{X}$
j	$j, 1$	X_{j1}
$j + k$	$j, 2$	X_{j2}
$j + 2k$	$j, 3$	X_{j3}
$j + (n - 1)k$	j, n	X_{jn}

With this new labeling, the variances of estimated means, totals, and proportions obtained from systematic sampling are as given in box 4.1.

The expressions shown in box 4.1 are equal to those of estimates obtained from simple random sampling multiplied by the factor $[1 + \delta_x(n - 1)]$. The parameter δ_x is called the **intraclass correlation coefficient** and is a measure of the homogeneity of elements *within* the k possible systematic samples, or clusters, that could theoretically have been selected from a population of $N = nk$ elements. Calculation of δ_x involves, for each cluster, the establishing of $\binom{n}{2}$ pairs of values (X_{ij}, X_{il}), which play the same role as do the pairs (X, Y) in the usual product-moment correlation coefficient. The difference is that deviations are computed about $(\bar{X}, \bar{X})$, where $\bar{X}$ is the mean of the X_{ij} over *all* observations in all possible systematic samples (i.e., the population mean). The summation

δ_x measures homogeneity within the k possible samples

Box 4.1 Variances of Population Estimates Under Systematic Sampling

Mean, x̄

$$\text{Var}(\bar{x}) = \left(\frac{\sigma_x^2}{n}\right)\left[1 + \delta_x(n-1)\right] \qquad (4.2)$$

Total, x′

$$\text{Var}(x') = \left(\frac{N^2\sigma_x^2}{n}\right)\left[1 + \delta_x(n-1)\right] \qquad (4.3)$$

Proportion, p_y

$$\text{Var}(p_y) = \left[\frac{P_y(1-P_y)}{n}\right]\left[1 + \delta_x(n-1)\right] \qquad (4.4)$$

where $n = N/k$ and

$$\delta_x = \frac{2\sum\limits_{i=1}^{k}\sum\limits_{j=1}^{n}\sum\limits_{\ell<j}(X_{ij}-\bar{X})(X_{i\ell}-\bar{X})}{nk(n-1)\sigma_x^2} \qquad (4.5)$$

In these equations N is the population size, n is the sample size, k is the sampling interval, X_{ij} is the jth element from the ith cluster, $X_{i\ell}$ is another element from the ith cluster ($\ell \neq j$), and the population notation is as defined in box 2.1.

---

in the numerator of equation (4.5) involves the cross product of these deviations over all pairs of points for each of the k possible systematic samples. This intraclass correlation coefficient can range from very small negative values, when the elements within each cluster tend to be very diverse or representative of the population of elements (this is called "heterogeneity"), to a maximum of one when the elements within each cluster are similar but differ from cluster to cluster (this is called "homogeneity").

It is clear from expressions (4.2), (4.3), and (4.4) that when δ_x is large, the variance of the mean, the total, or the proportion will be large. This can occur when the population's elements are arranged in a list demonstrating a high degree of periodicity. When δ_x equals zero, the resulting variances are the same as those of simple random sampling. This usually occurs when the population's elements are arranged in random order with respect to the variable under consideration. Finally, when δ_x is small and negative, the resulting variances will be smaller than those of simple random sampling. This can occur when the elements in the population are ordered with respect to the variable under study.

Let us now see what this all means by considering an example.

ILLUSTRATIVE EXAMPLE

Suppose that a list of appointments for a nurse practitioner is available to us and that we will take a sample of one in four of the patients seen by this nurse on a given day for purposes of estimating the average time spent per patient. Suppose that on the day in which the sample was to be taken, the nurse saw a total of 12 patients in the order shown in table 4.7

Table 4.7   Data for Nurse Practitioner's Visits (Unordered List)

Order of Visit	Time Spent with Patient (min)	Order of Visit	Time Spent with Patient (min)
1	15	7	49
2	34	8	40
3	35	9	25
4	36	10	46
5	11	11	33
6	17	12	14

Since we specify a one in four sample, the four possible samples are as shown in table 4.8.

Table 4.8   Four Possible Samples for Data of Table 4.7

SAMPLE 1		SAMPLE 2		SAMPLE 3		SAMPLE 4	
Patient	Time Spent	Patient	Time Spent	Patient	Time Spent	Patient	Time Spent
1	15	2	34	3	35	4	36
5	11	6	17	7	49	8	40
9	25	10	46	11	33	12	14
Total	51		97		117		90
Mean	17		32.33		39		30

The mean time $\bar{X}$ spent with the 12 patients is 29.583 min (minutes), with variance $\sigma_x^2 = 153.08$. The variance over all possible samples of the estimated mean time spent per patient is (see box 2.3)

$$\text{Var}(\bar{x}) = \tfrac{1}{4}\big[(17 - 29.583)^2 + (32.33 - 29.583)^2 + (39 - 29.583)^2$$
$$+ (30 - 29.583)^2\big] = 63.6$$

To show that this is equal to the expression given in relation (4.2), we will compute the necessary parameters. The intraclass correlation δ_x is (from box 4.1)

$$\delta_x = \frac{\begin{aligned}2[(15 - 29.583)(11 - 29.583) + (15 - 29.583)(25 - 29.583)\\ + (11 - 29.583)(25 - 29.583) + (34 - 29.583)(17 - 29.583)\\ + \cdots + (40 - 29.583)(14 - 29.583)]\end{aligned}}{(3)(4)(3 - 1)(153.08)}$$

$$= .1241$$

Then from equation (4.1), with $\sigma_x^2 = 153.08$, $n = 3$, and $\delta_x = .1241$, we have

$$\text{Var}(\bar{x}) = \left(\frac{153.08}{3}\right)[1 + .1241(3 - 1)] = 63.6$$

which agrees with what was found empirically.

Suppose now that the nurse scheduled appointments in such a way that the difficult patients requiring the most time would be seen first and the easier ones requiring less time would be seen later in the day. The list of appointments for the same patients discussed above might appear as shown in table 4.9.

Table 4.9   Data for Nurse Practitioner's Visits
(Monotonically Ordered List)

Order of Visit	Time Spent with Patient (min)	Order of Visit	Time Spent with Patient (min)
1	49	7	33
2	46	8	25
3	40	9	17
4	36	10	15
5	35	11	14
6	34	12	11

If we were to take a systematic sample of one in four patients from the list of appointments in table 4.9, we would obtain the four possible samples shown in table 4.10.

Since the procedure by which the sample was taken is a systematic sample of one in four elements, and since $N/k = \frac{12}{4} = 3$ is an integer, the sample mean is, as before, an unbiased estimate of the population mean; that is, $E(\bar{x}) = \bar{X} = 29.583$. The variance of

Table 4.10   Four Possible Samples for Data of Table 4.9

| SAMPLE 1 | | SAMPLE 2 | | SAMPLE 3 | | SAMPLE 4 | |
Patient	Time Spent	Patient	Time Spent	Patient	Time Spent	Patient	Time Spent
1	49	2	46	3	40	4	36
5	35	6	34	7	33	8	25
9	17	10	15	11	14	12	11
Total	101		95		87		72
Mean	33.67		31.67		29		24

the estimated mean $\bar{x}$ is

$$\text{Var}(\bar{x}) = \tfrac{1}{4}\big[(33.67 - 29.583)^2 + (31.67 - 29.583)^2 + (29 - 29.583)^2$$
$$+ (24 - 29.583)^2\big] = 13.13$$

Thus we see that in this situation—when the list of appointments is ordered—the systematic sampling procedure yields an estimated mean having a lower variance than that obtained from the same systematic sampling procedure when the list was not ordered. This makes sense intuitively, because the process of sampling systematically from a list that is ordered according to the level of the variable being measured ensures that every sample will have some elements having high values of the variable, some having low values, and some having moderate values. In other words, it would not be possible for any one particular sample to have a concentration of atypically high or atypically low values.

The intraclass correlation coefficient in this instance is equal to $-.371$, which is a negative number and considerably less than that obtained when the sampling was from the unordered list.

Let us now suppose that the nurse scheduled an easy patient followed by two moderately difficult patients followed by a very difficult patient (in terms of time required). The appointment list containing the same 12 patients might then appear as shown in table 4.11.

Table 4.11   Data for Nurse Practitioner's Visits (Periodicity in List)

Order of Visit	Time Spent with Patient (min)	Order of Visit	Time Spent with Patient (min)
1	11	7	35
2	17	8	46
3	36	9	15
4	49	10	25
5	14	11	33
6	34	12	40

Table 4.12   Four Possible Samples for Data of Table 4.11

| SAMPLE 1 | | SAMPLE 2 | | SAMPLE 3 | | SAMPLE 4 | |
Patient	Time Spent	Patient	Time Spent	Patient	Time Spent	Patient	Time Spent
1	11	2	17	3	36	4	49
5	14	6	34	7	35	8	46
9	15	10	25	11	33	12	40
Total	40		76		104		135
Mean	13.33		25.33		34.67		45

If we were to sample systematically one in four patients from the list in table 4.11, we would obtain the four possible samples listed in table 4.12.

Again the estimated mean is an unbiased estimate of the population mean. The variance of the distribution of estimated means is

$$\mathrm{Var}(\bar{x}) = \tfrac{1}{4}[(13.33 - 29.583)^2 + (25.33 - 29.583)^2 + (34.67 - 29.583)^2$$
$$+ (45 - 29.583)^2] = 136.41$$

The intraclass correlation coefficient δ_x in this situation is equal to .837. Thus in this situation the estimated mean has a much larger variance than it had in the other situations. The results we have obtained are summarized in table 4.13.

Table 4.13   Summary of Results for Four Types of Sampling

Sample Design	$Var(\bar{x})$	Intraclass Correlation Coefficient δ_x
systematic sampling, unordered list	63.6	.124
systematic sampling, monotonically ordered list	13.1	−.371
systematic sampling, periodicity in list	136.4	.837
simple random sampling	41.7	—

In the third systematic sampling situation—namely, that in which the nurse scheduled an easy patient followed by two moderately difficult patients followed by a very difficult one, in a continuing pattern—the variance of the estimated means was very high. The reason for this high variance is that the nurse's scheduling pattern involved a 1-in-4 periodicity that coincided with the periodicity in the sample selection, with the result that all the difficult patients were in the same sample and all the easy ones were in the same sample. Thus the sampling variability of estimated means was very high. This high variance contrasted with the low variance found when the appointments were made in order of increasing difficulty. As noted before, systematic sampling of this ordered list resulted in every possible sample having its share of difficult, moderate, and easy patients, so that the samples did not differ very much in the distribution of the variable being measured.

To generalize, systematic sampling from a list that is ordered in the variable being measured often results in estimates that have small sampling variance. On the other hand, if the list has periodicities in it that coincide with the periodicity in the sampling, the estimates could have very high variance and the survey estimates would in no way represent the population of interest.

If periodicities in list and sampling coincide, the estimates will have high variance

When a list is in "random order"—that is, there is no particular ordering or periodicity in the list—the variance in the estimated mean, total, or proportion obtained in systematic sampling is approximately that appropriate for simple random sampling. In other words,

$$\text{Var}(\bar{x}) \approx \left(\frac{\sigma_x^2}{n}\right)\left(\frac{N-n}{N-1}\right)$$

$$\text{Var}(p_y) \approx \left[\frac{P_y(1-P_y)}{n}\right]\left(\frac{N-n}{N-1}\right)$$

$$\text{Var}(x') \approx \left(\frac{N^2}{n}\right)(\sigma_x^2)\left(\frac{N-n}{N-1}\right)$$

For a list in random order the variances of the estimates are approximately equal to those for simple random sampling

Note that in the previous example the intraclass correlation coefficient δ_x was highest in the situation where there was a periodicity in the list. This result is understandable in light of the fact that δ_x measures homogeneity of elements with respect to the variable being measured. When the periodicity in the nurse's appointment list coincided with the periodicity in the sampling interval (e.g., when $k = 4$), all the difficult patients were in one sample and all the easy ones in another. This situation produced a homogeneity of patients within the same cluster, large differences between patients in different samples, a high intraclass correlation coefficient, and a high variance for the estimated mean.

4.5. A MODIFICATION THAT ALWAYS YIELDS UNBIASED ESTIMATES

We demonstrated earlier that systematic sampling of one in k elements does not yield unbiased estimates when the ratio N/k is not an integer, although the bias is likely to be small when N and k are reasonably large. In this section we present a method of taking a systematic sample of one in k elements that will *always* lead to unbiased estimates of population means, totals, and proportions. This method, however, requires prior knowledge of the population size N, and therefore it is only useful in those situations where N is known. We illustrate the method with an example.

The population size N must be known for this method

ILLUSTRATIVE EXAMPLE

Suppose that we wish to take a 1-in-6 sample from the list of 25 physicians in table 2.1 and that we know in advance of the sampling that there are 25 physicians on the list. Instead of taking a random number between 1 and 6 to start the systematic sampling, let us take a random number j between 1 and 25. We then divide j by 6 and determine the remainder. For example, if the random number is 9, then $\frac{9}{6} = 1\frac{3}{6}$, the remainder is 3, and we begin with the third physician. If the remainder is 1, we begin with the first physician; and so on. When there is no remainder, we begin with element k (e.g., 6 in this case).

Table 4.14   Distribution of Remainders and Samples for 25 Possible Random Numbers

Random Number, j	j/k	Remainder	Elements in Sample
1	$\frac{1}{6}$	1	1, 7, 13, 19, 25
2	$\frac{2}{6}$	2	2, 8, 14, 20
3	$\frac{3}{6}$	3	3, 9, 15, 21
4	$\frac{4}{6}$	4	4, 10, 16, 22
5	$\frac{5}{6}$	5	5, 11, 17, 23
6	$\frac{6}{6}$	0	6, 12, 18, 24
7	$\frac{7}{6}$	1	1, 7, 13, 19, 25
8	$\frac{8}{6}$	2	2, 8, 14, 20
9	$\frac{9}{6}$	3	3, 9, 15, 21
10	$\frac{10}{6}$	4	4, 10, 16, 22
11	$\frac{11}{6}$	5	5, 11, 17, 23
12	$\frac{12}{6}$	0	6, 12, 18, 24
13	$\frac{13}{6}$	1	1, 7, 13, 19, 25
14	$\frac{14}{6}$	2	2, 8, 14, 20
15	$\frac{15}{6}$	3	3, 9, 15, 21
16	$\frac{16}{6}$	4	4, 10, 16, 22
17	$\frac{17}{6}$	5	5, 11, 17, 23
18	$\frac{18}{6}$	0	6, 12, 18, 24
19	$\frac{19}{6}$	1	1, 7, 13, 19, 25
20	$\frac{20}{6}$	2	2, 8, 14, 20
21	$\frac{21}{6}$	3	3, 9, 15, 21
22	$\frac{22}{6}$	4	4, 10, 16, 22
23	$\frac{23}{6}$	5	5, 11, 17, 23
24	$\frac{24}{6}$	0	6, 12, 18, 24
25	$\frac{25}{6}$	1	1, 7, 13, 19, 25

Let us examine the distribution of remainders and samples for the 25 possible random numbers, which is shown in table 4.14. It is apparent that each sample does not have the same chance of being selected. For example, a remainder of 1 has a $\frac{5}{25}$ chance of occurring, since it occurs whenever random numbers 1, 7, 13, 19, and 25 are chosen. The other remainders have a $\frac{4}{25}$ chance of occurring (e.g., the remainder 5 occurs whenever random numbers 5, 11, 17, and 23 are chosen).

With this in mind, we examine the sampling distribution of estimated means shown in table 4.15.

Table 4.15   Sampling Distribution of Estimated Means from
Data of Tables 4.14 and 2.1

Elements in Sample	Estimated Mean No. of Visits, $\bar{x}$	Chance of Selection, π
1, 7, 13, 19, 25	12	$\frac{5}{25}$
2, 8, 14, 20	1	$\frac{4}{25}$
3, 9, 15, 21	4.25	$\frac{4}{25}$
4, 10, 16, 22	6.5	$\frac{4}{25}$
5, 11, 17, 23	3.5	$\frac{4}{25}$
6, 12, 18, 24	1.5	$\frac{4}{25}$

The mean $E(\bar{x})$ of the distribution of estimated mean household visits from this modified systematic sampling plan is (see box 2.4)

$$E(\bar{x}) = (12)(\tfrac{5}{25}) + (1)(\tfrac{4}{25}) + (4.25)(\tfrac{4}{25}) + (6.5)(\tfrac{4}{25}) + (3.5)(\tfrac{4}{25}) + (1.5)(\tfrac{4}{25})$$
$$= 5.08 = \bar{X}$$

Thus we see that this method, unlike the previously described one, leads to an unbiased estimate of the population mean even when N/k is not equal to an integer. Similarly, it leads to an unbiased estimate of population totals and proportions.

To generalize from the example, the modified method can be operationalized as follows:

1. Choose a random number between 1 and N, where N is the number of elements in the population.   *Steps in applying the modified method*

2. Compute the quotient j/k, where j is the random number selected and k is the sampling interval. Express this quotient as an integer plus a remainder (e.g., $\frac{23}{6} = 2\frac{5}{6}$, and the remainder is 5).

3. If the remainder is 0, take a systematic sample of one in k elements in the usual way, beginning with element k. If the remainder is nonzero (e.g., m), take a systematic sample of one in k elements in the usual way, beginning with element m.

4.6 ESTIMATION OF VARIANCES

As with all sampling methods, in order to construct confidence intervals, estimates of the standard errors of the sampling distributions are needed. In this section we demonstrate how estimates of standard errors are obtained in practice with systematic random sampling.

The variance of an estimated mean $\bar{x}$ from a systematic sample of one in k elements (assuming that N/k is an integer) is the average squared deviation over the k possible samples of the estimated mean from the true population mean. In other words, if $\bar{x}_i$ represents the mean value of $\mathscr{X}$ for the elements i, $i + k, i + 2k, \ldots, i + (n-1)k$, then the **variance of an estimated mean** $\bar{x}$ from a systematic sample of one in k elements is given by

For a systematic sample

$$\text{Var}(\bar{x}) = \frac{\sum\limits_{i=1}^{k} (\bar{x}_i - \bar{X})^2}{k} \qquad (4.6)$$

Let us compare this expression with the variance of the sampling distribution of the mean under simple random sampling, which is defined as

For a simple random sample

$$\text{Var}(\bar{x}) = \frac{\sum\limits_{i=1}^{M} (\bar{x}_i - \bar{X})^2}{M}$$

where M is the total number of possible samples. It is a marvelous property of simple random sampling that this variance can be determined simply by calculating σ_x^2, the variance of the original observations. That is,

In a simple random sample, if we know s_x^2, we can estimate $Var(\bar{x})$

$$\text{Var}(\bar{x}) = \left(\frac{N-n}{N-1}\right)\left(\frac{\sigma_x^2}{n}\right)$$

Of greater importance to the statistician is that, by estimating the variance σ_x^2 with the observations in a particular sample (i.e., s_x^2), the variance of $\bar{x}$ may be estimated as

$$\widehat{\text{Var}(\bar{x})} = \left(\frac{N-n}{N}\right)\left(\frac{s_x^2}{n}\right)$$

Hence, simply by knowing the variance of the observations in a particular sample, we can estimate the variance of the sampling distribution of the sample mean under simple random sampling.

Unfortunately, the same cannot be said of systematic sampling. In order to estimate the variance given in equation (4.6), it is necessary to have two or more of these $\bar{x}_i$ available to us. However, in our systematic sample the estimated mean $\bar{x}$ is simply one of the $\bar{x}_i$, with the particular one depending on which random number was chosen to start the sampling. We have no information from our sample concerning the variability of estimated means over all possible samples.

But in a systematic sample, calculating s^2 does not, in general, permit estimation of $Var(\bar{x})$

In practice, if we can assume that the list from which the systematic sample was taken represents a random ordering of the elements with respect to the variable being measured, then we often assume that the systematic sample is equivalent to a simple random sample. Therefore, the procedures developed for estimating the variances of estimates from simple random samples can be used. In other words, we estimate the population variance σ_x^2 by $\hat{\sigma}_x^2$, as given by

Assumption: the systematic sample is equivalent to a simple random sample

$$\hat{\sigma}_x^2 = \left(\frac{N-1}{N}\right)(s_x^2)$$

where

$$s_x^2 = \frac{\sum\limits_{i=1}^{n}(x_i - \bar{x})^2}{n-1}$$

and where the x_i's are the sample observations and $n = N/k$. The **estimated variance** of the estimated mean $\bar{x}$ from a systematic sample is then given by

$$\widehat{Var}(\bar{x}) = \left(\frac{\hat{\sigma}_x^2}{n}\right)\left(\frac{N-n}{N-1}\right) \tag{4.7}$$

Using this expression, we can then obtain confidence intervals for the population mean $\bar{X}$ in the usual way.

ILLUSTRATIVE EXAMPLE

Suppose that we take a 1-in-5 systematic sample of physicians from the list given in table 2.1 and that the initial random number chosen is 3. Table 4.16 lists the physicians in the sample along with their household visits.

Table 4.16   Systematic 1-in-5 Sample
Taken from Table 2.1

Physician in Sample	Number of Visits, x_i
3	1
8	0
13	6
18	0
23	0

Using the data in table 4.16, we have the following calculations (see box 2.2 and the equations given above):

$$\bar{x} = 1.4 \qquad n = 5 \qquad N = 25$$

$$s_x^2 = \tfrac{1}{4}[(1 - 1.4)^2 + (0 - 1.4)^2 + (6 - 1.4)^2 + (0 - 1.4)^2$$
$$+ (0 - 1.4)^2] = 6.8$$

$$\hat{\sigma}_x^2 = \left(\frac{24}{25}\right)(6.8) = 6.528$$

$$\widehat{Var(\bar{x})} = \left(\frac{6.528}{5}\right)\left(\frac{25 - 5}{24}\right) = 1.088$$

The upper and lower limits for a 95% confidence interval are given by (see box 3.3)

$$\bar{x} + (1.96)[\widehat{Var(\bar{x})}]^{1/2} = 1.4 + (1.96)(1.088)^{1/2} = 3.44$$
$$\bar{x} - (1.96)[\widehat{Var(\bar{x})}]^{1/2} = 1.4 - (1.96)(1.088)^{1/2} = -.64 = 0$$

(We use 0 for the lower limit since negative numbers make no sense in this example.) Thus the 95% confidence interval for the mean number of visits is 0 to 3.44.

This technique always yields unbiased variance estimates

If, in fact, the list were not in random order, the assumption of random ordering could lead to estimated variances of estimates that are either too low or too high, and the resulting confidence intervals could be misleading.

A modification of systematic sampling, called **repeated systematic sampling,** yields estimates of the variances of estimated means, proportions, and totals that are unbiased no matter what kind of ordering or periodicity exists in the list from which the sample is drawn. We will develop this procedure by using an example.

ILLUSTRATIVE EXAMPLE

For this example we will use the data shown in table 4.17.

Let us suppose that we wish to take a systematic sample of approximately 18 workers from the list of 162 workers for purposes of estimating the mean number of work days lost per worker from acute illnesses. Since $n = 18$ and $N = 162$, a systematic sample of one in nine workers would accomplish this. However, $18 = 6 \times 3$, and therefore we can obtain a sample of 18 workers by taking six systematic samples each containing three workers. In this case the sampling interval $k = 162/3 = 54$, and we would take six systematic samples of one in 54 workers. To do this, we first choose six random numbers between one and 54 (e.g., 2, 31, 46, 13, 34, 53), and then we choose systematic samples of one in 54 beginning with each random number. Our six samples are shown in table 4.18.

Table 4.17   Days Lost from Work Because of Acute Illness in
One Year Among 162 Employees in a Plant

Employee ID	Days Lost	Employee ID	Days Lost	Employee ID	Days Lost
1	7	55	8	109	1
2	6	56	2	110	7
3	10	57	9	111	9
4	11	58	9	112	6
5	3	59	8	113	6
6	8	60	6	114	3
7	0	61	5	115	4
8	5	62	3	116	2
9	8	63	9	117	5
10	4	64	6	118	10
11	7	65	3	119	10
12	13	66	3	120	15
13	4	67	4	121	5
14	5	68	9	122	5
15	2	69	5	123	6
16	0	70	8	124	3
17	7	71	5	125	9
18	17	72	11	126	9
19	5	73	5	127	6
20	6	74	9	128	5
21	1	75	8	129	4
22	7	76	7	130	1
23	9	77	6	131	1
24	3	78	4	132	11
25	8	79	3	133	3
26	9	80	9	134	5
27	4	81	5	135	9
28	8	82	5	136	5
29	4	83	3	137	1
30	17	84	5	138	15
31	6	85	4	139	2
32	9	86	0	140	10
33	9	87	11	141	8
34	5	88	3	142	2
35	8	89	4	143	6
36	5	90	11	144	14
37	8	91	0	145	10
38	5	92	6	146	8
39	8	93	1	147	7
40	0	94	9	148	9
41	3	95	6	149	1

Table 4.17 (*continued*)

Employee ID	Days Lost	Employee ID	Days Lost	Employee ID	Days Lost
42	5	96	0	150	2
43	3	97	3	151	6
44	6	98	6	152	4
45	11	99	0	153	6
46	6	100	12	154	3
47	5	101	11	155	1
48	5	102	6	156	8
49	0	103	1	157	0
50	8	104	3	158	3
51	1	105	2	159	2
52	10	106	5	160	8
53	7	107	3	161	0
54	9	108	12	162	15

Table 4.18   Data for Six Systematic Samples Taken from Table 4.17

Random Number	Elements of Sample	Days Lost	Estimated Mean, x_i
2	2	6	
	56	2	5.00
	110	7	
13	13	4	
	67	4	4.33
	121	5	
31	31	6	
	85	4	4.00
	139	2	
34	34	5	
	88	3	3.33
	142	2	
46	46	6	
	100	12	7.00
	154	3	
53	53	7	
	107	3	
	161	0	3.33

If we denote $\bar{x}_i$ as the estimated mean number of work days lost due to acute illness from the ith sample and m as the number of samples taken, then our **estimated mean** is

$$\bar{\bar{x}} = \frac{\sum\limits_{i=1}^{m} \bar{x}_i}{m} = \frac{5.00 + 4.33 + 4.00 + 3.33 + 7.00 + 3.33}{6} = 4.5$$

Since the estimated mean $\bar{\bar{x}}$ was obtained by taking a simple random sample of $m = 6$ means $\bar{x}_i$ from a population of $M = 54$ such means, we can use the theory of simple random sampling to obtain the estimate $\widehat{\text{Var}}(\bar{\bar{x}})$ of the variance of $\bar{\bar{x}}$:

$$\widehat{\text{Var}}(\bar{\bar{x}}) = \left(\frac{1}{m}\right) \frac{\sum\limits_{i=1}^{m} (\bar{x}_i - \bar{\bar{x}})^2}{m-1} \left(\frac{M-m}{M}\right)$$

where m is the number of samples taken and M is the total number of possible systematic samples. For this example we have

$$\frac{\sum\limits_{i=1}^{m} (\bar{x}_i - \bar{\bar{x}})^2}{m-1} = \frac{1}{5}[(5 - 4.5)^2 + (4.33 - 4.5)^2 + (4 - 4.5)^2$$
$$+ (3.33 - 4.5)^2 + (7 - 4.5)^2 + (3.33 - 4.5)^2] = 1.9$$

and

$$\widehat{\text{Var}}(\bar{\bar{x}}) = \left(\frac{1}{6}\right)(1.9)\left(\frac{54-6}{54}\right) = .2814$$

The 95% confidence interval is

$$\bar{\bar{x}} - (1.96)[\widehat{\text{Var}}(\bar{\bar{x}})]^{1/2} \leq \bar{X} \leq \bar{\bar{x}} + (1.96)[\widehat{\text{Var}}(\bar{\bar{x}})]^{1/2}$$
$$4.5 - (1.96)(.2814)^{1/2} \leq \bar{X} \leq 4.5 + (1.96)(.2814)^{1/2}$$
$$3.46 \leq \bar{X} \leq 5.54$$

A summary of the formulas needed for estimation procedures involving the population mean under repeated systematic sampling is shown in box 4.2. Expressions similar to those in box 4.2 can be constructed for population totals and proportions. In such expressions, $\bar{x}_i$, and $\bar{\bar{x}}$ of equation (4.9) would be replaced by x', and $\bar{x}'$ or by p_{yi} and $\bar{p}_y$ respectively.

The advantage of repeated systematic sampling over systematic sampling is that the variance and standard errors of the estimates can be estimated directly from the data. Its disadvantage is that it is necessary to go down the list more than once, whereas in systematic sampling one chooses the sample in one pass through the list. Also, in most instances periodicity will not be present in the

---

Box 4.2 Estimation Procedures for Population Mean Under Repeated Systematic Sampling

Point Estimate of Population Mean

$$\bar{\bar{x}} = \frac{\sum\limits_{i=1}^{m} \bar{x}_i}{m} \tag{4.8}$$

Estimated Variance

$$\widehat{\text{Var}}(\bar{\bar{x}}) = \left(\frac{1}{m}\right) \frac{\sum\limits_{i=1}^{m} (\bar{x}_i - \bar{\bar{x}})^2}{m-1} \left(\frac{M-m}{M}\right) \tag{4.9}$$

100(1 − α)% Confidence Intervals

$$\bar{\bar{x}} - z_{1-\alpha/2}\left[\widehat{\text{Var}}(\bar{\bar{x}})\right]^{1/2} \leq \bar{X} \leq \bar{\bar{x}} + z_{1-\alpha/2}\left[\widehat{\text{Var}}(\bar{\bar{x}})\right]^{1/2} \tag{4.10}$$

In these equations m is the number of systematic samples taken, each of size n', M is the total number of possible systematic samples and is equal to N/n' (N is the population size), $\bar{x}_i$ is the mean of observations in the ith systematic sample, $\bar{X}$ is the population mean, and $z_{1-\alpha/2}$ is the $100(1 - \alpha/2)$th percentile of the standard normal distribution.

---

data, and then simple random sampling formulas will provide appropriate confidence intervals.

4.7 HOW LARGE A SAMPLE DO WE NEED?

If we assume that the list from which the systematic sample is to be taken is in random order, we can assume that the situation is approximately that of simple random sampling. Then the methods for determining sample size that were developed in chapter 3 can be used.

Determining the required sample size beforehand may be very difficult

But if we are not willing to assume that the list is in random order, then the determination of sample size becomes a formidable problem. The reason for this is that the variance of estimates obtained from systematic sampling depends on the sampling interval. For example, a 1-in-4 systematic sample from a list of 100 elements yields a sample of 25 elements, whereas a 1-in-5 systematic sample from the same list yields a sample of 20 elements. However, the periodicity in the list may be such that the first sample yields estimates having larger variance than those obtained from the second sample, even though the first sample contains more elements than the second sample. Since we will not usually know the characteristics of the list before taking the sample, it will be difficult for us to determine an appropriate sampling interval, and hence the required sample size, beforehand.

In repeated systematic sampling it is possible to obtain some idea of the required sample size by taking a preliminary set of m' repeated systematic samples from the list, estimating parameters on the basis of the preliminary sample, and determining the **required number m of samples** on the basis of the next formula:

$$m = \frac{(z^2_{1-\alpha/2}) \left[\dfrac{\sum_{i=1}^{m'} (\bar{x}_i - \bar{\bar{x}})^2 \big/ (m'-1)}{(\bar{\bar{x}})^2} \right] \left(\dfrac{N}{n} \right)}{(\varepsilon^2) \left(\dfrac{N}{n} - 1 \right) + (z^2_{1-\alpha/2}) \left[\dfrac{\sum_{i=1}^{m'} (\bar{x}_i - \bar{\bar{x}})^2 \big/ (m'-1)}{(\bar{\bar{x}})^2} \right]} \qquad (4.11) \quad \textbf{\textit{For repeated systematic sampling}}$$

where ε, $z_{1-\alpha/2}$, n, and N are as defined before.

ILLUSTRATIVE EXAMPLE

Suppose we wish to sample the list of employees shown in table 4.17 for purposes of estimating the mean number of days lost from work due to acute illness and that to do so we will take repeated systematic samples of one in 81 employees. Suppose further that we wish to be virtually certain of estimating the mean number of days lost from work to within 20% of the true value and that we wish to determine how many systematic samples m of one in 81 workers are needed. Let us take a preliminary sample of six such samples for purposes of estimating m. We first choose six random numbers between 1 and 81 (e.g., 22, 48, 27, 61, 53, 10) and obtain the six samples given in table 4.19.

Table 4.19   Six Samples Taken from Table 4.17

Random Number	Workers in Sample	Estimated Mean Days Lost, $\bar{x}_i$
10	10, 91	2
22	22, 103	4
27	27, 108	8
48	48, 129	4.5
53	53, 134	6
61	61, 142	3.5

We then have the following calculations:

$$\bar{\bar{x}} = \frac{2 + 4 + 8 + 4.5 + 6 + 3.5}{6} = 4.67$$

$$\frac{\sum_{i=1}^{m'} (\bar{x}_i - \bar{\bar{x}})^2}{m' - 1} = \left(\frac{1}{6 - 1}\right)[(2 - 4.67)^2 + (4 - 4.67)^2 + (8 - 4.67)^2$$
$$+ (4.5 - 4.67)^2 + (6 - 4.67)^2 + (3.5 - 4.67)^2]$$
$$= 4.367$$

$$\varepsilon = .20 \qquad N = 162 \qquad n = 2 \qquad \frac{N}{n} = 81$$

From relation (4.11), then, we have

$$m = \frac{(9)\left[\dfrac{4.367}{(4.67)^2}\right](81)}{(.2)^2(81 - 1) + (9)\left[\dfrac{4.367}{(4.67)^2}\right]} = 29.18 \approx 30$$

Thus we would need approximately 30 systematic samples of one in 81 workers from the list to meet the specifications of the problem.

The formula for the required sample size in repeated systematic sampling is based on the fact that repeated systematic sampling of one in N/n elements from a list is equivalent to simple random sampling from a population of N/n elements, where the estimates obtained from each of the N/n samples are considered as the basic variables.

4.8 USING FRAMES THAT ARE NOT LISTS

So far, we have discussed systematic sampling primarily from the viewpoint of taking a 1-in-k sample from a list of elements. The list may either be available beforehand or be compiled during the sampling process. An example of the latter type of list would be the situation in which we may be sampling one of every five patients entering the emergency room of a hospital. There would be no list of patients available beforehand in this situation. An advantage of systematic sampling over other sampling schemes is that the sampling can be done even while the frame is being constructed.

Systematic sampling also can be done even when no list is available. For example, if a set of records is located in 12 file drawers, each having a depth of 26 in. (inches) and if a sample of 100 records is needed, we could take a systematic sample in the following way:

1. Compute the total length of filed records (e.g., $26 \times 12 = 312$ in.).

2. Divide the total length by the number of records to be sampled; denote this ratio by k (e.g., $k = 312/100 = 3.12$ in.).

3. Take a random number j between 0 and k (e.g., between 0.00 and 3.12; suppose that the number chosen is 1.19).

4. Using some kind of measuring device, take the record that is j units from the front of the first file drawer. Next, take the record that is a length of k units from the first record taken (it might be necessary to go to the next file drawer to choose that record). Continue this process until the end of the last drawer is reached. (In our example we first take the record that is 1.19 in. from the front of the first file drawer. Then we take as our next record the one that is 3.12 in. from the first one we took, and we continue taking records at every 3.12 in. until we come to the end of the last drawer.)

One way to take a systematic sample when no list is available

Another instance in which systematic sampling could be used without the existence of a list is in the sampling of geographical areas from a map. For example, suppose that we wish to estimate the average phosphate concentration of a river that is 250 mi (miles) long by taking a random sample of 100 specimens from the river. A simple method would be to divide the length of the river (250 mi) by the number of specimens needed (100) to obtain the sampling interval (2.5 mi). We could then choose a random number between 0 and 2.5 (e.g., 2.1) and locate the first sampling point 2.1 mi from the source of the river. (A second random number might be chosen corresponding to each point, indicating the distance from the shore at which the sample should be taken.) The second sample point would be 4.6 mi from the source (2.1 + 2.5); the third would be 7.1 mi from the source; and so forth. This procedure could be done quite easily with the use of a good map. An intuitively appealing advantage of systematic sampling in this instance is that it leads to samples being taken along the entire length of the river, so that it would be difficult to miss any spots of high phosphate levels.

An example for sampling geographical areas

SUMMARY

In this chapter we discussed systematic sampling, which may be the most widely used of all sampling procedures. Systematic sampling, unlike most other sampling procedures, does not require knowledge of the total number of sampling units in the population, and so the sampling can be performed at the same time as the sampling frame is being compiled.

Three methods of systematic sampling were discussed. One method leads to unbiased estimates only when the ratio N/k of the number of elements in the population to the sampling interval is an integer. The second method always leads to unbiased estimates but is of limited utility since it requires prior knowledge of N, the number of elements in the population. The third method, repeated systematic sampling, allows variances of the estimates and hence confidence intervals to be obtained.

EXERCISES

1. Suppose the local Childhood Lead Poisoning Prevention Council in a metropolitan area in western Tennessee undertakes the responsibility of determining the proportion of homes in a certain development of 120 homes with unsafe lead levels. Because of the great expense involved in performing spectrometric testing of interior walls, ceilings, floors, baseboards, cabinets, and other obvious lead hazards such as crib bars, as well as of exterior sidings, porches, and porch rails, it was decided to select a sample of the homes under study. A good, up-to-date frame exists for sampling purposes. This frame is a street list containing the address and owner of each home for each of the streets in the target area. It was decided to select a 1-in-3 systematic sample of homes. Let us assume that the only households with serious lead hazard problems are the 26th, 27th, 28th, and 29th on the list.

   (a) Suppose the random number 2 was chosen to start the sequence. Estimate the proportion of homes with lead hazards from the sample.

   (b) Obtain a 95% confidence interval for the proportion of homes with lead hazards. What assumption did you make?

   (c) What is the true variance of the distribution of the estimated proportion of lead hazardous homes? How does this compare with the variance estimated in part (b)?

   (d) Suppose that a simple random sample of 40 homes had been selected instead. What is the variance of the distribution of the estimated proportion of lead hazardous homes in this case? How does this value compare with the variance from a 1-in-3 systematic sample?

2. From the 120 homes of exercise 1, suppose a 1-in-5 systematic sample was taken and suppose the initial random number was 5.

   (a) Estimate the proportion of homes with lead hazards from this sample.

   (b) Obtain a 95% confidence interval for the proportion of homes with lead hazards.

   (c) What is the true variance of the distribution of the estimated proportion of lead hazardous homes? Compare this result with the estimated variance you used in part (b).

   (d) Suppose that instead of a 1-in-5 systematic sample, a simple random sample of the same number of homes is taken. What is the variance of the sampling distribution of the estimated proportion of lead hazardous homes obtained from this sampling scheme? How does it compare to that obtained from a 1-in-5 systematic sample?

3. Refer again to exercise 1. Suppose that instead of a 1-in-5 systematic sample, a total of 24 sample homes are obtained by repeated systematic sampling of one in 40 homes.

   (a) Suppose that the random numbers chosen are 3, 7, 12, 26, 31, 33, 38, and 40. Estimate the proportion of homes with lead hazards and obtain confidence intervals for the estimated proportion.

   (b) What is the estimated variance of the distribution of the estimated proportion of lead hazardous homes obtained from these eight systematic samples of one in 40 households? Compare this to the actual variance that arises from a 1-in-5 systematic sample, which you calculated in part (c) of exercise 2.

4. From the list of workers in table 4.17, use repeated systematic sampling to take a total sample of 18 workers for purposes of estimating the total number of work days lost due to acute illnesses by all workers and the proportion of workers having eight or more work days lost due to acute illnesses. Obtain 95% confidence intervals for each of these estimates. (Suppose the random numbers you choose are 4, 44, 29, 20, 27, and 5.)

5. Suppose a study is planned of the level of the pesticide dieldrin, which is believed to be a carcinogen, in a 7.5-mi stretch of a particular river. To assure

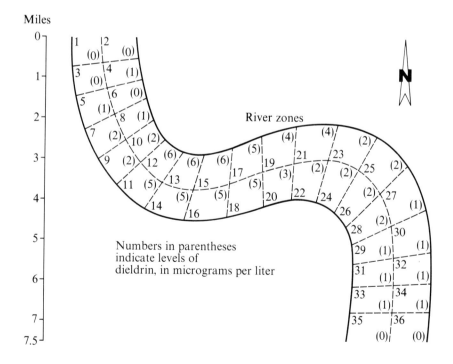

representativeness, a map of the river is divided into 36 zones, and a 1-in-4 systematic sample of these zones is to be selected. Water samples will be drawn by taking a boat out to the geographic center of the designated zone and drawing a grab sample of water from a depth of several centimeters below the surface level. The levels of dieldrin, in micrograms per liter, for each of these zones are shown in the accompanying map in parentheses.

(a) Compute the 90% confidence interval for the average level of dieldrin in this stretch of river.

(b) What advantages can you identify for this method of sampling the river over simple random sampling?

BIBLIOGRAPHY

For a more theoretically oriented discussion of systematic sampling, see the following textbook.

1. COCHRAN, W. G. *Sampling techniques.* 3d ed. New York: Wiley, 1977.

5
Stratification

Simple random sampling and systematic sampling, the two types of sampling discussed up to this point, each involve taking a sample from the population as a whole; neither requires identification of subdomains or subgroups before the sample is taken. Sometimes, however, the sampling frame can be partitioned into groups, or **strata,** and the sampling can be performed separately within each stratum. The resulting sampling design is called **stratified random sampling.**

A stratum is a subgroup of the population

In this chapter we introduce the basic concepts of stratification and define the population and sample characteristics of the strata. In the next chapter we will discuss the strategies that can be used for allocating the sample to strata for purposes of increasing the reliability of estimates.

5.1 WHAT IS A STRATIFIED RANDOM SAMPLE?

A **stratified random sample** is a sampling plan in which a population is divided into L mutually exclusive and exhaustive strata and a simple random sample of n_h elements is taken within each stratum h. The sampling is performed *independently* within each stratum. In essence, we can think of a stratified random sampling scheme as being L separate simple random samples.

Operationally, a stratified random sample is taken in the same way as a simple random sample, but the sampling is done separately within each stratum. If we let $N_1, N_2, \ldots, N_L$ represent the number of sampling units in each stratum and $n_1, n_2, \ldots, n_L$ represent the number of randomly selected sampling units

Taking the sample is similar to taking a simple random sample

91

in each stratum, then the total number of possible stratified random samples is equal to $\binom{N_1}{n_1} \cdot \binom{N_2}{n_2} \cdots \binom{N_L}{n_L}$, which is less than or equal to $\binom{N}{n}$, the total number of possible simple random samples.

For example, if we have three strata and $N_1 = 3$, $N_2 = 5$, and $N_3 = 6$, the total number of possible stratified random samples of $n_1 = 1$ element from stratum 1, $n_2 = 2$ elements from stratum 2, and $n_3 = 4$ elements from stratum 3 is

$$\binom{3}{1}\binom{5}{2}\binom{6}{4} = 450$$

The total number of simple random samples of seven elements from the 14 elements in the population is

$$\binom{14}{7} = 3432$$

The **probability** of an element being selected in the sample depends on the particular stratum into which the element is grouped and can be shown to be equal to n_h/N_h. In the example we just discussed, the probability of an element being selected is equal to $\frac{1}{3}$ for elements in stratum 1, $\frac{2}{5}$ for those in stratum 2, and $\frac{4}{6}$ for elements in stratum 3.

5.2 WHY STRATIFIED SAMPLING?

We use stratification when the population is composed of subgroups that should each be represented in the sample

Stratified random sampling is used in certain types of surveys because it combines the conceptual simplicity of simple random sampling with potentially significant gains in reliability. It is a convenient technique to use whenever we wish to obtain separate estimates for population parameters for each subdomain within an overall population and, in addition, wish to ensure that our sample is representative of the population. For example, suppose we wish to estimate the total number of beds in the hospitals of a certain state. We know that the majority of the hospitals are small or middle-sized and that there are only a few very large hospitals. We also know that these very large hospitals account for a substantial portion of the total number of beds.

Now suppose we decide to select a random sample of the hospitals in the state, determine the number of beds in each one so selected, and, using the methods of chapter 3, estimate the total number of beds in the entire state. The problem with this procedure is that there is a good chance that our sample may contain either too many or too few of the very large hospitals. As a result, the sample may not adequately represent the population.

One solution to this problem is to stratify the sampling units (hospitals), prior to sampling, into three groups on the basis of size (i.e., small, middle, large) and then select, using simple random sampling techniques, certain numbers of hospitals from each of the three groups. An estimate of the total number of beds can then be obtained from the combined results of the three strata. This is the essence of stratified sampling.

To illustrate the ideas and advantages of stratification, let us look at an example.

ILLUSTRATIVE EXAMPLE

Suppose that a road having a length of 24 mi traverses areas that can be classified as urban and rural and that the road is divided into eight segments each having a length equal to 3 mi. A sample of three segments is taken, and on each segment sampled special equipment is installed for purposes of counting the number of total motor vehicle miles traveled by cars and trucks on the segment during a particular year. In addition, a record of all accidents occurring on each sample segment during the year is kept.

The number of truck miles and the number of accidents in which a truck was involved during a certain period are given in table 5.1 for each segment.

Table 5.1   Truck Miles and Number of Accidents
Involving Trucks by Type of Road Segment

Segment	Type	Number of Truck Miles (× 1000)	Number of Accidents Involving Trucks
1	urban	6327	8
2	rural	2555	5
3	urban	8691	9
4	urban	7834	9
5	rural	1586	5
6	rural	2034	1
7	rural	2015	9
8	rural	3012	4

Suppose that we take a simple random sample of three segments for purposes of estimating the total number of truck miles traveled on the road. There are 56 possible samples of three segments from this population of eight segments. The sampling distribution of x', the estimated total truck miles traveled on the road, is given in table 5.2.

Estimates of the total number of truck miles obtained in this way range from 15,026.67 to 60,938.67, with the mean of the sampling distribution of x' equal to 34,054, the population total, and the standard error of x' equal to 10,536.9.

Now suppose that instead of taking a simple random sample of three segments from the population of eight segments, we first group the segments into two strata, one consisting of urban segments, the other consisting of rural segments, as shown in table 5.3.

Table 5.2   Sampling Distribution of x' for 56 Possible Samples of
Three Segments

Segments in Sample	x'	Segments in Sample	x'	Segments in Sample	x'	Segments in Sample	x'
(1, 2, 3)	46,861.33	(1, 4, 8)	45,794.67	(2, 4, 7)	33,077.33	(3, 5, 8)	35,437.33
(1, 2, 4)	44,576	(1, 5, 6)	26,525.33	(2, 4, 8)	35,736	(3, 6, 7)	33,973.33
(1, 2, 5)	27,914.67	(1, 5, 7)	26,474.67	(2, 5, 6)	16,466.67	(3, 6, 8)	36,632
(1, 2, 6)	29,109.33	(1, 5, 8)	29,133.33	(2, 5, 7)	16,416	(3, 7, 8)	36,581.33
(1, 2, 7)	29,058.67	(1, 6, 7)	27,669.33	(2, 5, 8)	19,074.67	(4, 5, 6)	30,544
(1, 2, 8)	31,717.33	(1, 6, 8)	30,328	(2, 6, 7)	17,610.67	(4, 5, 7)	30,493.33
(1, 3, 4)	60,938.67	(1, 7, 8)	30,277.33	(2, 6, 8)	20,269.33	(4, 5, 8)	33,152
(1, 3, 5)	44,277.33	(2, 3, 4)	50,880	(2, 7, 8)	20,218.67	(4, 6, 7)	31,688
(1, 3, 6)	45,472	(2, 3, 5)	34,218.67	(3, 4, 5)	48,296	(4, 6, 8)	34,346.67
(1, 3, 7)	45,421.33	(2, 3, 6)	35,413.33	(3, 4, 6)	49,490.67	(4, 7, 8)	34,296
(1, 3, 8)	48,080	(2, 3, 7)	35,362.67	(3, 4, 7)	49,440	(5, 6, 7)	15,026.67
(1, 4, 5)	41,992	(2, 3, 8)	38,021.33	(3, 4, 8)	52,098.67	(5, 6, 8)	17,685.33
(1, 4, 6)	43,186.67	(2, 4, 5)	31,933.33	(3, 5, 6)	32,829.33	(5, 7, 8)	17,634.67
(1, 4, 7)	43,136	(2, 4, 6)	33,128	(3, 5, 7)	32,778.67	(6, 7, 8)	18,829.33

Table 5.3   Two Strata for Data of Table 5.1

STRATUM 1 (URBAN SEGMENTS)		STRATUM 2 (RURAL SEGMENTS)	
Segment	Truck Miles (× 1000)	Segment	Truck Miles (× 1000)
1	6327	2	2555
3	8691	5	1586
4	7834	6	2034
		7	2015
		8	3012

We might now take a sample of one segment from stratum 1 and two segments from stratum 2 and estimate the total number of truck miles by the estimate x'_{str}, given by

$$x'_{str} = x'_1 + x'_2$$

where x'_1 = estimated number of truck miles in the three segments comprising stratum 1

x'_2 = estimated number of truck miles in the five segments comprising stratum 2

Conceptually, we consider each stratum as a subpopulation, sample independently within each subpopulation, and obtain an estimate for the population as a whole by aggregating the individual stratum estimates over all subpopulations or strata.

So if we take a simple random sample of one segment from stratum 1 and two segments from stratum 2, we obtain a total of $\binom{3}{1}\binom{5}{2} = 30$ possible samples. If we then use the estimation procedure given by the equation above for x'_{str}, we obtain the sampling distribution of x'_{str} shown in table 5.4.

The mean $E(x'_{str})$ of the sampling distribution of x'_{str} is equal to 34,054 (see box 2.3), which is the true population total. The standard error $SE(x'_{str})$ of the estimated total x'_{str}

Table 5.4   Sampling Distribution of x'_{str} for 30 Possible Samples of Three Segments

Stratum 1	*Stratum 2*	$x'_1 = 3\bar{x}_1$	$x'_2 = 5\bar{x}_2$	$x'_{str} = x'_1 + x'_2$
1	(2, 5)	18,981	10,352.5	29,333.5
1	(2, 6)	18,981	11,472.5	30,453.5
1	(2, 7)	18,981	11,425	30,406
1	(2, 8)	18,981	13,917.5	32,898.5
1	(5, 6)	18,981	9,050	28,031
1	(5, 7)	18,981	9,002.5	27,983.5
1	(5, 8)	18,981	11,495	30,476
1	(6, 7)	18,981	10,122.5	29,103.5
1	(6, 8)	18,981	12,615	31,596
1	(7, 8)	18,981	12,567.5	31,548.5
3	(2, 5)	26,073	10,352.5	36,425.5
3	(2, 6)	26,073	11,472.5	37,545.5
3	(2, 7)	26,073	11,425	37,498
3	(2, 8)	26,073	13,917.5	39,990.5
3	(5, 6)	26,073	9,050	35,123
3	(5, 7)	26,073	9,002.5	35,075.5
3	(5, 8)	26,073	11,495	37,568
3	(6, 7)	26,073	10,122.5	36,195.5
3	(6, 8)	26,073	12,615	38,688
3	(7, 8)	26,073	12,567.5	38,640.5
4	(2, 5)	23,502	10,352.5	33,854.5
4	(2, 6)	23,502	11,472.5	34,974.5
4	(2, 7)	23,507	11,425	34,927
4	(2, 8)	23,502	13,917.5	37,419.5
4	(5, 6)	23,502	9,050	32,552
4	(5, 7)	23,502	9,002.5	32,504.5
4	(5, 8)	23,502	11,495	34,997
4	(6, 7)	23,502	10,122.5	33,624.5
4	(6, 8)	23,502	12,615	36,117
4	(7, 8)	23,502	12,567.5	36,069.5

is equal to 3,297.6, which is much lower than the standard error of x', the equivalent estimate of the population total under simple random sampling. These results are summarized in table 5.5.

Table 5.5   Comparison of Results for Simple Random Sampling and Stratification

Sampling Design	Number of Elements in Sample	Number of Possible Samples	Mean of Distribution of Estimated Totals	Standard Error of Estimated Total	Range of Distribution of Estimated Totals
simple random sampling	3	56	34,054[a]	10,536.9	45,912
stratification	3[b]	30	34,054[a]	3,297.6	12,007

[a] This is also the population total.
[b] 1 from stratum 1 and 2 from stratum 2.

Intuitively we can see why the sampling plan based on stratification yielded an estimate having a lower standard error than the corresponding estimate based on simple random sampling. There are 56 possible values of the estimated total x' that can be obtained by simple random sampling, whereas stratification yields only 30 values of x'_{str}. Examination of the ranges of the two distributions shows that stratification eliminated those samples that resulted in extremely high or low estimates of the total. The three urban segments had high values and the five rural segments had low values of the characteristic being measured (truck miles). Stratification ensured that at least one urban segment and at least one rural segment would be selected in the sample, thus eliminating the possibility of extremely high and extremely low estimates of the total.

Advantages of stratification over simple random sampling

There are three major advantages of stratification over simple random sampling.

1. Given certain conditions, precision may be increased over simple random sampling (i.e., lower standard errors may result from the estimation procedure).

2. It is possible to obtain estimates for each of the strata that have been established by using simple random sampling theory for the particular stratum.

3. It may be just as easy, for either physical or administrative reasons, to collect information for a stratified sample as is possible for a simple random sample. In that case there is little to lose by taking a stratified sample since the resulting standard errors will rarely exceed those of simple random sampling.

The strategy employed for constructing strata involves two steps. First we determine the population parameter we are interested in estimating. Then we stratify the population with respect to another variable that is thought to be associated with the variable of interest. If our assumption of association is correct, this second step ensures that the strata are homogeneous with respect to the variable under consideration.

Strategy for constructing strata has two steps

For example, if we wish to estimate the number of beds in all hospitals in the state, we may choose to stratify the hospitals on the basis of floor space (which is information readily available for reasons of taxation), reasoning that hospitals with more space will have more beds. On the other hand, if we are interested in the average daily cost of a hospital bed to the patient, we might choose to stratify the hospitals according to their geographic location, reasoning that hospitals in economically thriving parts of the state can charge their patients more than can hospitals in economically depressed parts of the state.

In most practical situations it is difficult to stratify the population with respect to the variable under consideration, primarily for reasons of cost and practicality. More often the population is stratified in the most convenient manner by using administrative criteria (e.g., voting districts), geographic criteria (e.g., north, south, east, or west), or other natural criteria (e.g., sex or age). Stratification by convenience is not unreasonable, since it is not common for a modern survey to attempt to estimate a single parameter. Instead, much information is collected on each sampling unit and many parameters are of interest. Clearly, what might be an optimal stratification strategy for one variable, providing relatively homogeneous strata, may provide very heterogeneous strata with respect to another variable. It is important for the statistician to consider the scope of the data to be collected before deciding on an appropriate criterion for stratification. Such issues are sometimes discussed in reports of health surveys that use stratification (1, 2).

Often strata are constructed on the basis of convenience

The major disadvantage of stratified sampling is that it may take more time to select the sample than it would for simple random sampling. More time is involved because complete frames are necessary within each of the strata and each stratum must be sampled. You may wish to compare stratification to the strategy of cluster sampling (chapters 9–12), where major savings in time and cost may be possible. Nevertheless because of the advantages discussed above, stratification is a very powerful and widely used technique.

Stratification may be more time-consuming than simple random sampling

5.3 POPULATION CHARACTERISTICS FOR STRATA

Population characteristics for strata can be defined with the same type of notation that we used to define characteristics of a population in general. In this section we introduce notation that will be used throughout our discussion of sampling plans based on stratification.

Let us consider a population containing N elementary units that are grouped exclusively and exhaustively into L strata in such a way that stratum 1

Here is the notation we'll use

contains N_1 elementary units, stratum 2 contains N_2 elementary units, and stratum L contains N_L elementary units. In other words,

$$N = \sum_{h=1}^{L} N_h$$

is the **population size.**

Suppose we are considering a variable or characteristic $\mathcal{X}$ in the population. We use the notation $X_{h,i}$ to represent the **value of the characteristic** $\mathcal{X}$ for the ith elementary unit within stratum h. In other words, the elementary units within any particular stratum h are labeled from 1 to N_h.

ILLUSTRATIVE EXAMPLE

Suppose we are interested in estimating the average daily pharmaceutical cost per patient at a hospital. We decide to stratify the hospital into services (medical, surgical, ob-gyn, and all other services combined), and we define the elementary units as the patients on any given day.

Suppose that on a designated day there are 250 patients in the hospital, of which 100 are medical, 75 surgical, 50 ob-gyn, and 25 other services. Then using the notation introduced above, we have

$$N = 250, \quad N_1 = 100, \quad N_2 = 75, \quad N_3 = 50, \quad N_4 = 25$$

If $X_{h,i}$ designates the value of the variable $\mathcal{X}$ for the ith elementary unit within stratum h, then, for example, in stratum 2 we have

$X_{2,1} =$ the value of variable $\mathcal{X}$ for element 1 within stratum 2

$X_{2,2} =$ the value of variable $\mathcal{X}$ for element 2 within stratum 2

and so on, up to

$X_{2,75} =$ the value of variable $\mathcal{X}$ for element 75 within stratum 2

Elements within the other strata would be defined in a similar manner.

Here are some population parameters

We define population parameters for strata in a way that is similar to the way we defined general population parameters.

The **total** or aggregate amount of a variable $\mathcal{X}$ **within a stratum** h is denoted by X_{h+}. In other words,

$$X_{h+} = \sum_{i=1}^{N_h} X_{h,i}$$

The **total for the whole population** is given by the sum of the stratum totals, or

$$X = \sum_{h=1}^{L} \sum_{i=1}^{N_h} X_{h,i} = \sum_{h=1}^{L} X_{h+}$$

The **mean** level of a characteristic $\mathscr{X}$ **for a stratum** h is denoted by $\bar{X}_h$ and is given by

$$\bar{X}_h = \frac{\sum_{i=1}^{N_h} X_{h,i}}{N_h} = \frac{X_{h+}}{N_h}$$

The **mean** $\bar{X}$ of a variable $\mathscr{X}$ **for the entire population** is given by

$$\bar{X} = \frac{X}{N}$$

or its algebraic equivalent

$$\bar{X} = \frac{\sum_{h=1}^{L} N_h \bar{X}_h}{N} = \sum_{h=1}^{L} W_h \bar{X}_h$$

where

$$W_h = \frac{N_h}{N}$$

In other words, the mean $\bar{X}$ for the entire population is a **weighted average** of the individual stratum means $\bar{X}_h$, with weights ($W_h = N_h/N$) proportional to the number of elements in each stratum.

The **variance** σ_{hx}^2 of the distribution of a variable $\mathscr{X}$ among the elementary units **within a particular stratum** h is defined as the average squared deviation about the stratum mean and is given by

$$\sigma_{hx}^2 = \frac{\sum_{i=1}^{N_h} (X_{h,i} - \bar{X}_h)^2}{N_h}$$

Coefficients of variation and rel-variances are defined for each stratum in the same way as they were defined for a general population. The **coefficient of variation** for the distribution **within a particular stratum** h is given by

$$V_{hx} = \frac{\sigma_{hx}}{\bar{X}_h}$$

and the **rel-variance** is simply the square of the coefficient of variation.

For your convenience in later reference, the population parameters for stratified random sampling are summarized in box 5.1.

Box 5.1 Population and Strata Parameters for Stratified Random Sampling

WITHIN STRATUM   ENTIRE POPULATION

Total

$$X_{h+} = \sum_{i=1}^{N_h} X_{h,i} \qquad\qquad X = \sum_{h=1}^{L} \sum_{i=1}^{N_h} X_{h,i} = \sum_{h=1}^{L} X_{h+} \qquad (5.1)$$

Mean

$$\bar{X}_h = \frac{\sum_{i=1}^{N_h} X_{h,i}}{N_h} = \frac{X_{h+}}{N_h} \qquad\qquad \bar{X} = \frac{\sum_{h=1}^{L} N_h \bar{X}_h}{N} = \sum_{h=1}^{L} W_h \bar{X}_h = \frac{X}{N} \quad (5.2)$$

Proportion

$$P_{hy} = \frac{\sum_{i=1}^{N_h} Y_{h,i}}{N_h} \qquad\qquad P_y = \frac{\sum_{h=1}^{L} N_h P_{hy}}{N} = \sum_{h=1}^{L} W_h P_{hy} \qquad (5.3)$$

Variance

$$\sigma_{hx}^2 = \frac{\sum_{i=1}^{N_h} (X_{h,i} - \bar{X}_h)^2}{N_h} \qquad\qquad\qquad\qquad (5.4)$$

Relative Variance

$$V_{hx}^2 = \frac{\sigma_{hx}^2}{\bar{X}_h^2} \qquad\qquad\qquad\qquad (5.5)$$

In these definitions L is the number of strata, N_h is the population size in stratum h, N is the total population size, $X_{h,i}$ is the value of $\mathscr{X}$ for the ith element in stratum h, $Y_{h,i}$ indicates the presence or absence of some dichotomous attribute $\mathscr{Y}$ for the ith element in stratum h, and $W_h = N_h/N$ is the proportion of the total population belonging to stratum h.

Now let us see how these formulas can be used in practice.

ILLUSTRATIVE EXAMPLE

Consider a population of 14 families living on three city blocks. If we consider the families as elementary units, the blocks as strata, and family size as the characteristic $\mathcal{X}$, we might have the situation shown in table 5.6.

Table 5.6   Strata for a Population of 14 Families

BLOCK 1		BLOCK 2		BLOCK 3	
Family	Family Size	Family	Family Size	Family	Family Size
1	4	1	4	1	2
2	3	2	6	2	3
3	4	3	4	3	2
		4	7	4	2
		5	8	5	2
				6	3

In terms of the notation introduced above we have the following values of $\mathcal{X}$ for each stratum:

STRATUM 1, $N_1 = 3$ STRATUM 2, $N_2 = 5$ STRATUM 3, $N_3 = 6$

$$X_{1,1} = 4 \qquad X_{2,1} = 4 \qquad X_{3,1} = 2$$
$$X_{1,2} = 3 \qquad X_{2,2} = 6 \qquad X_{3,2} = 3$$
$$X_{1,3} = 4 \qquad X_{2,3} = 4 \qquad X_{3,3} = 2$$
$$\phantom{X_{1,3} = 4} \qquad X_{2,4} = 7 \qquad X_{3,4} = 2$$
$$\phantom{X_{1,3} = 4} \qquad X_{2,5} = 8 \qquad X_{3,5} = 2$$
$$\phantom{X_{1,3} = 4} \qquad \phantom{X_{2,5} = 8} \qquad X_{3,6} = 3$$

The totals of the variable $\mathcal{X}$ within each stratum h, using equation (5.1), are as follows:

$$X_{1+} = 4 + 3 + 4 = 11$$
$$X_{2+} = 4 + 6 + 4 + 7 + 8 = 29$$
$$X_{3+} = 2 + 3 + 2 + 2 + 2 + 3 = 14$$

The total for the entire population, again using equation (5.1), is

$$X = 11 + 29 + 14 = 54$$

The population means for the strata, using equation (5.2), are

$$\bar{X}_1 = \frac{11}{3} = 3.67 \qquad \bar{X}_2 = \frac{29}{5} = 5.8 \qquad \bar{X}_3 = \frac{14}{6} = 2.33$$

The population mean for the entire population, using equation (5.2), is

$$\bar{X} = \left(\frac{3}{14}\right)(3.67) + \left(\frac{5}{14}\right)(5.8) + \left(\frac{6}{14}\right)(2.33) = 3.857$$

The variances for the strata, using equation (5.4), are

$$\sigma_{1x}^2 = \frac{(4 - 3.67)^2 + (3 - 3.67)^2 + (4 - 3.67)^2}{3} = .222$$

$$\sigma_{2x}^2 = \frac{(4 - 5.8)^2 + (6 - 5.8)^2 + \cdots + (8 - 5.8)^2}{5} = 2.56$$

$$\sigma_{3x}^2 = \frac{(2 - 2.33)^2 + (3 - 2.33)^2 + \cdots + (3 - 2.33)^2}{6} = .222$$

The relative variances for the strata, using equation (5.5), are

$$V_{1x}^2 = \frac{.222}{(3.67)^2} = .0165 \qquad V_{2x}^2 = \frac{2.56}{(5.8)^2} = .0761 \qquad V_{3x}^2 = \frac{.222}{(2.33)^2} = .0409$$

5.4 SAMPLE CHARACTERISTICS FOR STRATA

Here is the notation we'll use

Within a particular stratum h, let us suppose that we have selected in some way a sample of n_h elements from the N_h elements in the stratum and that each sample element is measured with respect to some variable $\mathcal{X}$. For convenience we label the sample elements from 1 to n_h, and we let $x_{h,1}$ denote the value of the variable $\mathcal{X}$ for the sample element labeled "1," we let $x_{h,2}$ denote the value of $\mathcal{X}$ for the sample element labeled "2," and we let x_{h,n_h} denote the value for $\mathcal{X}$ for the sample element labeled "n_h." If a sample of n_h elements is taken within each stratum h, then the **total sample size** n is given by

$$n = \sum_{h=1}^{L} n_h$$

where L is the number of strata into which the population's elements have been grouped.

For instance, in the previous example, if we select one element from stratum 1, two elements from stratum 2, and four elements from stratum 3, we have

$$n_1 = 1, \qquad n_2 = 2, \qquad n_3 = 4$$

and

$$n = 1 + 2 + 4 = 7$$

If the four sample elements selected from stratum 3 are $X_{3,1}$, $X_{3,3}$, $X_{3,4}$, and $X_{3,6}$, then we have

$$x_{3,1} = X_{3,1} = 2 \qquad x_{3,3} = X_{3,4} = 2$$
$$x_{3,2} = X_{3,3} = 2 \qquad x_{3,4} = X_{3,6} = 3$$

Sample totals and **sample means for a particular stratum** h are given by, respectively,   *Here are some sample statistics*

$$x_{h+} = \sum_{i=1}^{n_h} x_{h,i}$$

and

$$\bar{x}_h = \frac{\sum_{i=1}^{n_h} x_{h,i}}{n_h} = \frac{x_{h+}}{n_h}$$

The **estimated total** x_h' **for a stratum** h is given by

$$x_h' = \frac{N_h x_{h+}}{n_h} = N_h \bar{x}_h$$

The **estimated population total** x_{str}' is given by

$$x_{str}' = \sum_{h=1}^{L} x_h'$$

The **estimated population mean** $\bar{x}_{str}$ is given by

$$\bar{x}_{str} = \frac{x_{str}'}{N}$$

which is algebraically equivalent to

$$\bar{x}_{str} = \frac{\sum_{h=1}^{L} N_h \bar{x}_h}{N} = \sum_{h=1}^{L} W_h \bar{x}_h$$

where W_h is defined as before. Thus we see that a population mean $\bar{X}$ is estimated from a stratified sample by taking a weighted average of the estimated stratum means, with weights W_h that are proportional to the number N_h of elements in the stratum.

For convenience in later reference, sample characteristics under stratified random sampling are summarized in box 5.2.

Box 5.2 Sample Statistics Under Stratified Random Sampling

WITHIN STRATUM	POPULATION PARAMETER ESTIMATE

Total

$$x'_h = \frac{N_h \sum_{i=1}^{n_h} x_{h,i}}{n_h} = \frac{N_h x_{h+}}{n_h} = N_h \bar{x}_h \qquad x'_{str} = \sum_{h=1}^{L} x'_h \qquad (5.6)$$

Mean

$$\bar{x}_h = \frac{\sum_{i=1}^{n_h} x_{h,i}}{n_h} = \frac{x_{h+}}{n_h} \qquad \bar{x}_{str} = \frac{x'_{str}}{N} = \frac{\sum_{h=1}^{L} N_h \bar{x}_h}{N} \qquad (5.7)$$

$$= \sum_{h=1}^{L} W_h \bar{x}_h$$

Proportion

$$p_{hy} = \frac{\sum_{i=1}^{n_h} y_{h,i}}{n_h} \qquad p_{y,str} = \frac{\sum_{h=1}^{L} N_h p_{hy}}{N} \qquad (5.8)$$

Variance

$$s_{hx}^2 = \frac{\sum_{i=1}^{n_h} (x_{h,i} - \bar{x}_h)^2}{n_h - 1} \qquad (5.9)$$

In these definitions L is the number of strata, N_h is the population size in stratum h, N is the total population size, $x_{h,i}$ is the value of $\mathcal{X}$ for the ith sample element in stratum h, $y_{h,i}$ indicates the presence or absence of some dichotomous attribute $\mathcal{Y}$ for the ith sample element in stratum h, and $W_h = N_h/N$ is the proportion of the total population belonging to stratum h.

In the next chapter we will see how these formulas can be used in practice.

SUMMARY

In this chapter we presented an overview of stratification. We introduced the concept of strata, and we defined what is meant by a stratified random sample. We discussed situations in which a stratified random sample might be appropriate and the advantages stratification has over simple random sampling as well as its major disadvantage. Finally, we presented the expressions that are used to determine the population parameters and sample statistics under stratified random sampling.

BIBLIOGRAPHY

The following articles present sample surveys in which stratification is used.

1. HEMPHILL, F. M. A sample survey of home injuries. *Public Health Reports* (1952) 67: 1026–1034.

2. HORVITZ, D. G. Sampling and field procedures of the Pittsburgh morbidity survey. *Public Health Reports* (1952) 67: 1003–1012.

The following publication presents additional discussions of stratification.

3. COCHRAN, W. G. *Sampling techniques.* 3d ed. New York: Wiley, 1977.

6

Stratified Random Sampling

In the previous chapter we introduced the concept of stratification and discussed the reasons why stratification is used as a strategy in designing sample surveys. We also introduced notation commonly used by statisticians in discussing population characteristics and estimation procedures appropriate for stratified sampling. In this chapter we will discuss one type of stratified sampling in considerable detail, namely, stratified random sampling.

6.1 ESTIMATION OF POPULATION PARAMETERS

Estimates of population means, proportions, and totals under stratified random sampling are obtained by computing weighted averages of the individual strata estimates and aggregating them. The formulas for these estimates were given in box 5.2. Now let us see how these formulas can be used by looking at an example.

ILLUSTRATIVE EXAMPLE

Consider the population of 14 families shown in table 5.6 (p. 101). Suppose we decide to take a sample of two families from stratum 1, two families from stratum 2, and four families from stratum 3. Then we have $n_1 = 2$, $n_2 = 2$, $n_3 = 3$, $N_1 = 3$, $N_2 = 5$, $N_3 = 6$, and $N = 14$. Suppose we select elements $X_{1,2}$ and $X_{1,3}$ from stratum 1 (i.e., $x_{1,1} = 3$ and $x_{1,2} = 4$), we select $X_{2,2}$ and $X_{2,5}$ from stratum 2 (i.e., $x_{2,1} = 6$ and $x_{2,2} = 8$), and we select $X_{3,1}$, $X_{3,2}$, $X_{3,4}$, and $X_{3,6}$ from stratum 3 (i.e., $x_{3,1} = 2$, $x_{3,2} = 3$, $x_{3,3} = 2$, and $x_{3,4} = 3$).

Using equation (5.6), we obtain the estimated total number of individuals on block 1:

$$x_1' = \frac{3(3 + 4)}{2} = 10.5$$

Similarly, we obtain $x_2' = 35$ and $x_3' = 15$.

Then by equation (5.6) the estimated total number of people in the population is

$$x_{str}' = 10.5 + 35 + 15 = 60.5$$

Using equation (5.7), we obtain the estimated mean number of individuals per family in block 1:

$$\bar{x}_1 = \frac{3 + 4}{2} = 3.5$$

Similarly, $\bar{x}_2 = 7$ and $\bar{x}_3 = 2.5$.

Then by equation (5.7) the estimated mean number of individuals per family is

$$\bar{x}_{str} = \frac{3(3.5)}{14} + \frac{5(7)}{14} + \frac{6(2.5)}{14} = 4.32$$

By equation (5.9) the variance in family size for stratum 1 is

$$s_{1x}^2 = \frac{(3 - 3.5)^2 + (4 - 3.5)^2}{1} = .5$$

Similarly, $s_{2x}^2 = 2$ and $s_{3x}^2 = .33$.

If we let

$$y_{h,i} = \begin{cases} 0 & \text{if family size is less than 4} \\ 1 & \text{if family size is 4 or more} \end{cases}$$

then by equation (5.8) we have

$$p_{1y} = \frac{0 + 1}{2} = .5$$

Similarly, $p_{2y} = 1$ and $p_{3y} = 0$.

6.2 SAMPLING DISTRIBUTIONS OF ESTIMATES

Since a stratified random sample consists of L simple random samples, which are drawn separately and independently within each stratum, and since the estimated population mean, total, or proportion is a linear combination of the individual stratum means, totals, or proportions obtained from the sample, it follows that the mean of the sampling distribution of any of these estimated values is equal to the corresponding linear combination of population parameters. In other words, population means, totals, and proportions, when estimated as indicated in relations (5.7), (5.6), and (5.8), are, under stratified random sampling, unbiased estimates of the corresponding population means, totals, and proportions.

The estimates are unbiased

Means and standard errors of population estimates are given in the next box.

Box 6.1 Means and Standard Errors of Population Estimates Under Stratified Random Sampling

Mean

$$E(\bar{x}_{\text{str}}) = \frac{\sum\limits_{h=1}^{L} (N_h)E(\bar{x}_h)}{N} = \frac{\sum\limits_{h=1}^{L} N_h \bar{X}_h}{N} = \bar{X}$$

$$\text{SE}(\bar{x}_{\text{str}}) = \left[\sum_{h=1}^{L} (N_h^2)\left(\frac{\sigma_{hx}^2}{n_h}\right)\left(\frac{N_h - n_h}{N_h - 1}\right) \middle/ N^2 \right]^{1/2}$$

(6.1)

Total

$$E(x'_{\text{str}}) = \sum_{h=1}^{L} E(x'_h) = \sum_{h=1}^{L} X_{h+} = X$$

$$\text{SE}(x'_{\text{str}}) = N[\text{SE}(\bar{x}_{\text{str}})] = \left[\sum_{h=1}^{L} (N_h^2)\left(\frac{\sigma_{hx}^2}{n_h}\right)\left(\frac{N_h - n_h}{N_h - 1}\right) \right]^{1/2}$$

(6.2)

Proportion

$$E(p_{y,\text{str}}) = \frac{\sum\limits_{h=1}^{L} N_h P_{hy}}{N} = \frac{\sum\limits_{h=1}^{L} Y_{h+}}{N} = P_y$$

$$\text{SE}(p_{y,\text{str}}) = \left\{ \sum_{h=1}^{L} (N_h^2)\left[\frac{P_{hy}(1 - P_{hy})}{n_h}\right]\left(\frac{N_h - n_h}{N_h - 1}\right) \middle/ N^2 \right\}^{1/2}$$

(6.3)

The population notation used in these formulas is defined in box 5.1, and n_h is the sample stratum size.

Let us see how these formulas are used by looking at an example.

ILLUSTRATIVE EXAMPLE

In the example used earlier in which the strata are three city blocks (p. 101), the elementary units are families and the variable $\mathcal{X}$ is family size. We took a stratified random sampling of two families from stratum 1, two from stratum 2, and four from stratum 3. Then we have $n_1 = 2$, $n_2 = 2$, $n_3 = 4$, $N_1 = 3$, $N_2 = 5$, $N_3 = 6$, $\sigma_{1x}^2 = .222$, $\sigma_{2x}^2 = 2.56$, $\sigma_{3x}^2 = .222$, $P_1 = .67$, $P_2 = 1.00$, and $P_3 = 0$, where P_i is the proportion of families in the ith stratum with four or more persons. Using equation (6.1), we have

$$
SE(\bar{x}_{str}) = \left\{ \left[(3^2)\left(\frac{.222}{2}\right)\left(\frac{3-2}{3-1}\right) + (5^2)\left(\frac{2.56}{2}\right)\left(\frac{5-2}{5-1}\right) \right. \right.
$$
$$
\left. \left. + (6^2)\left(\frac{.222}{4}\right)\left(\frac{6-4}{6-1}\right) \right] \middle/ 14^2 \right\}^{1/2}
$$
$$
= .359
$$

$$
SE(x'_{str}) = (14)(.359) = 5.03
$$

From relation (6.3) we have

$$
SE(p_{y,\,str}) = \left\{ \left[(3^2)\left(\frac{.67(1-.67)}{2}\right)\left(\frac{3-2}{3-1}\right) + (5^2)\left(\frac{1(1-1)}{2}\right)\left(\frac{5-2}{5-1}\right) \right. \right.
$$
$$
\left. \left. + (6^2)\left(\frac{0(1-0)}{4}\right)\left(\frac{6-4}{6-1}\right) \right] \middle/ 14^2 \right\}^{1/2}
$$
$$
= .0504
$$

where y is the attribute of having a family size of four or more persons.

6.3 ESTIMATION OF STANDARD ERRORS

Under stratified random sampling the standard errors of estimated means, totals, and proportions can be estimated by substituting, into relations (6.1), (6.2), and (6.3), $\hat{\sigma}_{hx}^2$ for σ_{hx}^2 or p_{hy} for P_{hy}, where

$$
\hat{\sigma}_{hx}^2 = \frac{(N_h - 1)s_{hx}^2}{N_h} \qquad (6.4) \quad \textbf{\textit{Estimated population variance}}
$$

$$
s_{hx}^2 = \frac{\sum\limits_{i=1}^{n_h}(x_{h,i} - \bar{x}_h)^2}{n_h - 1} \qquad (6.5) \quad \textbf{\textit{Sample variance}}
$$

and p_{hy} is the observed proportion of elements in the stratum having attribute y. The resulting estimated standard errors are given in the next box.

Box 6.2 Estimated Standard Errors Under Stratified Random Sampling

Mean

$$\widehat{SE}(\bar{x}_{str}) = \left[\sum_{h=1}^{L} (N_h^2) \left(\frac{s_{hx}^2}{n_h} \right) \left(\frac{N_h - n_h}{N_h} \right) \Big/ N^2 \right]^{1/2} \qquad (6.6)$$

Total

$$\widehat{SE}(x'_{str}) = \left[\sum_{h=1}^{L} (N_h^2) \left(\frac{s_{hx}^2}{n_h} \right) \left(\frac{N_h - n_h}{N_h} \right) \right]^{1/2} \qquad (6.7)$$

Proportion

$$\widehat{SE}(p_{y,str}) = \left\{ \sum_{h=1}^{L} (N_h^2) \left[\frac{p_{hy}(1 - p_{hy})}{n_h - 1} \right] \left(\frac{N_h - n_h}{N_h} \right) \Big/ N^2 \right\}^{1/2} \qquad (6.8)$$

where N is the population size, N_h is the population stratum size, n_h is the sample stratum size, s_{hx} is as defined in equation (5.9), and p_{hy} is the observed proportion of elements in the stratum having attribute y.

Now let us see how we can use some of these formulas.

ILLUSTRATIVE EXAMPLE

For the illustrative example considered in section 6.1, we have the following:

$\bar{x}_1 = 3.5$	$x'_1 = 10.5$	$s_{1x}^2 = .5$	$\hat{\sigma}_{1x}^2 = .33$
$\bar{x}_2 = 7$	$x'_2 = 35$	$s_{2x}^2 = 2$	$\hat{\sigma}_{2x}^2 = 1.6$
$\bar{x}_3 = 2.5$	$x'_3 = 15$	$s_{3x}^2 = .33$	$\hat{\sigma}_{3x}^2 = .2083$

The last column was obtained by using equation (6.4).

As shown in the example in section 6.1, the estimate x'_{str} of the total number of persons X on the three blocks is, from equation (5.6),

$$x'_{str} = 10.5 + 35 + 15 = 60.5$$

with standard error, from relation (6.7), estimated by

$$\widehat{SE}(x'_{str}) = \left[(3^2)\left(\frac{.5}{2}\right)\left(\frac{3-2}{3}\right) + (5^2)\left(\frac{2}{2}\right)\left(\frac{5-2}{5}\right) + (6^2)\left(\frac{.33}{4}\right)\left(\frac{6-4}{6}\right) \right]^{1/2} = 4.09$$

Thus a 95% confidence interval for X, the population total, is given by

$$x'_{str} - (1.96)[\widehat{SE}(x'_{str})] \le X \le x'_{str} + (1.96)[\widehat{SE}(x'_{str})]$$
$$60.5 - (1.96)(4.09) \le X \le 60.5 + (1.96)(4.09)$$
$$52.48 \le X \le 68.52$$

Clearly this interval covers the true population total $X = 54$.

In a manner similar to that in the example above, estimates may be obtained for standard errors of estimated means and proportions, which can be used in obtaining approximate confidence intervals.

6.4 ESTIMATION OF CHARACTERISTICS OF SUBGROUPS

In chapter 3 we showed that under simple random sampling estimated means, totals, and proportions for subgroups are unbiased estimates of the corresponding population means, totals, and proportions for the subgroups. This is not necessarily true under stratified random sampling, as is shown in the next example.

ILLUSTRATIVE EXAMPLE

Let us consider the data given in table 6.1.

Table 6.1   Retail Prices of 20 Capsules of a Tranquilizer in All Pharmacies in Two Communities (Strata)

| | COMMUNITY 1 | | | COMMUNITY 2 | |
Pharmacy	Type[a]	Price of Drug	Pharmacy	Type[a]	Price of Drug
1	C	$5.00	1	I	$6.75
2	I	4.50	2	I	6.25
3	I	6.00	3	C	6.00
4	I	5.50	4	C	5.50
5	C	4.50			
6	C	4.75			
7	C	4.95			

[a] I = independent, C = chain.

If we let $\bar{X}_I$ denote the average price among the five independent pharmacies in the combined two communities, we see that $\bar{X}_I = \$5.80$. Suppose we take a stratified random sample of six pharmacies from stratum 1 and three pharmacies from stratum 2 for purposes of estimating $\bar{X}_I$. Suppose also that we do not know before the sampling whether a given pharmacy is an independent or an affiliate of a chain.

Our estimate $\bar{x}_{I,\text{str}}$ of $\bar{X}_I$ is given by

$$\bar{x}_{I,\text{str}} = \frac{\displaystyle\sum_{h=1}^{2} N_h \bar{x}_{Ih}}{N}$$

where $\bar{x}_{Ih}$ is the estimated mean for the independent pharmacies obtained in the sample taken in stratum h.

There are seven possible samples of six pharmacies that can be taken in stratum 1, and there are four possible samples of three pharmacies that can be taken in stratum 2. These samples and the estimated mean for each sample are listed in table 6.2.

Table 6.2   Possible Samples for the Stratified Random Sample

SAMPLES FROM STRATUM 1		SAMPLES FROM STRATUM 2	
Pharmacies in Sample	$\bar{x}_{I1}$	Pharmacies in Sample	$\bar{x}_{I2}$
1, 2, 3, 4, 5, 6	$5.33	1, 2, 3	$6.50
1, 2, 3, 4, 5, 7	5.33	1, 2, 4	6.50
1, 2, 3, 4, 6, 7	5.33	1, 3, 4	6.75
1, 2, 3, 5, 6, 7	5.25	2, 3, 4	6.25
1, 2, 4, 5, 6, 7	5.00		
1, 3, 4, 5, 6, 7	5.75		
2, 3, 4, 5, 6, 7	5.33		

There are $\binom{7}{6}\binom{4}{3} = 28$ possible values of $\bar{x}_{I,\text{str}} = (7\bar{x}_{I1} + 4\bar{x}_{12})/11$. The sampling distribution of $\bar{x}_{I,\text{str}}$ is shown in table 6.3.

Table 6.3   Sampling Distributing for $\bar{x}_{I,\text{str}}$

$\bar{x}_{I,\text{str}}$	f	$\bar{x}_{I,\text{str}}$	f
$5.755	8	$6.023	2
5.846	4	5.795	1
5.665	4	5.614	1
5.705	2	5.636	1
5.545	2	6.114	1
5.455	1	5.932	1
Total			28

The mean $E(\bar{x}_{I,\text{str}})$ of the distribution of $\bar{x}_{I,\text{str}}$ over the 28 possible samples is equal to $5.76, which is not equal to $5.80, the value of $\bar{X}_I$, the mean price over the five independent pharmacies in the two communities.

In the example above we have demonstrated empirically that for stratified random sampling the estimate $\bar{x}_{I,\text{str}}$ of the population mean $\bar{X}_I$ for a subgroup within the population is not necessarily an unbiased estimate of $\bar{X}_I$. The reason for this lies in the fact that the individual stratum sample means $\bar{x}_{hI}$ for the subgroup I are weighted in the construction of $\bar{x}_{I,\text{str}}$ by N_h/N, the proportion of all elements in the population belonging to stratum h, rather than by the proportion of all subgroup I elements belonging to stratum h. If N_{Ih} denotes the number of elements in stratum h belonging to the subgroup I and if N_I denotes the total number of elements in the population belonging to subgroup I (i.e., $N_I = \sum_{h=1}^{L} N_{Ih}$), then it is not necessarily true that N_{Ih}/N_I is equal to N_h/N. That is, the elements in subgroup I are not necessarily allocated to the various strata in the same proportions as are the elements of the population as a whole. It is for this reason that the estimate $\bar{x}_{I,\text{str}}$ is not necessarily an unbiased estimate of $\bar{X}_I$. If the proportions N_{Ih}/N_I were known, then they could be used as weights in constructing an unbiased estimate of $\bar{X}_I$. Generally, however, they are not known.

Estimates for population parameters of subgroups are not necessarily unbiased

For the same reasons as given above, the sample proportion $p_{Iy,\text{str}}$ and the estimated total $x'_{I,\text{str}}$ are not, in general, unbiased estimates of P_{Iy} and X_I for subgroups under stratified random sampling.

Estimation of characteristics of subgroups of a population under stratified random sampling is generally done by *ratio estimation* procedures, which will be discussed in the next chapter.

6.5 ALLOCATION OF SAMPLE TO STRATA

Once we decide to use stratified random sampling, and once we specify the total number n of sample elements, the next important decision we must make is that of **allocation,** or specification of how many elements are to be taken from each stratum under the constraint that a total of n elements is to be taken over all strata. As we will see in this section, the standard errors of the estimated population parameters may be reduced considerably if careful thought is given to allocation.

Equal Allocation

In equal allocation the same number of elements are sampled from each stratum. In other words, for each stratum h, the **sample size** is given by

The samples selected from each stratum are of equal size

$$n_h = \frac{n}{L}$$

Except in rather unusual circumstances, this type of allocation yields no particular advantage over other types of allocation, and we will not discuss it further.

Proportional Allocation: Self-weighting Samples

n_h/N_h is the same for each stratum

In proportional allocation the sampling fraction n_h/N_h is specified to be the same for each stratum, which implies also that the overall sampling fraction n/N is the fraction taken from each stratum. In other words, the **number of elements** taken from each stratum, n_h, is given by

$$n_h = (N_h)\left(\frac{n}{N}\right) \tag{6.9}$$

Under proportional allocation the **estimated population mean** $\bar{x}_{\text{str}}$, as given in relation (5.7), reduces to the form

$$\bar{x}_{\text{str}} = \frac{\sum\limits_{h=1}^{L} \sum\limits_{i=1}^{n_h} x_{h,i}}{n} \tag{6.10}$$

which is a considerably simpler expression than the one given in expression (5.7).

You do not need to keep track of strata in computing $\bar{x}_{str}$ in proportional allocation

Let us compare the formula for $\bar{x}_{\text{str}}$ under proportional allocation with the general formula for an estimated population mean under stratified random sampling. We see that in the general formula [relation (5.7)] the value $x_{h,i}$ of characteristic $\mathcal{X}$ for a sample element is multiplied by the ratio $N_h/(n_h N)$, which is not necessarily the same for each stratum. Thus in order to obtain $\bar{x}_{\text{str}}$ it is not necessary to keep track of the stratum to which each sample element belongs. On the other hand, relation (6.10) indicates that for proportional allocation each sample element is multiplied by the same constant, $1/n$, irrespective of the stratum to which the element belongs. Estimates of this type are known as **self-weighting estimates.**

The advantage of proportional allocation is its simplicity

This technique of proportional allocation greatly simplifies the amount of bookkeeping involved in the data processing and hence reduces computational expenses. In large surveys in which much information is collected on each sampled individual, proportional allocation is often used because of its simplicity, even if it is not the optimal design in terms of precision of estimates. Also, since this estimate corresponds to the sample mean under simple random sampling, packaged statistical programs may be used to perform the data processing, because the formulas for calculations in these packages are usually based on the assumption of simple random sampling.

We note that a stratified sample allocated proportionately will be self-weighting only if the proportion of sampled individuals *who respond* is the same within each stratum. Nonresponse, particularly where the nonresponse rate differs from stratum to stratum, can drastically affect the validity of the estimate given in expression (6.10). For this reason, methods of handling nonresponse, as discussed in chapter 13, are critically important.

Nonresponse may affect the estimate $\bar{x}_{str}$

Now let us look at an example of proportional allocation.

ILLUSTRATIVE EXAMPLE

Consider the data in table 6.4, which shows the number of general hospitals located in four

Table 6.4   General Hospitals in Illinois by Geographic Stratum, 1971[a]

Stratum	No. of General Hospitals
1	44
2	116
3	48
4	47
Total	255

[a] Data compiled from a study evaluating emergency medical care in Illinois conducted at the University of Illinois School of Public Health. At the time of the writing of this text, the study had not yet been published.

strata, where a stratum is comprised of one or more geographical regions within Illinois. Suppose we wish to take a stratified random sample of 51 hospitals from among the 255 hospitals in the population, and we wish to use proportional allocation. Then letting $N = 255$ and $n = 51$, we have, from relation (6.9),

$$n_1 = (44)\left(\frac{51}{255}\right) = 8.8 \approx 9$$

$$n_2 = (116)\left(\frac{51}{255}\right) = 23.2 \approx 23$$

$$n_3 = (48)\left(\frac{51}{255}\right) = 9.6 \approx 10$$

$$n_4 = (47)\left(\frac{51}{255}\right) = 9.4 \approx 9$$

Thus we would take nine elements (hospitals) from stratum 1, 23 from stratum 2, ten from stratum 3, and nine from stratum 4.

The sampling fractions within each stratum are

$$\frac{n_1}{N_1} = \frac{9}{44} = .2045 \qquad \frac{n_2}{N_2} = \frac{23}{116} = .1983$$

$$\frac{n_3}{N_3} = \frac{10}{48} = .2083 \qquad \frac{n_4}{N_4} = \frac{9}{47} = .1915$$

The slight differences in sampling fractions among the strata are due to the fact that the required allocation given by relation (6.9) does not necessarily yield integer values. Thus the n_h taken are those specified by (6.9) but rounded up or down to the nearest integer. These minor differences among sampling fractions are generally ignored in constructing the estimates, and the sample is treated as if it were exactly a self-weighting sample. Note that $\sum_{h=1}^{4} n_h = n$.

In proportional allocation the **variance** $\mathrm{Var}(\bar{x}_{str})$ **of an estimated mean** $\bar{x}_{str}$, obtained from relation (6.10) with n_h set equal to $N_h(n/N)$, becomes

$$\mathrm{Var}(\bar{x}_{str}) = \left(\frac{N - n}{N^2}\right) \sum_{h=1}^{L} \left(\frac{N_h^2}{N_h - 1}\right)\left(\frac{\sigma_{hx}^2}{n}\right) \tag{6.11}$$

If all the N_h are reasonably large, this expression reduces to the approximation given by

$$\mathrm{Var}(\bar{x}_{str}) \approx \left(\frac{\sigma_{wx}^2}{n}\right)\left(\frac{N - n}{N}\right) \tag{6.12}$$

where

Variance among elements in a stratum

$$\sigma_{wx}^2 = \frac{\sum_{h=1}^{L} N_h \sigma_{hx}^2}{N} \tag{6.13}$$

The **sample estimate** of $\mathrm{Var}(\bar{x}_{str})$ is given by

$$\widehat{\mathrm{Var}}(\bar{x}_{str}) = \left(\frac{N - n}{N^2}\right) \sum_{h=1}^{L} (N_h)\left(\frac{s_{hx}^2}{n}\right)$$

Note that relation (6.12) has a form that is very similar to the formula for the variance of an estimated mean $\bar{x}$ under simple random sampling. The formula for the standard error was given in box 3.1, and the square of this quantity, the variance, is given as

$$\mathrm{Var}(\bar{x}) = \left(\frac{\sigma_x^2}{n}\right)\left(\frac{N - n}{N - 1}\right) \tag{6.14}$$

The difference between the two formulas is that for proportional allocation in stratified random sampling, the population variance σ_x^2 is replaced by σ_{wx}^2, which is a weighted average of the individual variances σ_{hx}^2 of the distribution of $\mathcal{X}$ among elements within each stratum. The weights in σ_{wx}^2 are proportional to N_h, the number of elements in each stratum.

Comparison of relations (6.12) and (6.14) indicates that stratified random sampling with proportional allocation will yield an estimated mean having lower variance than that obtained from simple random sampling whenever σ_{wx}^2 is less than σ_x^2. But note that, as in analysis of variance methodology, the population variance σ_x^2 may be partitioned into the two components

$$\sigma_x^2 = \sigma_{bx}^2 + \sigma_{wx}^2$$

Partitioning of σ_x^2

where

$$\sigma_{bx}^2 = \frac{\sum_{h=1}^{L} N_h(\bar{X}_h - \bar{X})^2}{N} \qquad (6.15)$$

Variance among stratum means

and σ_{wx}^2 is as given by relation (6.13). Thus the ratio of the variance of the estimated mean $\bar{x}$ under simple random sampling to that of $\bar{x}_{\text{str}}$, the estimated mean under stratified random sampling, is given by

$$\frac{\text{Var}(\bar{x})}{\text{Var}(\bar{x}_{\text{str}})} = \frac{\sigma_{bx}^2 + \sigma_{wx}^2}{\sigma_{wx}^2} = 1 + \frac{\sigma_{bx}^2}{\sigma_{wx}^2} \qquad (6.16)$$

Ratio of variances

This ratio is always greater than or equal to 1, and the extent to which it differs from 1 depends on the size of the ratio $\sigma_{bx}^2/\sigma_{wx}^2$. When $\sigma_{bx}^2/\sigma_{wx}^2$ is large, the estimated mean under stratified random sampling with proportional allocation will have a smaller variance than the corresponding estimate under simple random sampling. The component σ_{bx}^2 represents the **variance among the stratum means,** whereas the component σ_{wx}^2 represents the **variance among elements** within the same stratum.

If all the stratum means $\bar{X}_h$ are of the same order of magnitude, then little or nothing is gained from using stratified random sampling rather than simple random sampling. On the other hand, if the stratum means are very different, it is likely that considerable reduction in the variance of an estimated mean can be obtained by use of stratified random sampling rather than simple random sampling. This makes sense intuitively, because the purpose of stratification is to group the elements, in advance of the sampling, into strata on the basis of their similarity with respect to the values of a variable or a set of variables. If the elements within each stratum have very similar values of the variable being measured, then it would be dfficult to obtain a "bad" sample, since each stratum is represented in the sample. A reliable estimate could then be obtained by sampling a small number of elements within each stratum. On the other

If the stratum means are similar, then little is gained by using stratified random sampling rather than simple random sampling

hand, if the stratum means are very similar, then there is no point to stratification, and the extra effort required to take a stratified sample would not result in an improved estimate.

For convenience, formulas for estimates of population parameters under proportional allocation are summarized in the next box.

Box 6.3 Estimates of Population Parameters Under Proportional Allocation

Under proportional allocation [i.e., $n_h = (N_h/N)n$] the following formulas are used for estimating population parameters.

Mean

$$\bar{x}_{str} = \frac{\sum\limits_{h=1}^{L} \sum\limits_{i=1}^{n_h} x_{h,i}}{n}$$

$$\widehat{Var}(\bar{x}_{str}) = \left(\frac{N-n}{N^2}\right) \sum\limits_{h=1}^{L} (N_h) \left(\frac{s_{hx}^2}{n}\right)$$

Total

$$x'_{str} = (N) \left(\frac{\sum\limits_{h=1}^{L} \sum\limits_{i=1}^{n_h} x_{h,i}}{n}\right)$$

$$\widehat{Var}(x'_{str}) = (N^2) \left(\frac{N-n}{N^2}\right) \sum\limits_{h=1}^{L} (N_h) \left(\frac{s_{hx}^2}{n}\right)$$

Proportion

$$p_{y,str} = \frac{\sum\limits_{h=1}^{L} \sum\limits_{i=1}^{n_h} y_{h,i}}{n}$$

$$\widehat{Var}(p_{y,str}) = \left(\frac{N-n}{N^2}\right) \sum\limits_{h=1}^{L} (N_h) \left[\frac{p_{hy}(1-p_{hy})}{n-1}\right]$$

All quantities in these expressions are as defined in box 5.2.

Now let us look at an example that investigates whether stratification is likely to result in an estimate having lower variance than one obtained from simple random sampling.

ILLUSTRATIVE EXAMPLE

Let us suppose that we wish to estimate the average number of hospital admissions for major trauma conditions per county among 82 counties in Illinois having general hospitals. A sample of counties will be taken, and the admissions records of all hospitals in the sample counties will be reviewed for major trauma admissions. If it is reasonable to assume that there may be a strong correlation between the number of hospital beds among general hospitals within a county and the total number of admissions for major trauma conditions, then it would make sense to stratify by number of hospital beds. So this is the sampling plan that is chosen. In table 6.5 counties in Illinois are grouped into two strata on the

Table 6.5   Strata for Number of Hospital Beds by County Among Counties in Illinois (Excluding Cook County) Having General Hospitals

| | STRATUM 1 (1–399 BEDS) | | | | | | STRATUM 2 (400 OR MORE BEDS) | |
County	No. of Beds	County	No. of Beds	County	No. of Beds		County	No. of Beds
1	216	23	103	45	144		1	823
2	170	24	262	46	210		2	1343
3	252	25	105	47	160		3	908
4	38	26	80	48	204		4	648
5	170	27	54	49	200		5	1043
6	179	28	66	50	195		6	1325
7	31	29	54	51	140		7	1123
8	40	30	50	52	96		8	690
9	295	31	50	53	108		9	519
10	336	32	165	54	121		10	1118
11	166	33	200	55	61		11	522
12	121	34	113	56	63		12	715
13	280	35	64	57	104		13	851
14	188	36	100	58	150		14	552
15	35	37	58	59	48		15	470
16	134	38	54	60	48		16	1187
17	63	39	82	61	69		17	980
18	280	40	35	62	79			
19	75	41	204	63	75			
20	142	42	42	64	32			
21	293	43	72	65	39			
22	152	44	39					

basis of number of hospital beds. Stratum 1 consists of those counties having 1–399 beds, and stratum 2 consists of those having 400 beds or more.

From table 6.5 we calculate the following:

$$\bar{X}_1 = 123.91 \qquad \sigma^2_{1x} = 6,131.63 \qquad N_1 = 65$$
$$\bar{X}_2 = 871.59 \qquad \sigma^2_{2x} = 77,287.92 \qquad N_2 = 17$$
$$\bar{X} = 278.92 \qquad \sigma^2_x = 112,751.93 \qquad N = 82$$

(where $\mathscr{X}$ = the number of beds).

From relations (6.15) and (6.13) we have

$$\sigma^2_{bx} = \frac{65(123.91 - 278.92)^2 + 17(871.59 - 278.92)^2}{82} = 91,868.39$$

$$\sigma^2_{wx} = \frac{65(6,131.63) + 17(77,287.92)}{82} = 20,883.54$$

Thus from relation (6.16) the ratio of the variances, $\text{Var}(\bar{x})/\text{Var}(\bar{x}_{str})$, is

$$\frac{\text{Var}(\bar{x})}{\text{Var}(\bar{x}_{str})} = 1 + \frac{91,868.39}{20,883.54} = 5.40$$

Therefore, we conclude that in terms of reduction of the variance of an estimated mean, stratification is likely to be of great benefit in this situation if, in fact, admissions for multiple trauma and number of beds are related, since the variance under stratification is less than 20% of the variance under simple random sampling.

Optimum Allocation

Often proportional allocation is not the type of allocation that will result in an estimated mean, proportion, or total having the lowest variance among all possible ways of allocating a total sample of n elements among the L strata. It can be shown that the allocation of n sample units into each stratum that will yield an estimated mean, total, or proportion having minimum variance is given by

This allocation scheme yields estimates having minimum variance

$$n_h = \left(\frac{N_h \sigma_{hx}}{\sum_{h=1}^{L} N_h \sigma_{hx}} \right)(n) \qquad (6.17)$$

ILLUSTRATIVE EXAMPLE

Let us use the data in table 6.5 and assume a close relationship between number of beds and number of admissions for major trauma. From relation (6.17), the following allocation of 25 sample elements will produce the estimated mean having the lowest variance:

$$n_1 = \left(\frac{65\sqrt{6131.63}}{65\sqrt{6131.63} + 17\sqrt{77,287.92}}\right)(25) = 12.96 \approx 13$$

$$n_2 = \left(\frac{17\sqrt{77,287.92}}{65\sqrt{6131.63} + 17\sqrt{77,287.92}}\right)(25) = 12.04 \approx 12$$

Thus the optimal allocation of the 25 sample elements is 13 elements from stratum 1 and 12 elements from stratum 2. Proportional allocation would have specified that 20 elements be taken from stratum 1 and 5 elements from stratum 2.

The standard error of an estimated mean under stratified random sampling with optimal allocation is given by relation (6.1), which is valid in general for any type of allocation under statified random sampling. For the data in table 6.5, using number of beds as the characteristics of interest, we have, for optimal allocation from equation (6.1),

$$\text{SE}(\bar{x}_{\text{str}}) = \left\{\left[(65)^2\left(\frac{6131.63}{13}\right)\left(\frac{65-13}{65-1}\right) + (17)^2\left(\frac{77,287.92}{12}\right)\left(\frac{17-12}{17-1}\right)\right]\bigg/82\right\}^{1/2}$$

$$= 18.09$$

For proportional allocation we have, taking the square root of the expression in equation (6.11),

$$\text{SE}(\bar{x}_{\text{str}}) = \left[\left(\frac{82-25}{82^2}\right)\left\{\left(\frac{65^2}{64}\right)\left(\frac{6131.63}{25}\right) + \left(\frac{17^2}{16}\right)\left(\frac{77,287.92}{25}\right)\right\}\right]^{1/2} = 24.71$$

Thus we see that for these data the estimated mean under optimal allocation has a standard error considerably lower than that of the estimated mean under proportional allocation.

From relation (6.17) we see that the optimal number of sample elements to be taken from a given stratum is proportional to N_h, the total number of elements in the stratum, and to σ_{hx}, the standard deviation of the distribution of the variable $\mathscr{X}$ among all elements in the stratum. This makes sense intuitively. The population mean $\bar{X}$, which we are trying to estimate, is equal to $\sum_{h=1}^{L} N_h\bar{X}_h/N$, or, in other words, $\bar{X}$ is a weighted average of the individual stratum means $\bar{X}_h$, with weights that are proportional to the total number of elements in the stratum. Since the strata that have the largest number of elements are the most important in determining the population mean, it makes sense that they would also be most important in estimating it from a sample. If the distribution of characteristic $\mathscr{X}$ among elements in a particular stratum has a small standard deviation, then only a small number of sample elements are required to yield a reliable estimate of a stratum parameter relative to the number required to estimate a parameter in a stratum in which the distribution of $\mathscr{X}$ has a large standard deviation. This fact is taken into consideration in the formula for

Under optimal allocation the sample size assigned to a stratum is large if the number of observations or the variability of the observations in a particular stratum is large

optimal allocation, since the sample allocation, as given by relation (6.17), is proportional to the size of the standard deviation σ_{hx}. Also note that if the distribution of $\mathscr{X}$ within each stratum has the same standard deviation, then optimal allocation as given by relation (6.17) reduces to proportional allocation as given by relation (6.9).

Optimal Allocation and Economics

Suppose now that the cost of sampling an elementary unit is not the same for each stratum. Then the **total cost** C of taking a sample of n_1 elements from stratum 1, n_2 elements from stratum 2, and so on is given by

$$C = \sum_{h=1}^{L} n_h C_h$$

where C_h is the cost of sampling an elementary unit in stratum h.

For a given sample size n, the allocation that will yield an estimate having the lowest variance per unit cost is given by

Optimal allocation per unit cost

$$n_h = \frac{(n)(N_h \sigma_{hx}/\sqrt{C_h})}{\sum\limits_{h=1}^{L} N_h \sigma_{hx}/\sqrt{C_h}} \qquad (6.18)$$

Similarly, if the total cost of taking the sample is fixed at C, the allocation that will yield estimated means having the lowest standard error at fixed cost C is given by

For fixed total cost

$$n_h = \frac{C(N_h \sigma_{hx}/\sqrt{C_h})}{\sum\limits_{h=1}^{L} N_h \sigma_{hx} \sqrt{C_h}} \qquad (6.19)$$

Both relations (6.18) and (6.19) choose sample sizes n_h that are directly proportional to N_h and σ_{hx} and inversely proportional to the cost C_h of sampling an element in a particular stratum.

Now let us look at an example of optimum allocation taking cost into consideration.

ILLUSTRATIVE EXAMPLE

Let us suppose that a corporation has 260,000 accident reports available over a period of time and that a sample survey is being contemplated for purposes of estimating the average number of days of work lost per accident. Of the 260,000 accident reports, 150,000 are coded and 110,000 are uncoded. The coded forms could be processed on the computer directly, whereas the uncoded forms must first be coded before processing. Approximately $5,000 is available for taking the sample and coding and processing the data. With this in mind, it is desired to find the best way of allocating the sample elements among coded and uncoded forms.

In the terminology of stratified sampling we have

$$N_1 = 150{,}000 \text{ coded forms (stratum 1)}$$
$$N_2 = 110{,}000 \text{ uncoded forms (stratum 2)}$$
$$C = \$5{,}000$$

Let us suppose that the cost of sampling and processing sample forms is equal to $.16 for a coded form and $.49 for an uncoded form; that is,

$$C_1 = \$.16 \quad \text{and} \quad C_2 = \$.49$$

If we assume that the standard deviation of the distribution of days lost from work is twice as large among uncoded reports as among coded reports (i.e., $\sigma_{1x} = \sigma_{2x}/2$), then from relation (6.19) we have

$$n_1 = \frac{(5{,}000)(150{,}000)(\sigma_{2x}/2)/\sqrt{.16}}{(150{,}000)(\sigma_{2x}/2)(\sqrt{.16}) + (110{,}000)(\sigma_{2x})(\sqrt{.49})} \approx 8{,}762$$

$$n_2 = \frac{(5{,}000)(110{,}000)(\sigma_{2x})/\sqrt{.49}}{(150{,}000)(\sigma_{2x}/2)(\sqrt{.16}) + (110{,}000)(\sigma_{2x})(\sqrt{.49})} \approx 7{,}343$$

Thus we would take a sample of 8,762 coded reports and 7,343 uncoded reports.

We can verify that the total cost of the sampling is equal to $5,000 by substituting the values for C_1, C_2, n_1, and n_2 into the relation for C:

$$C = (8{,}762)(.16) + (7{,}343)(.49) = \$5{,}000$$

We note that in order to determine the optimal allocation, it is not necessary to know the actual values of the σ_{hx}. If we can express each σ_{hx} in terms of one of them (e.g., σ_{h^*x}), as was done in the example discussed above, then σ_{h^*x} appears as a common factor in both the numerator and denominator and therefore can be canceled.

One problem often encountered in optimal allocation, either with or without costs being taken into consideration, is that the optimal sample size n_h may be greater than N_h, the total number of elements in the stratum. When this occurs, we set n_h equal to N_h for each stratum having optimal allocation greater than N_h. Then we reallocate the remaining sample to the other strata as specified by the algorithm for obtaining optimal allocation.

What to do if optimal n_h is greater than N_h

For example, let us consider the summary data from three strata as given below:

Stratum	N_h	σ_{hx}
1	100	50
2	110	10
3	120	5

If we wish to allocate a total sample of 140 elements to each stratum by using optimum allocation, we have, by relation (6.17),

$$n_1 = 104, \qquad n_2 = 23, \qquad n_3 = 13$$

We would then take $n_1 = N_1 = 100$ and allocate the four remaining elements originally allocated to stratum 1 to strata 2 and 3 according to relation (6.17) as follows:

$$n_2 = \left[\frac{(110)(10)}{(110)(10) + (120)(5)} \right](4) = 2.6 \approx 3$$

$$n_3 = \left[\frac{(120)(5)}{(110)(10) + (120)(5)} \right](4) = 1.4 \approx 1$$

Thus the final optimum allocation is

$$n_1 = 100, \qquad n_2 = 26, \qquad n_3 = 14$$

How to select the best allocation scheme for the survey

In the planning of a sample survey for which stratified random sampling is indicated, it is often a good strategy to calculate the optimal allocation for the most important variables in the survey. If the allocation differs among the variables, some compromise allocation might be considered (such as the mean of the optimal n_h over all variables of importance). Also, proportional allocation should be given some consideration. If the standard errors anticipated under proportional allocation are not much higher than those anticipated under optimal allocation, then the simplicity and convenience of proportional allocation may offset the small reduction in standard error under optimal allocation, and proportional allocation may be the best choice.

6.6 STRATIFICATION AFTER SAMPLING

A sample design in which the sampling plan is that of simple random sampling but the estimation procedure is that appropriate for stratified random sampling can sometimes produce estimates having standard errors that are not much higher than those obtained by stratified random sampling. The advantage of this design is that it eliminates the inconvenience, or impossibility, of grouping the elements into strata in advance of the sampling. This type of design has been considered by Hansen, Hurwitz, and Madow (2) and Cochran (1), among others. It is known as **stratification after sampling,** or **poststratification.**

For example, it might be of interest to estimate the proportion of premature births in a given hospital during the past year. It is known from past experience that the prematurity rate among blacks is higher than the corresponding rate for whites. However, to stratify the entire set of hospital records by racial group would be impractical, since racial group is recorded in the record and all records would have to be inspected to do such stratification prior to the sampling. However, if the total number of blacks and the total number of whites who have entered the hospital during the year for deliveries is known (as it may well be by the hospital administration), a simple random sample may be stratified after the sampling to improve the precision of the estimate.

Let $\bar{x}_{pstr}$ and $Var(\bar{x}_{pstr})$ represent the **estimate of the poststratified sample mean** and the **variance of its sampling distribution,** respectively. Then

$$\bar{x}_{pstr} = \sum_{i=1}^{L} \left(\frac{N_h}{N}\right)(\bar{x}_h)$$

$$Var(\bar{x}_{pstr}) = \left(\frac{\sigma_{wx}^2}{n}\right)\left(\frac{N-n}{N-1}\right) + \left(\frac{1}{n}\right)\left[\sum_{h=1}^{L} (\sigma_{hx}^2)\left(1 - \frac{N_h}{N}\right)\left(\frac{1}{\bar{n}L}\right)\left(\frac{N-n}{N-1}\right)\right]$$

$$(6.20)$$

where $\bar{n} = n/L$ is the average of sample elements per stratum.

The first term in relation (6.20) is simply the variance of an estimated mean under stratified sampling with proportional allocation. The second term increases the variance and reflects the fact that the n_h in the resulting sample are random variables that may not arise the same proportion of the time as they would under stratified sampling with proportional allocation. In any case, this second term will be small when $\bar{n}$ is large (say, greater than 20).

Since σ_{hx}^2 and σ_{wx}^2 are not known, they are estimated by

$$\hat{\sigma}_{hx}^2 = \left(\frac{N_h - 1}{N_h}\right)(s_{hx}^2)$$

$$\hat{\sigma}_{wx}^2 = \sum_{h=1}^{L} \left(\frac{N_h}{N}\right)(\hat{\sigma}_{hx}^2) = \sum_{h=1}^{L} \left(\frac{N_h - 1}{N}\right)(s_{hx}^2)$$

Hence the **sample estimate** of $Var(\bar{x}_{pstr})$ is given by

$$\widehat{Var}(\bar{x}_{pstr}) = \left(\frac{1}{n}\right)\left[\sum_{h=1}^{L} \left(\frac{N_h - 1}{N}\right)(s_{hx}^2)\right]\left(\frac{N-n}{N-1}\right)$$

$$+ \left(\frac{1}{n}\right)\left[\sum_{h=1}^{L} \left(\frac{N_h - 1}{N_h}\right)\left(\frac{N - N_h}{N}\right)(s_{hx}^2)\right]\left(\frac{1}{\bar{n}L}\right)\left(\frac{N-n}{N-1}\right)$$

$$(6.21)$$

Expressions similar to (6.20) can be derived for the variance of the poststratified total and proportion, as well as for the estimated variances from the sample information.

Now let us look at an example of how poststratification can be useful in reducing sampling error.

ILLUSTRATIVE EXAMPLE

A veterinarian is interested in studying the annual veterinary costs of his clientele (who own either cats or dogs). From a separate record system he knows that he sees 850 dogs and 450 cats regularly in his practice (these are numbers of animals, not numbers of visits). He knows that the information on type of animal (i.e., dog or cat) is contained in the medical records but that it would take too much time to sort all the records into strata defined by animal type. So he decides to select a simple random sample and then poststratify. He regards the stratification process as necessary since he knows that, on the average, it costs more to keep dogs healthy than to keep cats healthy. He samples 50 records, recording the total amount of money spent (including medication) by the owners of the animals he saw over the past two years. The sampling results are given in table 6.6.

Table 6.6   Sample Data of Veterinarian's Survey

Sample Animal Number	Animal Type	No. of Visits	Total Expenses	Sample Animal Number	Animal Type	No. of Visits	Total Expenses
1	dog	4	$45.14	26	dog	4	$48.30
2	dog	5	50.13	27	dog	5	54.64
3	cat	2	27.15	28	cat	3	21.45
4	dog	3	45.80	29	cat	3	10.71
5	cat	1	23.39	30	dog	4	60.57
6	cat	2	8.24	31	dog	6	53.37
7	dog	6	61.22	32	dog	5	40.52
8	cat	2	29.90	33	dog	4	50.26
9	dog	5	56.57	34	cat	2	15.23
10	dog	4	42.39	35	dog	4	42.02
11	cat	2	27.24	36	dog	5	32.78
12	cat	3	22.17	37	cat	2	30.21
13	dog	6	39.67	38	cat	1	27.54
14	dog	4	40.52	39	dog	6	52.03
15	dog	4	39.48	40	dog	5	54.47
16	cat	1	7.14	41	dog	5	46.88
17	dog	4	61.82	42	cat	2	23.77
18	cat	2	39.88	43	dog	3	52.48
19	cat	2	16.89	44	dog	2	60.49
20	dog	3	55.31	45	dog	2	53.70
21	dog	2	63.19	46	dog	2	46.39
22	dog	2	45.11	47	dog	2	53.24
23	dog	3	66.20	48	cat	1	14.18
24	cat	3	17.16	49	dog	3	41.52
25	cat	3	28.55	50	dog	2	39.26

Now suppose that this sample of 50 animals is to be used to estimate the average biannual expense of owning a dog or cat. Then we have the following calculations (refer to boxes 2.2 and 3.1):

$$\bar{x} = \frac{45.14 + 50.13 + \cdots + 39.26}{50} = 39.73$$

$$s_x^2 = \frac{(45.14 - 39.73)^2 + \cdots + (39.26 - 39.73)^2}{50 - 1} = 256.68$$

$$\widehat{SE}(\bar{x}) = \left[\left(\frac{1300 - 50}{1300 - 1}\right)\left(\frac{256.68}{50}\right)\right]^{1/2} = \sqrt{4.936} = 2.222$$

Hence the 95% confidence interval estimate of the population mean $\bar{X}$ is given by

$$\bar{x} - (1.96)[\widehat{SE}(\bar{x})] \leq \bar{X} \leq \bar{x} + (1.96)[\widehat{SE}(\bar{x})]$$

$$39.73 - (1.96)(2.222) \leq \bar{X} \leq 39.73 + (1.96)(2.222)$$

$$35.38 \leq \bar{X} \leq 44.08$$

Let us now use the known stratum totals in a poststratification process to obtain a more precise estimate of $\bar{X}$. The veterinarian knows that the total number of dogs in his files is $N_1 = 850$ and the total number of cats is $N_2 = 450$. Stratifying the 50 animals in the sample given in table 6.6 into dogs and cats yields $n_1 = 32$ dogs and $n_2 = 18$ cats in the sample. Then we have (refer to box 2.2)

$$\bar{x}_1 = \frac{45.14 + 50.13 + \cdots + 39.26}{32} = 49.86$$

$$\bar{x}_2 = \frac{27.15 + 23.39 + \cdots + 14.18}{18} = 21.71$$

$$s_{1x}^2 = \frac{(45.14 - 49.86)^2 + \cdots + (39.26 - 49.86)^2}{31} = 70.22$$

$$s_{2x}^2 = \frac{(27.15 - 21.71)^2 + \cdots + (14.18 - 21.71)^2}{17} = 75.00$$

$$\bar{x}_{pstr} = \left(\frac{850}{1300}\right)(49.86) + \left(\frac{450}{1300}\right)(21.71) = 40.12$$

$$\widehat{Var}(\bar{x}_{pstr}) = \left(\frac{1}{50}\right)\left[\left(\frac{850 - 1}{1300}\right)(70.22) + \left(\frac{450 - 1}{1300}\right)(75.00)\right]\left(\frac{1300 - 50}{1300 - 1}\right)$$

$$+ \left(\frac{1}{50}\right)\left[\left(\frac{850 - 1}{850}\right)\left(\frac{1300 - 850}{1300}\right)(70.22)\right.$$

$$+ \left.\left(\frac{450 - 1}{450}\right)\left(\frac{1300 - 450}{1300}\right)(75.00)\right]\left[\frac{1}{(25)(2)}\right]\left(\frac{1300 - 50}{1300 - 1}\right)$$

$$= 1.408$$

$$\widehat{SE}(\bar{x}_{pstr}) = \sqrt{1.408} = 1.19$$

Hence the 95% confidence interval estimate of the population mean $\bar{X}$ is given, via post-stratification, as

$$\bar{x}_{pstr} - (1.96)[\widehat{SE}(\bar{x}_{pstr})] \leq \bar{X} \leq \bar{x}_{pstr} + (1.96)[\widehat{SE}(\bar{x}_{pstr})]$$
$$40.12 - (1.96)(1.19) \leq \bar{X} \leq 40.12 + (1.96)(1.19)$$
$$37.79 \leq \bar{X} \leq 42.45$$

We see that by poststratifying the originally selected random sample, the veterinarian obtained a much narrower confidence interval than the one calculated for the original simple random sample.

Poststratification works well when stratification works well

We note that poststratification will only be profitable (in terms of smaller standard errors) when the established strata are homogeneous with respect to the variable of interest. In other words, poststratification will work well when stratification works well. In addition, the method cannot be carried out unless the stratum totals are known. However, when the sample is taken from human populations, it is often possible to use available census data to obtain a good enough guess of the stratum totals to make using the method advantageous.

6.7 HOW LARGE A SAMPLE IS NEEDED?

Suppose that we wish to determine the number of elements needed to be $100(1 - \alpha)\%$ certain of obtaining, from stratified random sampling, an estimated mean $\bar{x}_{str}$ that differs from the true mean $\bar{X}$ by no more than $100\varepsilon\%$. This formulation is equivalent to that discussed earlier for simple random sampling and systematic sampling. The formula (valid for reasonably large N_h) for the required n is as follows:

Sample size needed

$$n \approx \frac{\left(\dfrac{z_{1-\alpha/2}^2}{N^2}\right)\left(\displaystyle\sum_{h=1}^{L} \dfrac{N_h^2 \sigma_{hx}^2}{\pi_h \bar{X}^2}\right)}{\varepsilon^2 + \left(\dfrac{z_{1-\alpha/2}^2}{N^2}\right)\left(\displaystyle\sum_{h=1}^{L} \dfrac{N_h^2 \sigma_{hx}^2}{\bar{X}^2}\right)} \tag{6.22}$$

where

$$\pi_h = \frac{n_h}{n}$$

Relation (6.22) is valid for any type of allocation.

We can see from inspection of relation (6.22) that its use requires more knowledge about parameters of the distribution than is likely to be available or than can be guessed with any degree of confidence. For this reason relation (6.22) is unlikely to be of much help in actual practice.

If one assumes proportional allocation, then relation (6.22) reduces to the form

$$n \approx \frac{N z_{1-\alpha/2}^2 (\sigma_{wx}^2 / \bar{X}^2)}{z_{1-\alpha/2}^2 (\sigma_{wx}^2 / \bar{X}^2) + N\varepsilon^2} \qquad (6.23)$$

Assuming proportional allocation

where σ_{wx}^2 is as defined in expression (6.13).

Note that relation (6.23) is similar to expression (3.15) for the sample size required for estimation of a sample mean under simple random sampling (box 3.4). The only difference between the two expressions is that V_x^2 (which is equal to $\sigma_x^2/\bar{X}^2$) in equation (3.15) is replaced by $\sigma_{wx}^2/\bar{X}^2$ in relation (6.23). If we have some idea concerning the order of magnitude of V_x^2, the relative variance of the distribution of variable $\mathscr{X}$ in the population, and if in addition we have some idea of the ratio $\gamma = \sigma_{bx}^2/\sigma_{wx}^2$, then since $\sigma_x^2 = \sigma_{bx}^2 + \sigma_{wx}^2$, relation (6.23) becomes

$$n \approx \frac{[z_{1-\alpha/2}^2 N/(1+\gamma)](V_x^2)}{[z_{1-\alpha/2}^2 V_x^2/(1+\gamma)] + N\varepsilon^2} \qquad (6.24)$$

Let us look at an example to see how relation (6.24) might be used in practice.

ILLUSTRATIVE EXAMPLE

Suppose that we are planning to take a sample of the members of a health maintenance organization (HMO) for purposes of estimating the average number of hospital episodes per person. The sample will be selected from membership lists grouped according to age (under 45 years, 45–64 years, 65 years and over). Let us suppose that the distributions of hospital episodes are available from national data (such as the NCHS Health Interview Survey) and are as given in table 6.7.

Suppose further that the number of HMO members in each age group is as follows:

Age group 1: $N_1 = 600$

Age group 2: $N_2 = 500$

Age group 3: $N_3 = 400$

Table 6.7   Distribution of Hospital Episodes Per Person Per Year

Age Group	Average No. of Hospital Episodes	Variance of Distribution of Hospital Episodes
1: under 45	.164	.245
2: 45–64	.166	.296
3: 65 years and over	.236	.436

If we assume that the results found on the national level are likely to be true also for the HMO members, then the anticipated mean number of hospital episodes per person is, from equation (5.2),

$$\bar{X} = \frac{(600)(.164) + (500)(.166) + (400)(.236)}{1500} = .184$$

The anticipated variance component σ_{bx}^2 is, from equation (6.15),

$$\sigma_{bx}^2 = \frac{(600)(.164 - .184)^2 + (500)(.166 - .184)^2 + (400)(.236 - .184)^2}{1500}$$

$$= .0009891$$

The anticipated variance component σ_{wx}^2 is, from equation (6.13),

$$\sigma_{wx}^2 = \frac{(600)(.245) + (500)(.296) + (400)(.436)}{1500} = .31293$$

Finally, the anticipated values of σ_x^2, V_x^2, and γ are

$$\sigma_x^2 = .0009891 + .31293 = .31392$$

$$V_x^2 = \frac{.31392}{(.184)^2} = 9.27$$

$$\gamma = \frac{.0009891}{.31293} = .00316$$

Now using relation (6.24), we can calculate the estimated number of subjects needed to be virtually certain of estimating the mean number of hospital episodes to within 20% of the true mean under stratified sampling with proportional allocation:

$$n \approx \frac{[(9)(1500)/(1 + .00316)](9.27)}{[(9)(9.27)/(1 + .00316)] + 1500(.20)^2} = 872$$

The number n_h allocated to each stratum would then be as follows:

$$n_1 = (600)\left(\frac{872}{1500}\right) = 349$$

$$n_2 = (500)\left(\frac{872}{1500}\right) = 291$$

$$n_3 = (400)\left(\frac{872}{1500}\right) = 232$$

If we wish to use optimal allocation assuming equal stratum costs, the required sample size could be estimated by first determining the optimal π_h from national estimates and then computing the required n from relation (6.23). This would be done as follows.

First, compute the optimal π_h (which is equal to $N_h\sigma_{hx}/\sum_{h=1}^{L} N_h\sigma_{hx}$) based on the national data:

$$\pi_1 = \frac{600\sqrt{.245}}{600\sqrt{.245} + 500\sqrt{.296} + 400\sqrt{.436}} = .356$$

$$\pi_2 = \frac{500\sqrt{.296}}{600\sqrt{.245} + 500\sqrt{.296} + 400\sqrt{.436}} = .327$$

$$\pi_3 = \frac{400\sqrt{.436}}{600\sqrt{.245} + 500\sqrt{.296} + 400\sqrt{.436}} = .317$$

Next, compute the required n based on relation (6.22) with $\varepsilon = .20$:

$$n \approx \frac{\left[\dfrac{9}{(1500)^2}\right]\left[\dfrac{(600)^2(.245)}{(.356)(.184)^2} + \dfrac{(500)^2(.296)}{(.327)(.184)^2} + \dfrac{(400)^2(.436)}{(.317)(.184)^2}\right]}{(.2)^2 + \left[\dfrac{9}{(1500)^2}\right]\left[\dfrac{600(.245)}{(.184)^2} + \dfrac{500(.296)}{(.184)^2} + \dfrac{400(.436)}{(.184)^2}\right]} = 860$$

Finally, the sample of 860 necessary to achieve $\varepsilon = .20$ with virtual certainty is allocated to the strata by multiplying 396 by the appropriate π_h:

$$n_1 = n\pi_1 = 860(.356) = 306$$
$$n_2 = n\pi_2 = 860(.327) = 281$$
$$n_3 = n\pi_3 = 860(.317) = 273$$

Note that the required sample size is smaller under optimal allocation as compared to that required under proportional allocation.

SUMMARY

In this chapter we developed the concepts of stratification. In particular, we discussed estimation of population means, totals, and proportions under stratified random sampling, along with methods of allocation of sample to strata. Finally, we presented methods of estimating the required sample size under stratified random sampling.

EXERCISES

1. A sample survey of households in a community containing 1500 households is to be conducted for purposes of determining the total number of persons over 18 years of age in the community who have one or more permanent

teeth (other than third molars) missing. Since this variable is thought to be correlated with age and income, the strata shown in the accompanying table are formed by using available population data. A stratified random sample of 100 families is to be taken.

Stratum	AGE (YEARS) Mean	Standard Deviation	ANNUAL FAMILY INCOME (× $1000) Mean	Standard Deviation	No. of Families
1	30	15	15	5	300
2	32	15	7	3	500
3	25	10	15	3	100
4	27	10	8	2	600

(a) Specify in algebraic detail how the estimate of the total number of persons having one or more missing teeth is to be constructed.

(b) Determine the number of families to be taken from each stratum if proportional allocation is used.

(c) Determine the number of families to be taken from each stratum if optimal allocation is used based on annual family income.

(d) Determine the number of families to be taken from each stratum if optimal allocation is used based on age.

(e) How would you allocate the sample to strata taking into consideration both age and annual family income?

(f) What is the variance of the distribution of annual family income for the entire population?

(g) Suppose the number of persons over 18 having missing teeth in a family is highly correlated with family income. Is stratified random sampling with proportional allocation likely to yield an estimate having lower variance than that obtained from a simple random sample of the same number of households?

2. Let us suppose that the data from table 3.8 (p. 52) were obtained from a stratified random sample of the 1200 workers in the plant in which the working force was stratified according to exposure to pulmonary stressors (high, medium, low) and proportional allocation was used to allocate the sample.

(a) How many workers in the population are there in each stratum?

(b) Estimate the mean forced vital capacity among the workers in the plant.

How does this estimate differ from the mean that would be calculated under the assumption that the sample was obtained by simple random sampling?

(c) Obtain a 95% confidence interval for the population mean.

(d) What is the gain from stratified random sampling over what would be obtained from simple random sampling?

3. Let us suppose that a household survey is to be taken for purposes of estimating characteristics of families having female household heads. Since it is not known in advance of the survey which families have female heads, the sample households will be screened and those sample households with female heads will be given a detailed interview. It is anticipated that the cost of screening a household is $5.00 and of interviewing a household having a female head is $25.00. The population is stratified into three strata according to the latest census information on the proportion of households having female heads. The strata are shown in the accompanying table. Assume that the variance of the characteristics being measured is the same in each stratum and that a total budget of $5000 is allowed for the field work. How many households in each stratum should be sampled?

Stratum	No. of Households	Percentage of Households Having Female Head
1	10,000	25%
2	20,000	15%
3	5,000	10%

4. Consider the 40 workers presented in table 3.8 to be a simple random sample from the 1200 workers in the plant.

(a) Compute a 90% confidence interval for the population mean forced vital capacity.

(b) Suppose it is known, prior to analyzing the data, that the 1200 workers were distributed as follows:

$$N_1 = 1000 \quad \text{(number with high exposure)}$$
$$N_2 = 100 \quad \text{(number with medium exposure)}$$
$$N_3 = 100 \quad \text{(number with low exposure)}$$

Poststratify the original simple random sample of table 3.8 and construct a 90% confidence interval for the population mean forced vital capacity.

(c) Compare the intervals of parts (a) and (b). Which is larger? Why?

BIBLIOGRAPHY

The following textbooks present additional discussions of stratification.

1. COCHRAN, W. G. *Sampling techniques*, 3d ed. New York: Wiley, 1977.

2. HANSEN, M. H.; HURWITZ, W. N.; and MADOW, W. G. *Sample survey methods and theory*, Vols. 1 and 2. New York: Wiley, 1953.

The following publications present sample survey in which stratification is used.

3. HEMPHILL, F. M. A sample survey of home injuries. *Public Health Reports* (1952) 67: 1026–1034.

4. HORVITZ, D. G. Sampling and field procedures of the Pittsburgh morbidity survey. *Public Health Reports* (1952) 67: 1003–1012.

7

Ratio Estimation

In this chapter we introduce the concept of a ratio $\bar{x}/\bar{y}$ of two sample means $\bar{x}$ and $\bar{y}$. This ratio serves as an estimate of the ratio $\bar{X}/\bar{Y}$ of the means of two variables $\mathcal{X}$ and $\mathcal{Y}$ in a population. But, more importantly, it also serves as a device for obtaining a more accurate estimate of a population total X than can be obtained from the estimate x' determined by simple inflation of a sample total x by N/n, the inverse of the sampling fraction. This method is called **ratio estimation,** and the estimates are called **ratio estimates.**

To begin, let us look at an example of ratio estimation.

ILLUSTRATIVE EXAMPLE

Let us consider a community having eight community areas. Suppose that we desire to estimate the ratio R of total pharmaceutical expenses X to total medical expenses Y among all persons in the community. To do this, a simple random sample of two community areas is to be taken and every household in each sample community area is to be interviewed.

With this sampling design the elements are community areas, and the ratio X/Y of total pharmaceutical to total medical expenses can be estimated by r, where $r = x/y$, the ratio obtained from the sample. Let us suppose that the data for the eight community areas are as given in table 7.1.

Table 7.1   Pharmaceutical Expenses and Total Medical Expenses
Among All Residents of Eight Community Areas

Community Area	Total Pharmaceutical Expenses, X_i	Total Medical Expenses, Y_i
1	$ 10,000	$ 30,000
2	5,000	20,000
3	7,500	30,000
4	20,000	60,000
5	15,000	45,000
6	17,500	52,000
7	17,000	68,000
8	15,000	45,000
Total	$107,000	$350,000

Now suppose, for example, that community areas 2 and 5 are selected in the sample. Then we have

$$x = 5,000 + 15,000 = 20,000$$
$$y = 20,000 + 45,000 = 65,000$$

and

$$r = \frac{x}{y} = \frac{20,000}{65,000} = .308$$

Thus the ratio of total pharmaceutical expenses to total medical expenses as estimated from this sample is equal to .308.

7.1 RATIO ESTIMATE UNDER SIMPLE RANDOM SAMPLING

*Expressions for the population ratio **R** and the sample ratio estimate **r***

The example above can be generalized as follows: Suppose that we have a simple random sample of n elements from a population of N elements and that we wish to estimate the **ratio** R of two population totals X and Y. Clearly R is given by

$$R = \frac{X}{Y}$$

or, equivalently, by

$$R = \frac{\bar{X}}{\bar{Y}}$$

The ratio R can be **estimated by** r, as given by

$$r = \frac{x'}{y'}$$

or by the two algebraically equivalent forms

$$r = \frac{x}{y} \quad \text{and} \quad r = \frac{\bar{x}}{\bar{y}}$$

The estimate r is called a ratio estimate because both the numerator $\bar{x}$ and the denominator $\bar{y}$ of r are subject to sampling variation.

Now let us return to the example presented in the introduction to the chapter to see whether an estimated ratio is an unbiased estimate.

ILLUSTRATIVE EXAMPLE

In the example given above there are $\binom{8}{2} = 28$ possible simple random samples of two elements from the population of eight elements. These possible samples are listed in table 7.2 along with the values of x, y, and r obtained from each sample.

Table 7.2   Possible Samples of Two Elements from the Population of Eight Elements (Table 7.1)

Community Areas in Sample	x	y	r	Community Areas in Sample	x	y	r
1, 2	15,000	50,000	.300	3, 5	22,500	75,000	.300
1, 3	17,500	60,000	.292	3, 6	25,000	82,000	.305
1, 4	30,000	90,000	.333	3, 7	24,500	98,000	.250
1, 5	25,000	75,000	.333	3, 8	22,500	75,000	.300
1, 6	27,500	82,000	.335	4, 5	35,000	105,000	.333
1, 7	27,000	98,000	.276	4, 6	37,500	112,000	.335
1, 8	25,000	75,000	.333	4, 7	37,000	128,000	.289
2, 3	12,500	50,000	.250	4, 8	35,000	105,000	.333
2, 4	25,000	80,000	.313	5, 6	32,500	97,000	.335
2, 5	20,000	65,000	.308	5, 7	32,000	113,000	.283
2, 6	22,500	72,000	.313	5, 8	30,000	90,000	.333
2, 7	22,000	88,000	.250	6, 7	34,500	120,000	.288
2, 8	20,000	65,000	.308	6, 8	32,500	97,000	.335
3, 4	27,500	90,000	.306	7, 8	32,000	113,000	.283

The sampling distribution of the estimated ratio r has a mean $E(r)$ and a standard error $SE(r)$ given by*

$$E(r) = \left(\frac{1}{28}\right)(.300 + .292 + \cdots + .283) = .3054$$

$$SE(r) = \left(\frac{1}{\sqrt{28}}\right)[(.300 - .3054)^2 + (.292 - .3054)^2$$

$$+ \cdots + (.283 - .3054)^2]^{1/2} = .0268$$

The true value of R from table 7.1 is

$$R = \frac{107,000}{350,000} = .3057$$

An estimated ratio is not always an unbiased estimate   The difference between the mean $E(r)$ of the sampling distribution of the estimated ratio r and the true population ratio R is real and not due to rounding error. Thus we see that an estimated ratio r is not necessarily an unbiased estimate of a population ratio R. However, in most situations the bias in an estimated ratio r is small, and estimates of this form are widely used.

Note that in order to calculate $SE(r)$ in the example above, it was necessary to generate all possible samples and compute the standard error of the sampling distribution. Of course, in actual practice we do not generate the entire sampling distribution. However, unlike other estimates (such as means, totals, and proportions) we have considered so far in this text, the estimated ratio r has both numerator and denominator subject to sampling variability; thus an exact expression for its standard error cannot be derived. However, it has been suggested by Hansen, Hurwitz, and Madow (1) that if the coefficient of variation $V(\bar{y})$ of the denominator $\bar{y}$ of r (using the form $r = \bar{x}/\bar{y}$) is less than or equal to .05, then the **standard error** $SE(r)$ of r can be approximated by the following form:

$$SE(r) \approx \left(\frac{R}{\sqrt{n}}\right)(V_x^2 + V_y^2 - 2\rho_{xy}V_xV_y)^{1/2}\left(\frac{N-n}{N-1}\right)^{1/2} \qquad (7.1)$$

where ρ_{xy} is the **correlation coefficient** between x and y, as defined by

$$\rho_{xy} = \frac{\sum\limits_{i=1}^{N}(X_i - \bar{X})(Y_i - \bar{Y})\Big/N}{\sigma_x\sigma_y} \qquad (7.2)$$

---

* To find the mean and standard error of the sampling distribution of r, we follow the same procedure as that used with $\bar{x}$, x', or p_y in box 2.3.

Let us do some calculations for the example we have been working with.

ILLUSTRATIVE EXAMPLE

For the data given in table 7.1 we have the following population parameters [refer to the expressions in box 2.1 and to equations (2.7) and (7.2)]:

$$\sigma_x = 4{,}941.85 \qquad \bar{X} = 13{,}375 \qquad R = .3057$$

$$\sigma_y = 15{,}270.48 \qquad \bar{Y} = 43{,}750 \qquad V_x = .3695$$

$$N = 8 \qquad \rho_{xy} = .9272 \qquad V_y = .3490$$

For the data of table 7.2, the coefficient of variation of the denominator $\bar{y}$ of r is

$$V(\bar{y}) = \left(\frac{1}{\bar{Y}}\right)\left(\frac{\sigma_y}{\sqrt{n}}\right)\left(\frac{N-n}{N-1}\right)^{1/2} = \left(\frac{1}{43{,}750}\right)\left(\frac{15{,}270.48}{\sqrt{2}}\right)\left(\frac{8-2}{8-1}\right)^{1/2} = .2285$$

Calculation with equation (7.1) gives

$$SE(r) \approx \left(\frac{.3057}{\sqrt{2}}\right)[(.3695)^2 + (.3490)^2 - 2(.9272)(.3695)(.3490)]^{1/2}\left(\frac{8-2}{8-1}\right)^{1/2}$$

$$= .0277$$

compared to the exact value of .0268. Since the coefficient of variation of $\bar{y}$ is greater than .05, the approximation given by equation (7.1) should not normally be used for $SE(r)$. However, in this case it seems to work well.

Now consider selecting samples of size $n = 7$ from the given population. The exact distribution of r for samples of $n = 7$ elements is shown in table 7.3

Table 7.3   Samples of Seven Elements from the Population of Table 7.1

Sample	x	y	r
1, 2, 3, 4, 5, 6, 7	92,000	305,000	.3016
1, 2, 3, 4, 5, 6, 8	90,000	282,000	.3191
1, 2, 3, 4, 5, 7, 8	89,500	298,000	.3003
1, 2, 3, 4, 6, 7, 8	92,000	305,000	.3016
1, 2, 3, 5, 6, 7, 8	87,000	290,000	.3000
1, 2, 4, 5, 6, 7, 8	99,500	320,000	.3109
1, 3, 4, 5, 6, 7, 8	102,000	330,000	.3091
2, 3, 4, 5, 6, 7, 8	97,000	320,000	.3031

The exact standard error SE(r) of r obtained by enumerating all possible samples is equal to .0063.

Calculations show that

$$V(\bar{y}) = \left(\frac{1}{43,750}\right)\left(\frac{15,270.48}{\sqrt{7}}\right)\left(\frac{8-7}{8-1}\right)^{1/2} = .0499$$

Therefore, since $V(\bar{y}) = .0499 \le .05$, we expect the approximation of equation (7.1) to provide a good approximation to the true value of SE(r). This calculation is as follows:

$$SE(r) \approx \left(\frac{.3057}{\sqrt{7}}\right)[(.3695)^2 + (.3490)^2 - 2(.9272)(.3695)(.3490)]^{1/2}\left(\frac{8-7}{8-1}\right)^{1/2}$$

$$= .0061$$

Thus we see that the approximation (7.1) agrees very closely in this example with the exact standard error of r.

The standard error of an estimated ratio can be estimated from the data by replacing $\hat{\sigma}_x^2$ for σ_x^2, $\hat{\sigma}_y^2$ for σ_y^2, $\hat{\rho}_{xy}$ for ρ_{xy}, $\bar{x}$ for $\bar{X}$, $\bar{y}$ for $\bar{Y}$, and r for R in relation (7.1). The resulting **estimate** $\widehat{SE}(r)$ is given by

$$\widehat{SE}(r) = \left(\frac{r}{\sqrt{n}}\right)(\hat{V}_x^2 + \hat{V}_y^2 - 2\hat{\rho}_{xy}\hat{V}_x\hat{V}_y)^{1/2}\left(\frac{N-n}{N-1}\right)^{1/2} \qquad (7.3)$$

where

$$\hat{V}_x^2 = \left(\frac{N-1}{N}\right)\left(\frac{s_x^2}{\bar{x}^2}\right)$$

$$\hat{V}_y^2 = \left(\frac{N-1}{N}\right)\left(\frac{s_y^2}{\bar{y}^2}\right)$$

$$\hat{\rho}_{xy} = \frac{\sum\limits_{i=1}^{n}(x_i - \bar{x})(y_i - \bar{y})}{(n-1)s_x s_y}$$

Generally this approximation will only be used when $(s_y/\sqrt{n}\bar{y})[(N-n)/N]^{1/2}$, the estimated coefficient of variation of the denominator of r, is less than .05.

For convenience, formulas that can be used for ratio estimation are summarized in the next box.

Box 7.1 Formulas for Ratio Estimation Under Simple Random Sampling

POPULATION PARAMETERS

$$R = \frac{X}{Y} = \frac{\bar{X}}{\bar{Y}}$$

$$SE(r) \simeq \left(\frac{R}{\sqrt{n}}\right)(V_x^2 + V_y^2 - 2\rho_{xy}V_xV_y)^{1/2}\left(\frac{N - n}{N - 1}\right)^{1/2}$$

SAMPLE ESTIMATES

$$r = \frac{x'}{y'} = \frac{x}{y} = \frac{\bar{x}}{\bar{y}}$$

$$\widehat{SE}(r) = \left(\frac{r}{\sqrt{n}}\right)(\hat{V}_x^2 + \hat{V}_y^2 - 2\hat{\rho}_{xy}\hat{V}_x\hat{V}_y)^{1/2}\left(\frac{N - n}{N - 1}\right)^{1/2}$$

A $100(1 - \alpha)\%$ confidence interval may be constructed as

$$r - z_{1-\alpha/2}\widehat{SE}(r) \le R \le r + z_{1-\alpha/2}\widehat{SE}(r)$$

V_x and V_y are as defined in equation (2.7). X, $\bar{X}$, σ_x^2, Y, $\bar{Y}$, and σ_y^2 are as defined in box 2.1. ρ_{xy} is as defined in equation (7.2). x, $\bar{x}x'$, y, $\bar{y}y'$, s_x^2, and s_y^2 are as defined in box 2.2. Then

$$\hat{V}_x^2 = \left(\frac{N - 1}{N}\right)\left(\frac{s_x^2}{\bar{x}^2}\right)$$

$$\hat{V}_y^2 = \left(\frac{N - 1}{N_.}\right)\left(\frac{s_y^2}{\bar{y}^2}\right)$$

$$\hat{\rho}_{xy} = \frac{\sum\limits_{i=1}^{n} (x_i - \bar{x})(y_i - \bar{y})}{(n - 1)s_xs_y}$$

Now let us do some calculations.

ILLUSTRATIVE EXAMPLE

Suppose we take the sample consisting of community areas 1, 2, 3, 4, 5, 6, 8 from table 7.1. We calculate $s_y = 14,103.36$, $\bar{y} = 40,285.71$, and $(s_y/\sqrt{n}\bar{y})[(N - n)/N]^{1/2} = .0468$, which is less than .05. Thus we expect approximation (7.3) to provide a good estimate of the standard error of the estimated ratio r. For this example we have

$$r = .3191 \qquad \hat{\rho}_{xy} = .9900$$
$$s_x = 5,482.66 \qquad s_y = 14,103.36$$
$$\bar{x} = 12,857.14 \qquad \bar{y} = 40,285.71$$
$$\hat{V}_x^2 = .1591 \qquad \hat{V}_y^2 = .1072$$

Then we obtain

$$\widehat{SE}(r) = \left(\frac{.3191}{\sqrt{7}}\right)[.1591 + .1072 - 2(.9900)(\sqrt{.1591})(\sqrt{.1072})]^{1/2}\left(\frac{8 - 7}{8 - 1}\right)^{1/2}$$

$$= .0040$$

as compared to the true population value of SE(r), which is .0063. This discrepancy is not surprising, since estimated variances are known to be highly variable.

Estimated ratios are important when enumeration units are not the same as elementary units

The estimated ratio r is, in general, a biased estimate of R. However, when sample sizes are reasonably large, the bias is generally small, and approximate confidence intervals for the unknown population ratio R can be constructed by use of the estimated standard error $\widehat{SE}(r)$ of r.

Estimates of ratios are important in sample surveys, especially when the enumeration units are not the same as the elementary units. For example, if a simple random sample of households is taken for purposes of estimating the mean number of days lost from work per person because of acute illnesses, a ratio estimate of the form discussed above could be used, with the numerator being number of days lost per household and the denominator being number of persons per household. Both the numerator and denominator would be subject to sampling variability.

In an earlier section (3.5) we discussed the estimation of population means for subgroups of a population under simple random sampling. The estimate appropriate for this situation is a special case of an estimated ratio, where the denominator is the number of members of the subgroup in the sample. If the sampling plan is that of a simple random sample of elements, this form of ratio estimate is an unbiased estimate of the appropriate subgroup mean.

7.2 RATIO ESTIMATION OF TOTALS UNDER SIMPLE RANDOM SAMPLING

The estimates of totals or aggregates discussed so far have been obtained from simple inflation of a sample total by the ratio N/n. We have discussed the fact that estimates x' of this type are unbiased estimates, and we have developed an expression for the standard error of such estimates and the methodology for constructing approximate confidence intervals for the unknown population total X under simple random sampling. Sometimes, however, we are in a position to use additional information available to us for purposes of constructing a different estimator of a population total, one which is based on an estimated ratio, so that the resulting estimator has a smaller mean square error than the simple inflation estimate x'.

Let us investigate this idea by looking at an example.

An estimated ratio of a population total can be used to obtain an estimate of the population total with a smaller MSE than was possible using previously discussed methods

---

ILLUSTRATIVE EXAMPLE

Let us suppose that a village comprises six census tracts having the 1980 population given in table 7.4. The school enrollment (considered unknown in advance of the survey) is also given in table 7.4.

Table 7.4 Population (1980 Census) and Present School Enrollment by Census Tract

Census Tract	1980 Population	Present School Enrollment[a]
1	6,657	2,269
2	4,057	1,324
3	3,642	952
4	5,320	1,558
5	4,480	1,352
6	5,880	1,796
Total	30,036	9,251

[a] Unknown until the schools are surveyed.

Let us suppose that we wish to estimate the total present school enrollment by taking a simple random sample of two census tracts and ascertaining the school enrollment in each sample tract by surveying each school within the tract, counting heads, and inflating the sample totals by N/n as discussed in chapter 3. The $\binom{6}{2} = 15$ possible samples are listed in table 7.5 along with the values of x', the estimated total.

Table 7.5   Possible Samples of Two Schools Taken from Data
of Table 7.4

Schools in Sample	Estimated School Enrollment, x'	Schools in Sample	Estimated School Enrollment, x'
1, 2	10,779	2, 6	9,360
1, 3	9,663	3, 4	7,530
1, 4	11,481	3, 5	6,912
1, 5	10,863	3, 6	8,244
1, 6	12,195	4, 5	8,730
2, 3	6,828	4, 6	10,062
2, 4	8,646	5, 6	9,444
2, 5	8,028		

From our results on simple random sampling, we know that the estimated total x' is an unbiased estimate of the population total. The standard error of x' (computed by enumerating all the samples listed above and referring to box 2.3) is

$$SE(x') = 1,568.4577$$

Instead of using the estimate x' as we did in the example above, we can estimate the total school enrollment X by using the data on 1980 population that is available for each census tract. Each sample of census tracts enables us not only to estimate total school enrollment from the sample but also to estimate the total population from the sample. Suppose we use the following notation:

Y = the total number of persons in the population

Y_i = the number of persons in census tract i

y_i = the number of persons in sample tract i

$y = \sum\limits_{i=1}^{n} y_i =$ the total number of persons in the sample census tracts

Then the estimated population total y' is given by

$$y' = \left(\frac{N}{n}\right)(y)$$

where

N = the total number of tracts

n = the number of sample tracts

Each sample gives us an estimate x' of X and y' of Y. But since Y is known to us from census data, then it might make sense, if school enrollment and population size are strongly correlated, to assume that the estimator x' might differ from X in the same proportion that the estimator y' differs from Y, that is, $X/x' = Y/y'$. This motivates the use of an **estimator** x'' of X given by

$$x'' = \left(\frac{x'}{y'}\right)(Y) \qquad (7.4)$$

or its algebraic equivalent

$$x'' = rY \qquad (7.5)$$

where r is an estimated ratio.

Further insight into this estimator is evident by writing it as follows:

$$x'' = \left(\frac{Y}{y'}\right)(x')$$

If the estimated population size y' is less than the known true total Y, then y' underestimates Y. We would also expect that the estimate x' obtained from the same sample underestimates to a similar extent the true unknown total X, since X and Y are correlated. But note that the ratio Y/y' would be greater than one in this case, and x'' would be greater than the simple inflation estimator x'. The opposite occurs when y' is greater than Y. Thus we see that even for particularly bad samples (i.e., those that yield values of x' that differ greatly from X in absolute value) the ratio Y/y' would adjust for this, and the estimator x'' would not differ from X as much as x' does.

Let us examine all these ideas in some examples.

ILLUSTRATIVE EXAMPLE

For samples of $n = 2$ census tracts taken from the population shown in table 7.4, let us investigate the sample values of x' and x''. These values are listed in table 7.6.

Table 7.6   Values of x' and x'' for the Samples in Table 7.5

Sample	x'	x''	Sample	x'	x''
1, 2	10,779	10,073	2, 6	9,360	9,431
1, 3	9,663	9,394	3, 4	7,530	8,412
1, 4	11,481	9,597	3, 5	6,912	8,520
1, 5	10,863	9,766	3, 6	8,244	8,668
1, 6	12,195	9,739	4, 5	8,730	8,919
2, 3	6,828	8,879	4, 6	10,062	8,995
2, 4	8,646	9,231	5, 6	9,444	9,127
2, 5	8,028	9,415			

We see from the sampling distribution shown in table 7.6 that the mean $E(x'')$, the standard error $SE(x'')$, and the mean square error $MSE(x'')$ are (refer to box 2.3)

$$E(x'') = \frac{10{,}073 + 9{,}394 + \cdots + 9{,}127}{15} = 9{,}211.07$$

$$SE(x'') = \left[\frac{(10{,}073 - 9{,}211.07)^2 + (9{,}394 - 9{,}211.07)^2 + \cdots + (9{,}127 - 9{,}211.07)^2}{15}\right]^{1/2} = 466.38$$

$$MSE(x'') = Var(x'') + B^2(x'') = 217{,}512.33 + (9{,}211.07 - 9{,}251)^2$$
$$= 219{,}106.73$$

Since the simple inflation estimate x' is an unbiased estimate of X, its MSE is equal to its variance:

$$MSE(x') = Var(x') = (1568.4577)^2 = 2{,}460{,}059.56$$

Thus even though x'' is a biased estimate of X, its mean square error in this example is much less than that of x'.

ILLUSTRATIVE EXAMPLE

The data from table 5.1 (p. 93) can also be used to illustrate estimation of a total by a ratio. If we wish to estimate the total number X of truck miles driven from a simple random sample of $n = 3$ segments, we can estimate the ratio r of truck miles to accidents involving trucks from the sample. If the total number Y of accidents involving trucks is known for the entire road, the estimate x'' can be constructed. For example, if segments 1, 3, and 4 are sampled, we have the following calculations (refer to boxes 3.1 and 7.1):

$$x' = (\tfrac{8}{3})(6{,}327 + 8{,}691 + 7{,}834) = 60{,}938.67$$
$$= \text{simple inflation estimate of truck miles driven}$$

$$y' = (\tfrac{8}{3})(8 + 9 + 9) = 69.33$$
$$= \text{simple inflation estimate of number of accidents involving trucks}$$

$$r = \frac{x'}{y'} = 878.9230$$

$$= \text{estimated ratio of truck miles driven to accidents involving trucks}$$

$Y = 50$ is known; hence

$$x'' = -Y = 878.9230(50) = 43{,}946.15 \text{ truck miles}$$

which is closer to the true total ($X = 34{,}054$) than is the simple inflation estimate x'.

The estimate x'' is of the form rY, where r is an estimated ratio and Y is a known population total. Hence it follows that its **standard error** $SE(x'')$ is equal to $Y[SE(r)]$, which can be approximated by the following expression provided that $V(\bar{y})$, the coefficient of variation of $\bar{y}$, is less than .05:   *Formulas for ratio estimation of totals*

$$SE(x'') = \left(\frac{YR}{\sqrt{n}}\right)(V_x^2 + V_y^2 - 2\rho_{xy}V_xV_y)^{1/2}\left(\frac{N-n}{N-1}\right)^{1/2} \qquad (7.6)$$

Likewise, an **estimate** $\widehat{SE}(x'')$ of $SE(x'')$ can be obtained from data by substituting $\widehat{SE}(r)$ [relation (7.3)] for $SE(r)$ in expression (7.6), as given below:

$$\widehat{SE}(x'') = \left(\frac{Yr}{\sqrt{n}}\right)(\hat{V}_x^2 + \hat{V}_y^2 - 2\hat{\rho}_{xy}\hat{V}_x\hat{V}_y)^{1/2}\left(\frac{N-n}{N-1}\right)^{1/2} \qquad (7.7)$$

Expression (7.7) can be used to obtain approximate confidence intervals for an unknown total X, provided that $\hat{V}(\bar{y})$, the estimated coefficient of variation of $\bar{y}$, is less than .05.

Let us look at another example.

ILLUSTRATIVE EXAMPLE

If segments 1, 3, and 4 are sampled in the data from table 5.1, we have the sample data given in table 7.7.

Table 7.7   Sample Data from Table 5.1

Segment in Sample	No. of Truck Miles, x_i	No. of Accidents Involving Trucks, y_i
1	6,327	8
3	8,691	9
4	7,834	9

We then have the following summary statistics:

$n = 3$	$\bar{x} = 7{,}617.33$	$s_x = 1{,}196.80$	$\hat{V}_x^2 = .0245$
$N = 8$	$\bar{y} = 8.67$	$s_y = .5774$	$\hat{V}_y^2 = .004435$
$\hat{\rho}_{xy} = .9337$	$Y = 50$	$r = 878.5848$	$x'' = 43{,}929.24$

The estimated coefficient of variation $\hat{V}(\bar{y})$ is*

$$\hat{V}(\bar{y}) = \left(\frac{s_y}{\sqrt{n\bar{y}}}\right)\left(\frac{N-n}{N}\right)^{1/2} = \left[\frac{.5774}{\sqrt{3(8.67)}}\right]\left(\frac{8-3}{8}\right)^{1/2} = .0304$$

Since $\hat{V}(\bar{y}) < .05$, expression (7.7) can be used to estimate the standard error of x'', as follows:

$$\widehat{SE}(x'') = \left[\frac{(50)(878.5848)}{\sqrt{3}}\right]$$

$$\times [.0245 + .004435 - 2(.9337)(\sqrt{.0245})(\sqrt{.004435})]^{1/2}\left(\frac{8-3}{8-1}\right)^{1/2}$$

$$= 2{,}085.89$$

We then have the following 95% confidence interval for the estimated total number of truck miles driven:

$$x'' - (1.96)[\widehat{SE}(x'')] \le X' \le x'' + (1.96)[\widehat{SE}(x'')]$$

$$43{,}929.24 - (1.96)(2{,}085.89) \le X' \le 43{,}929.24 + (1.96)(2{,}085.89)$$

$$39{,}840.90 \le X' \le 48{,}017.43$$

Note that for this particular sample the 95% confidence interval does not cover the true population total.

7.3 COMPARISON OF RATIO ESTIMATE WITH SIMPLE INFLATION ESTIMATE

Let us assume that the approximation to the standard error of the ratio estimate of a total under simple random sampling, given by relation (7.6), is valid and that the bias in the ratio estimate can be ignored. Then we can evaluate whether a ratio estimate x'' is likely to result in an improved estimate of a total over a simple inflation estimate x' by examining the ratio of the variance of x'' to the variance of x', as follows:

We compare the ratio of the variances

$$\frac{\text{Var}(x'')}{\text{Var}(x')} = \frac{V_x^2 + V_y^2 - 2\rho_{xy}V_xV_y}{V_x^2}$$

---

* The formula for $V(\bar{y})$ is given in equation (3.7). Substituting $(\hat{V}_y^2)^{1/2}$ as given in box 7.1 into formula (3.7), we obtain

$$\hat{V}(\bar{y}) = \left(\frac{\hat{V}_y}{\sqrt{n}}\right)\left(\frac{N-n}{N-1}\right)^{1/2} = \left[\left(\frac{N-1}{N}\right)^{1/2}\left(\frac{s_y^2}{\bar{y}^2}\right)^{1/2}\middle/\sqrt{n}\right]\left(\frac{N-n}{N-1}\right)^{1/2}$$

$$= \left(\frac{s_y}{\sqrt{n\bar{y}}}\right)\left(\frac{N-n}{N}\right)^{1/2}$$

since

$$\text{Var}(x'') = Y^2\text{Var}(r)$$

$$= (Y^2)\left(\frac{R^2}{n}\right)(V_x^2 + V_y^2 - 2\rho_{xy}V_xV_y)\left(\frac{N-n}{N-1}\right)$$

$$\text{Var}(x') = \left(\frac{N^2}{n}\right)(\sigma_x^2)\left(\frac{N-n}{N-1}\right)$$

$$= \left(\frac{N^2}{n}\right)(\bar{X}^2V_x^2)\left(\frac{N-n}{n-1}\right) = \left(\frac{X^2}{n}\right)(V_x^2)\left(\frac{N-n}{N-1}\right)$$

It follows that x'' will have smaller variance than x' whenever

$$V_x^2 + V_y^2 - 2\rho_{xy}V_xV_y < V_x^2$$

or, equivalently, whenever

$$\frac{V_y}{V_x} < 2\rho_{xy} \tag{7.8}$$

Whenever this statement is true, Var(x'') < Var(x')

Thus for fixed values of coefficients of variation of $\mathscr{X}$ and $\mathscr{Y}$ in the population, the greater the correlation between $\mathscr{X}$ and $\mathscr{Y}$, the more likely it is that a total estimated by x'' will have lower variance than when estimated by x', the simple inflation estimate.

7.4 APPROXIMATION TO STANDARD ERROR OF RATIO-ESTIMATED TOTAL

A special situation of interest occurs when the relationship between X and Y can be represented reasonably closely by a straight line through the origin. In other words, suppose that the relationship between X and Y can be expressed by the **regression model**

$$X_i = \beta Y_i + \varepsilon_i \tag{7.9}$$

where β is the **slope** of the regression line of X on Y and

$$\sum_{i=1}^{N} \varepsilon_i = 0$$

Then the expression for ρ_{xy} becomes

$$\rho_{xy} = \frac{\sum_{i=1}^{N} (\beta Y_i + \varepsilon_i - \beta\bar{Y})(Y_i - \bar{Y})\Big/N}{\sigma_x\sigma_y}$$

$$= \frac{\beta\sum_{i=1}^{N} (Y_i - \bar{Y})^2 + \sum_{i=1}^{N} \varepsilon_i(Y_i - \bar{Y})}{N\sigma_x\sigma_y}$$

If the expression $\sum_{i=1}^{N} c_i(Y_i - \bar{Y})$ is close to zero (which it will be if the model represented above fits the data well), then ρ_{xy} is approximately equal to the expression

$$\rho_{xy} \approx \frac{\beta \sum_{i=1}^{N} (Y_i - \bar{Y})^2}{N \sigma_x \sigma_y}$$

Since it follows from expression (7.9) that $\beta = \bar{X}/\bar{Y}$ and since

$$\sum_{i=1}^{N} (Y_i - \bar{Y})^2 = N\sigma_y^2$$

we have

$$\rho_{xy} \approx \frac{\bar{X}\sigma_y}{\bar{Y}\sigma_x} = \frac{V_y}{V_x} \tag{7.10}$$

This gives us, from relation (7.6), the following **approximation to the standard error** of x'', the total estimated from a ratio:

$$SE(x'') \approx \left(\frac{YR}{\sqrt{n}}\right)(V_x^2 - V_y^2)^{1/2} \left(\frac{N-n}{N-1}\right)^{1/2} \tag{7.11}$$

which can be **estimated** from the data by the expression

$$\widehat{SE}(x'') \approx \left(\frac{Yr}{\sqrt{n}}\right)(\hat{V}_x^2 - \hat{V}_y^2)^{1/2} \left(\frac{N-n}{N-1}\right)^{1/2} \tag{7.12}$$

The approximations above are especially useful since they do not involve the correlation coefficient in explicit form.

For the example given earlier in which 3 segments were sampled, assuming that the regression is linear and passes through the origin, the estimated standard error $\widehat{SE}(x'')$, as given by approximation (7.12), is

$$\widehat{SE}(x'') = \left[\frac{(50)(878.5848)}{\sqrt{3}}\right](.0245 - .004435)^{1/2} \left(\frac{8-3}{8-1}\right)^{1/2} = 3036.33$$

which is larger than the standard error that was obtained from relation (7.7).

7.5 DETERMINATION OF SAMPLE SIZE

In order to be $(1 - \alpha) \times 100\%$ confident that an estimated ratio r or a ratio-estimated total x'' is within $\varepsilon\%$ of its true value, the approximate **sample size** needed is given by

$$n = \frac{(z_{1-\alpha/2})^2 N(V_x^2 + V_y^2 - 2\rho_{xy}V_xV_y)}{(z_{1-\alpha/2})^2(V_x^2 + V_y^2 - 2\rho_{xy}V_xV_y) + (n-1)\varepsilon^2} \tag{7.13}$$

If the parameters in expression (7.13) can be either guessed or estimated from preliminary data, a sample size can be determined.

SUMMARY

In this chapter we developed the basic concepts of ratio estimation, a technique often used to estimate population ratios as well as population totals. Ratio estimation can be used with any sampling plan, and when used to estimate totals, it often produces estimates that have lower standard errors than those produced by alternative estimation procedures. Particular emphasis was given in this chapter to ratio estimation under simple random sampling. For this type of sampling we discussed the sampling distributions of ratio estimates and presented methods for estimating standard errors for determining sample sizes and for constructing confidence intervals.

EXERCISES

1. The accompanying table, based on a simple random sample of 33 families from a community of 600 families, gives the family size, weekly net family income, and weekly cost of medical expenditures including pharmaceuticals. The community contains 2700 persons.

Family Number	Family Size	Weekly Net Income	Weekly Medical Expenses
1	2	$186	$14.30
2	3	186	20.80
3	3	261	22.70
4	5	195	30.50
5	4	174	41.20
6	7	276	28.20
7	2	264	24.20
8	4	237	30.00
9	2	249	24.20
10	5	186	44.40
11	3	189	13.40
12	6	186	19.80
13	4	180	29.40
14	4	225	27.10
15	2	270	22.20
16	5	225	37.70
17	3	207	22.60
18	4	249	36.00
19	2	255	20.60

Family Number	Family Size	Weekly Net Income	Weekly Medical Expenses
20	4	219	27.70
21	2	198	25.90
22	5	174	23.30
23	3	231	39.80
24	4	207	16.80
25	7	195	37.80
26	3	231	34.80
27	3	207	28.70
28	6	285	63.00
29	2	231	19.50
30	2	207	21.60
31	6	207	18.20
32	4	201	20.10
33	2	189	20.70

(a) Estimate and give a 95% confidence interval for the average weekly expenditure per family.

(b) Estimate and give a 95% confidence interval for the average weekly medical expenditure per person. Justify your method of estimation.

(c) Estimate and give a 95% confidence interval for the average proportion of family income spent on medical expenses.

(d) Estimate and give a 95% confidence interval for the total weekly medical expenses paid by the community.

(c) Estimate and give a 95% confidence interval for the average proportion of family income spent on medical expenses for families whose weekly net income is less than $200. Do the same for those whose net income is greater than $200 per week.

BIBLIOGRAPHY

The following textbook contains a more detailed discussion of ratio estimation.

1. HANSEN, M. H.; HURWITZ, W. N.; and MADOW, W. G. *Sample survey methods and theory.* Vols. 1 and 2. New York: Wiley, 1953.

8

Network Sampling, Synthetic Estimation, and Randomized Response

In the previous chapters we developed many of the basic concepts of sampling theory and survey methodology. Many issues that are considered of current importance to health professionals engaged in sample surveys can be understood from what we have developed thus far. In this chapter we consider three such issues: the estimation of rare events or rare population elements by sample survey, the estimation of characteristics for local populations from sample surveys conducted in larger populations, and the extraction of information that is considered sensitive to the respondents. All three of these issues have been the subject of much research over the past decade, and all can be understood from the concepts developed in the previous chapters.

Three current issues are considered

8.1 ESTIMATION OF RARE EVENTS: NETWORK SAMPLING

We have shown that modification of a basic simple random sampling plan without alteration of the estimation procedure (e.g., stratified random sampling with proportional allocation) can sometimes lead to estimates that have smaller sampling errors than those obtained through simple random sampling. We have also discussed how a simple random sampling plan using a modified estimation procedure (e.g., ratio estimation) can also lead to estimates with lower sampling errors. In a similar way, in this section we will show how modification of a counting rule can lead to estimates that have lower sampling errors than what would have been obtained through conventional counting rules.

The method of this section involves modification of a counting rule

153

*A counting rule
links enumeration
units to elementary
units*

A counting rule is an algorithm that links enumeration units (or listing units) to elementary units. For example, in a sample survey of households conducted to estimate total births that occur in the population during a specified time period, an obvious counting rule is to allow births to be reported in the household of the parents of the newborn. Such a counting rule links each element (e.g., birth) to one and only one enumeration unit (e.g., household). However, an alternative counting rule might allow births to be reported in the household of the grandparents of the newborn as well as in the household of the parents. This counting rule would then allow an element to be linked to more than one listing unit.

A counting rule that allows an element to be linked to only one enumeration unit is called a **conventional counting rule.** A counting rule that allows an element to be linked to more than one enumeration unit is called a **multiplicity counting rule.** Sample designs that use multiplicity counting rules are called **network samples.** Network samples have received considerable attention over the past decade, especially in the health sciences and especially in situations involving rare events or characteristics. Let us investigate this design through an example.

ILLUSTRATIVE EXAMPLE

Let us consider a county that has 100 identified primary health care providers. Suppose that we are interested in conducting a sample survey of ten health care providers in order to estimate the total number of persons who were treated for skin cancer during a particular time period. This process would be a simple one if every patient had been treated by one and only one health provider. However, a person with skin cancer may be treated by several providers (e.g., internist, surgeon, radiologist, physical therapist, etc.). Thus in designing the sample survey we must specify a counting rule that allows us to link the elements (i.e., persons treated for skin cancer) with more than one enumeration unit (i.e., health care providers).

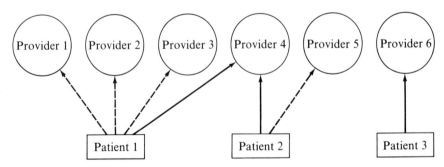

Figure 8.1   Network Sample for Health Care Providers and Skin Cancer Patients

Let us suppose that three persons were treated for skin cancer during the year. Person 1 was treated by four physicians (physicians 1, 2, 3, and 4); person 2 was treated by two physicians (physicians 4 and 5); and person 3 was treated by one physician (physician 6). We then have the network linking health care providers with skin cancer patients that is shown in figure 8.1. The solid lines in the figure indicate the *first* provider (chronologically) who treated the patient.

If we use a conventional counting rule—such as linking patients with the first provider who treated them—then patients 1 and 2 would be reported by provider 4 and patient 3 would be reported by provider 6; the other 98 providers would report no patients. If we let X_i be the number of patients reported by the ith provider according to this counting rule, then $X_4 = 2$, $X_6 = 1$, and the remaining $X_i = 0$. For a simple random sample of $n = 10$ health care providers, we see, by enumerating all samples, that the estimator $x' = (100/10)x$ has the following distribution:

x'	0	10	20	30
Relative Frequency	.8091	.0909	.0909	.0091

The mean $E(x')$ of the distribution of x' is equal to 3 (the true population total), and the standard error $SE(x')$ of x' is equal to 6.681. Notice that in more than 80% of the samples, no patients would be found and the estimate x' would be equal to 0.

Referring to the example above, suppose now that we use a counting rule that allows a patient to be reported by *any* health provider treating the patient. This is a multiplicity rule since it allows a patient to be reported by more than one provider. Since those patients who were treated by more than one provider have a greater chance of being selected than those treated by only one provider, a modified estimation procedure must be used to obtain an unbiased estimator of the total. This is done by defining for each enumeration unit i (e.g., health care provider) the following variable x_i^*, given by

A modified estimation procedure is used

$$x_i^* = \sum_{j=1}^{m} \frac{\delta_{ij}}{s_j}$$

where

$m =$ total number of elements (patients) identified in the sample

$\delta_{ij} = \begin{cases} 1 \text{ if the } i\text{th enumeration unit (provider } i) \\ \quad \text{ is linked to the } j\text{th element by the counting rule} \\ 0 \text{ otherwise} \end{cases}$

$s_j =$ the number of enumeration units linked to element j (called the **multiplicity** of element j)

The s_j's are extra information that must be obtained from the sample enumeration units (if possible) or, in some cases, from some other source, such as the elements themselves. We note that this process of obtaining the multiplicities might add considerably to the cost of the survey.

For simple random samples of health care providers from a population of N such providers, the **estimated total** x'_{mult} is given by

$$x'_{mult} = \left(\frac{N}{n}\right)(X^*)$$

where X^* is the **sample total** of the x_i^*.

Let us return to our example.

ILLUSTRATIVE EXAMPLE

Referring to the previous example, let us use a counting rule that allows a patient to be reported by any health provider treating the patient. Then for the sample shown in figure 8.1 we have

$$s_1 = 4, \qquad s_2 = 2, \qquad s_3 = 1$$
$$x_1^* = \tfrac{1}{4}, \qquad x_2^* = \tfrac{1}{4}, \qquad x_3^* = \tfrac{1}{4}, \qquad x_4^* = \tfrac{1}{4} + \tfrac{1}{2} = \tfrac{3}{4}, \qquad x_5^* = \tfrac{1}{2}, \qquad x_6^* = 1$$

Table 8.1 gives the distribution of x'_{mult} for simple random samples of $n = 10$ of the $N = 100$ health care providers in this example.

Table 8.1   Distribution of x'_{mult}

x'_{mult}	Relative Frequency[a]
0	.5223
2.5	.1843
5.0	.0807
7.5	.08132
10	.08251
12.5	.03076
15.0	.01003
17.5	.00839
20.0	.00192
22.5	.00074
25	.00019
27.5	.00001
30.0	.000003

[a] Obtained from combination theory.

The mean $E(x'_{mult})$ and the standard error $SE(x'_{mult})$, as calculated from the distribution shown in table 8.1 (and using expressions 2.24 given in box 2.4), are

$$E(x'_{mult}) = 3 = X \qquad \text{and} \qquad SE(x'_{mult}) = 4.13$$

Thus we see that for this example the estimated total x'_{mult} is not only an unbiased estimator of the population total X but has in this case a much smaller standard error than x', the estimated total obtained from the conventional counting rule.

The theory of network sampling is discussed in greater detail in articles by Sirken (9, 10). It has been shown to be especially useful in estimating the incidence or prevalence of attributes that occur in less than 3% of the population (i.e., "rare events"). For example, it has been used to estimate the number of births and marriages occurring in a population during a specified time period (8) as well as the prevalence of such diseases as cystic fibrosis (10) and diabetes (11). It has been extended to stratification (10, 9), ratio estimation (12), and cluster sampling (4). *Network sampling is used for rare events*

Multiplicity counting rules can improve the reliability of an estimate because they often increase the yield of a sample. For instance, in the example used above approximately 81% of all samples of size $n = 10$ would yield no patients with skin cancer if a conventional counting rule were used, whereas only about 52% of all samples would yield no skin cancer patients under the multiplicity rule. Under the multiplicity rule the network of health providers eligible to report skin cancer patients is doubled from 3 to 6 (see figure 8.1). *Network sampling can improve reliability of an estimate*

8.2 ESTIMATION OF CHARACTERISTICS FOR LOCAL AREAS: SYNTHETIC ESTIMATION

The planning of health and social services in the United States is often done on a subnational geographic basis, using areas such as groups of states, individual states, groups of counties, standard metropolitan statistical areas (SMSAs), or others. It is therefore of considerable importance to have valid and reliable estimates of health and social characteristics for these local areas so that planning decisions can be made on the basis of good baseline data. *Planning of health services is often based on local area statistics*

On the other hand, such estimates for local areas are often not easily obtainable. Although estimates of births, deaths, marriages, and divorces can be obtained for local areas through the vital statistics registration system, estimates of morbidity, disability, and utilization of services are often not available on a local basis. The major reason for the lack of local area health data lies in the fact that most health data are collected from a system of nationwide surveys conducted by the National Center for Health Statistics (NCHS). This system of health surveys can provide reliable and valid estimates for the *Local area characteristics are often not available*

United States as a whole and for large geographic subnational regions (i.e., Northeast, North Central, South, West). But limitations in the sample size and in the design of these surveys make them unsuitable for production of good estimates for the relatively small local areas that often serve as planning units.

Nationwide health surveys are not usually suitable sources for data because of the way strata are constructed

The major characteristic of the designs of these nationwide surveys that makes them unsuitable for production of small-area estimates is the way the strata are constructed. For example, in the Health Interview Survey (HIS)—which is a nationwide household interview survey yielding estimates of morbidity, disability, and utilization of health services—strata consist of one or more counties or SMSAs grouped according to similar demographic characteristics. For example, an HIS stratum might include three counties: one from Iowa, one from Nebraska, and one from Kansas. Only one of these three would be selected in the sample to represent the entire stratum. Estimates for the United States are obtained by aggregating such stratum estimates over all the strata. However, it is virtually impossible to piece together estimates for such areas as states, cities, or health-planning areas, which are generally not combinations of HIS strata.

Synthetic estimation uses data from nationwide surveys

One method of using data from nationwide health surveys for purposes of obtaining estimates for small areas that has found some acceptance—mainly because of its simplicity and intuitive appeal—is called **synthetic estimation.** This procedure obtains small-area estimates of characteristics by combining nationwide estimates of the characteristics specific to population groups with estimates of the proportional distribution within the small-area population into these same population groups. The groups are chosen on the basis both of their relevance to the characteristic being estimated and of the availability of small-area population data specific to the group.

More formally, a **synthetic estimate** $\tilde{\bar{x}}_a$ of the mean level $\bar{X}_a$ of characteristic $\mathscr{X}$ for area a is given by

$$\tilde{\bar{x}}_a = \sum_{k=1}^{K} \hat{P}_{ak} \bar{x}'_k$$

where, for $k = 1, 2, \ldots, K$, $\bar{x}'_k$ is the **estimated nationwide mean level of** characteristic $\mathscr{X}$ for persons in group k obtained from the nationwide survey and $\hat{P}_{ak}$ is the **estimated proportion** of all persons in area a who are in group k. The $\hat{P}_{ak}$ are estimates of local population proportions generally obtained from a U.S. census or from local agencies. K represents the total number of population groups chosen for study.

Synthetic estimation is similar to to poststratification

We see that the synthetic estimate $\tilde{\bar{x}}_a$ has some characteristics that are very similar to the estimates developed in the discussion of poststratification in chapter 6 (although there are also important differences). The similarity to poststratification lies in the fact that both methods combine means specific to groups that are not strata with population proportions appropriate for the groups. The major difference lies in the fact that the group specific means $\bar{x}'_k$

used in constructing a synthetic estimate are constructed from data obtained primarily from individuals outside the small area.

As mentioned earlier, synthetic estimation has found some acceptance because it is a more feasible alternative, in terms of resources and costs, to conducting a survey in the small area for which estimates are desired. Statistical properties of synthetic estimates have been investigated by Gonzalez and Hoza (2) and Levy and French (6). They are biased estimates, with **bias** given by

Synthetic estimates are biased

$$B(\tilde{\bar{x}}_a) = \sum_{k=1}^{K} \hat{P}_{ak}(\bar{X}_k - \bar{X}_{ak})$$

where, for $k = 1, 2, \ldots, K$, $\bar{X}_k$ is the mean level of characteristic $\mathscr{X}$ on the national level for group k and $\bar{X}_{ak}$ is the mean level of characteristic $\mathscr{X}$ for individuals in area a who are in group k.

Since synthetic estimates are generally based on large sample sizes, their sampling errors often are small, and hence their accuracy depends largely on the magnitude of their bias. Note that the bias in a synthetic estimate is a weighted average of the differences between the mean for a group on the nationwide level and that for the same group in the small area.

Their sampling errors are small

A more thorough discussion of synthetic estimation and other methods of obtaining small-area estimates can be found in an article by Levy (5).

8.3 EXTRACTION OF SENSITIVE INFORMATION: RANDOMIZED RESPONSE TECHNIQUES

In many sample surveys information of a sensitive nature must be extracted from individuals selected in the sample. For example, in a study of family-planning practices it might be necessary to ask questions concerning contraceptive practices or history of abortions. To some individuals such questions might be threatening or embarrassing. In order to avoid an excess of refusals or misleading responses, a method called **randomized response** has been developed, originally by Warner (13), and has been used with some success in many surveys.

The randomized response technique in its most basic form presents the respondent with two questions, a sensitive question and an innocuous question. The respondent is then given some randomizing device such as a bag containing red and white chips and told to select a chip from the bag without letting the interviewer see it. If a red chip is selected, the respondent is instructed to answer "yes" or "no" to the innocuous question. If the white chip is selected, the respondent is to answer "yes" or "no" to the sensitive question. The interviewer then records the respondent's answer without knowing which question is being answered.

The technique involves two questions, one sensitive and one innocuous

The rationale behind this method is that the respondent will be more willing to answer the sensitive question truthfully if he or she feels that the

*The interviewer
does not know
which question is
answered*

interviewer does not know whether the response is to the sensitive or to the innocuous question. To illustrate, the respondent might be given the following flashcard:

1. Have you ever cheated on your income tax return?
2. Is the last digit in your Social Security number an odd number (1, 3, 5, 7, 9)?

After being told to respond to question 1 if a red chip is chosen and to question 2 if a white chip is chosen, the respondent responds "yes" or "no" without indicating to the interviewer which question is being answered.

If both the composition of the randomizing device and the theoretical probability of answering "yes" to the innocuous question are known, an **estimate** can be obtained **of the proportion** of individuals in the population who have the attribute specified in the sensitive question from the total proportion of respondents for whom a "yes" response is recorded. This estimate is given by

$$\hat{P}_1 = \frac{p^* - P_2(1 - \theta)}{\theta}$$

where $\hat{P}_1$ is the **estimated proportion** in the population who have the attribute specified by the sensitive question; p^* is the **proportion of "yes" responses** obtained in the survey; P_2 is the **theoretical probability** of answering "yes" to the innocuous question; and θ is the **probability** of answering the sensitive question (e.g., the proportion of red chips in the bag).

ILLUSTRATIVE EXAMPLE

In the example given above, suppose that the bag contained 75% red chips and that the last digit of an individual's Social Security number is equally likely to end in an odd digit as in an even digit. Then we have θ and P_2 given by

$$\theta = \tfrac{3}{4} = .75 \quad \text{and} \quad P_2 = \tfrac{1}{2} = .50$$

Suppose that 40% of all respondents answered "yes." In other words, $p^* = .40$. Then the estimated proportion $\hat{P}_1$ of persons who cheat on income tax returns is

$$\hat{P}_1 = \frac{.40 - .50(1 - .75)}{.75} = .367$$

Thus we would estimate that 36.7% of all individuals cheat on their income tax returns.

Because the responses to the innocuous question in a sense waste information, randomized response techniques generally require larger sample sizes than conventional surveys to meet specified standards of reliability. Also, it is possible to obtain negative estimates by this method.

The technique requires large sample sizes

A more detailed exposition of this method is given in papers by Abernathy, Greenberg, and Horvitz (1), and some elaborations of this technique are discussed by I-Cheng, Chow, and Rider (3).

SUMMARY

In this chapter we discussed some issues of current importance to health survey practitioners that can be understood from the concepts developed in chapters 1–7. In particular, we discussed the problems of estimation of rare events, estimation of characteristics for small areas, and extraction of sensitive information. Methods of solving these three problems were presented—namely, network sampling, synthetic estimation, and randomized response techniques, respectively. All three methods are products of research efforts originating in the 1960s, are based on relatively simple concepts, and are finding increasing acceptance.

BIBLIOGRAPHY

The following publications provide examples from the health sciences that use the techniques discussed in this chapter.

1. ABERNATHY, J. R.; GREENBERG, B. G.; and HORVITZ, D. G. Estimates of induced abortion in urban North Carolina. *Demography* (1970) 7: 19–29,

2. GONZALEZ, M. E., and HOZA, C. Small-area estimation with applications to unemployment and housing estimates. *Journal of the American Statistical Association* (1978) 73: 7–15.

3. I-CHENG, C.; CHOW, L. P.; and RIDER, R. V. The randomized response technique as used in the Taiwan outcome of pregnancy study. *Studies in Family Planning*, A publication of the Population Council (1972) 3: 265–269.

4. LEVY, P. S. Simple cluster sampling with multiplicity. *Proceedings of the American Statistical Association, Social Statistics Section* (1977): 963–966.

5. LEVY, P. S. Small-area estimation—synthetic and other procedures, 1968–1978. *Proceedings of the Workshop on Synthetic Estimates for Small Areas*, National Institute of Drug Abuse, Research Monograph 24. U.S. Government Printing Office, Washington, D.C. 1969.

6. LEVY, P. S., and FRENCH, D. *Synthetic estimation of state health characteristics based on the health interview survey*. Vital and Health Statistics,

Series 2, No. 75, DHEW publication No. (PHS) 78–1349, Washington, DC: U.S. Government Printing Office, 1977.

7. LEVY, P. S. Optimum allocation in stratified random network sampling for estimating the prevalence of attributes in rare populations. *Journal of the American Statistical Association* (1978) 72: 758–763.

8. NATHAN, G.; SCHMELZ, U. O.; and KENVIN, J. *Multiplicity study of marriages and births in Israel*, Vital and Health Statistics, Series 2, No. 70, Rockville, MD: National Center for Health Statistics, 1977.

9. SIRKEN, M. G. Household surveys with multiplicity, *Journal of the American Statistical Association* (1970) 65: 257–266.

10. SIRKEN, M. G. Stratified sample surveys with multiplicity, *Journal of the American Statistical Association* (1972) 67: 224–227.

11. SIRKEN, M. G.; INDERFURTH, G. P.; BURNHAM, C. E.; and DANCHIK, K. M. Household sample survey of diabetes: Design effects of counting rules. *Proceedings of the American Statistical Association, Social Statistics Section* (1975): 659–663.

12. SIRKEN, M. G., and LEVY, P. S. Multiplicity estimation of proportions based on ratios of random variables. *Journal of the American Statistical Association* (1974) 69: 68–73.

13. WARNER, S. L. Randomized response: A survey technique for eliminating evasive answer bias. *Journal of the American Statistical Association* (1965) 60: 63–69.

9

Cluster Sampling: Introduction and Overview

The sampling techniques discussed in previous chapters all require sampling frames that list the individual enumeration units (or listing units). Sometimes, however, especially in sample surveys of human populations, it is not feasible—and perhaps not even possible—to compile sampling frames that list all enumeration units for the entire population. On the other hand, sampling frames can often be constructed that identify groups or *clusters* of enumeration units without listing explicitly the individual enumeration units. Sampling can be performed from such frames by taking a sample of the clusters, obtaining a list of enumeration units only for those clusters that have been selected in the sample, and then selecting a sample of the enumeration units. These sample designs are known as *cluster samples* and are widely used in practice. In this chapter we introduce some basic concepts of cluster sampling, and in the following three chapters we will discuss some specific techniques of cluster sampling that are widely used.

We use cluster sampling when we cannot easily obtain a list of all enumeration units

To illustrate the process of cluster sampling and to contrast it with designs based on direct sampling of enumeration units, let us consider a simple example.

ILLUSTRATIVE EXAMPLE

Suppose that we wish to select a sample of households in a medium-size city for purposes of investigating utilization of health services among residents of the city. If an up-to-date city directory that lists all households in the city is available, it can serve as a sampling frame from which the sample can be selected. However, if such a directory or some other list of households is not available, it would be very expensive in terms of person-hours to construct such a sampling frame.

It might be relatively easy, however, to construct a list of city blocks. For many cities maps that identify and label each city block are available from the U.S. Bureau of the Census. This list of city blocks can then serve as a sampling frame. Each city block can be considered as a cluster of households, and every household in the city would be associated with a particular block. The sample of households can be taken by first taking a sample of blocks and then, within each of the blocks selected in the sample, listing each household. From this resulting list of households the final sample of households can be drawn. Note that it is necessary to list only those households that are on the blocks selected in the sample of blocks.

9.1 WHAT IS CLUSTER SAMPLING?

The term **cluster,** when used in sample survey methodology, can be defined as any sampling unit with which one or more listing units can be associated. This unit can be geographic, temporal, or spatial in nature. Some examples of clusters that might occur in practice are shown in table 9.1

Table 9.1   Some Practical Examples of Clusters

Cluster	Listing Unit	Elementary Unit	Application
1. city block	household	person	estimation of total persons in a city having hypertension
2. county	hospital	patient	estimation of the proportion of all hospital patients discharged dead in a particular state
3. school	classroom	student	estimation of mean scholastic achievement among students in a school district
4. batch of syringes	individual syringe	individual syringe	estimation of the proportion of all syringes having defects
5. page of text	line of text	word	estimation of total number of words in a book
6. file drawer	file folder	account	estimation of total number of accounts that are overdue
7. calendar week	calendar day	calendar day	estimation of proportion of all days having maximum ozone levels above some level

For purposes of further illustration let us consider the second example of a cluster shown in the table. If we wish to estimate the proportion of all hospitalized patients discharged dead in a particular state during a particular year, we might first list all counties in the state and take a sample of counties from this list. For each of the counties selected in the sample we might then list all hospitals in the county and select a sample of individual hospitals. Finally, for each hospital selected in the sample we would obtain the total number of persons admitted during the year and the total discharged dead. From these data the proportion discharged dead can be estimated for the entire state.

For the seventh example of a cluster shown in the table, a list consisting of 52 calendar weeks can be compiled and a sample of weeks can be selected from this list. For each of the weeks selected in the sample, a sample of days can be taken, and on each sample day ozone measurements can be made.

The relationship between clusters and listing units is very similar to that between listing units and elementary units. A cluster has listing units associated with it in the same way that a listing unit has elementary units associated with it. As we will see later, cluster sampling is a hierarchical kind of sampling in which the elementary units are often at least two steps removed from the original sampling of clusters.

Now that we have introduced the concept of clusters, we can define **cluster sampling** broadly as any sampling plan that uses a frame consisting of clusters of listing units. With this definition of cluster sampling in mind, we list below some important features of cluster sampling.

Some important features of cluster sampling

1. *The process by which a sample of listing units is selected might be stepwise.* For example, if city blocks are clusters and households are listing units, there might be two steps involved in selecting the sample households. The first step might entail selecting a sample of blocks, and the second step might entail selecting a sample of households within each of the blocks selected at the first step. In sampling terminology these steps are called **stages,** and sampling plans are often categorized in terms of the number of stages involved. For example, a *single-stage cluster sample* is one in which the sampling is done in only one step. That is, once the sample of clusters is selected, every listing unit within each of the selected clusters is included in the sample.

An example of multistage sampling

In many surveys covering large geographical areas, several stages of sampling are often involved. For example, an immunization survey of school-children in a state might entail five stages. First, we take a sample of counties within the state. Second, we take a sample of townships or other minor civil divisions within each of the counties that were selected at the first stage. Third, we take a sample of school districts within each of the townships selected at the second stage. Fourth, we take a sample of schools within each of the school districts selected at the third stage. Fifth, we take a sample of classrooms within each of the schools selected at the fourth stage. And finally, we take every child within the classrooms selected at the fifth stage. In this example the children are the elementary units and the classrooms are the listing units. There are five stages of sampling involving four types of clusters: counties, townships, school districts, and schools. In sample designs involving more than two stages the clusters used at the first stage of sampling are generally referred to as **primary sampling units,** or, in abbreviated form, as PSUs.

2. Clusters can be selected by a variety of sampling techniques. For example, we can select a sample of clusters by simple random sampling or by systematic sampling. We can group the clusters into strata and take a stratified random sample of clusters.

All the techniques described previously can be used

When clusters are selected by simple random sampling, the term **simple cluster sampling** is generally used to describe the sampling design. More specifically, the term **simple one-stage cluster sampling** is used to categorize sample designs in which there is one stage of sampling and the clusters are selected by simple random sampling. Similarly, **simple two-stage cluster sampling** is used to describe sampling designs in which the clusters are selected at the first stage by simple random sampling; the listing units are selected at the second stage independently within each sample cluster, also by simple random sampling; and the fraction of listing units chosen at the second stage is the same for each sample cluster. Simple one-stage cluster sampling will be discussed in chapter 10, and simple two-stage cluster sampling will be discussed in chapters 11 and 12.

Another type of cluster sampling design often used in practice is called **sampling with probability proportional to size,** or PPS sampling. This type of sampling, which is discussed in chapter 12, is one in which the clusters are not selected by simple random sampling.

3. More than one sampling frame might be involved in the process. To illustrate this situation, we refer back to the example above in which an immunization survey of schoolchildren in a state is taken by a five-stage procedure. The sampling frame at the first stage is a list of all counties in the state. The sampling frame at the second stage is a list of townships or other minor civil divisions within each of the counties selected at the first stage. The sampling frame at the third stage is a list of all school districts located within those townships or minor civil divisions selected at the second stage. At the fourth stage of sampling the sampling frame is a list of schools within each of the school districts chosen at the third stage. Finally, the sampling frame used at the fifth stage is a list of classrooms within each of the schools sampled at the fourth stage.

In multistage sampling each stage has its own sampling frame

4. After the first stage of sampling, the sampling frame is compiled from only those clusters chosen in the sample. Once the sample clusters are selected at the first stage, the listing of second-stage sampling units is compiled only for the sample clusters. Likewise, if there are more than two stages of sampling, sampling units at any later stage are listed only for those sampling units selected at the previous stage. Since the listing of clusters or of listing units is often an expensive field operation, listing costs are often much lower for cluster sampling designs than for other designs.

9.2 WHY IS CLUSTER SAMPLING WIDELY USED?

The two most important reasons cluster sampling is so widely used in practice, especially in sample surveys of human populations and in sample surveys covering large geographical areas, are *feasibility* and *economy*.

Cluster sampling is often the only feasible method of sampling because the only sampling frames readily available for the target population are lists of clusters. This is especially true in surveys of human populations for which the household serves as the listing unit. It is almost never feasible in terms of time and resources to compile a list of households for any sizable population (e.g., the United States, a state, or even a city) for the sole purpose of conducting a survey. However, lists of blocks or other geographical units can be compiled relatively easily, and these can serve as the sampling frame.

Cluster sampling may be the only feasible method

Cluster sampling is often the most economical form of sampling. Not only are listing costs almost always lowest for cluster sampling but also traveling costs are often lowest. For example, if a cluster is a geographic unit such as a census tract, then once households are selected within sample tracts, the cost of traveling within the sample tracts from household to household is relatively low. Thus a cluster sample of households within a few sample census tracts involves considerably less travel than a simple random sample of the same number of households spread over many more census tracts.

Cluster sampling may cost less than other designs

Cluster sampling may be advantageous in surveys of institutions such as hospitals. It is often very expensive and time-consuming to enlist an institution into a study. For example, to obtain permission from a hospital adminstration to take a sample of patient records from the hospital may entail a great deal of effort, some public relations expertise, and sometimes even a great deal of influence. Therefore, once access is gained into hospital records, it is often worthwhile to sample many records rather than just a few.

To illustrate further how cluster sampling can lower the costs of a sample survey, let us consider the following example.

ILLUSTRATIVE EXAMPLE

Suppose that scattered throughout a particular county there are five housing developments for senior citizens, and each of these developments contains 20 apartments. Suppose that a sample of ten apartments is to be selected for purposes of estimating the total number of senior citizens in these developments who have need for the services of a visiting nurse. Further, let us suppose that the households are the listing units and that the major field costs of the survey involve listing and interviewing tasks.

In order to list all the apartments in a housing development, let us suppose that a member of the field staff would have to travel to the development and jot down the names of the families from mailboxes. Assume that it would take .5 hour to travel to the development and 3 minutes to list each household, or $3 \times 20 = 60$ minutes to list all households in the development. We then estimate that it would take 1.5 person-hours to list an entire development (1 hour of listing plus .5 hour of travel) and 7.5 person-hours (1.5 person-hours per development × 5 developments) to list all five developments.

Suppose that it takes 15 minutes (.25 hour) to interview each household selected in the sample. Then the interviewing costs in person-hours for a particular development are equal to .25 times the number of households selected in the development plus the cost of traveling to the development (.5 person-hour per trip).

Let us now compare two sampling designs with respect to the interviewing and listing costs for a sample of ten households. The first design is simple random sampling, and let us assume that households from four of the developments are chosen in the sample. The second design is a simple two-stage cluster sample of ten households, five households from each of two developments. The listing and interviewing costs for each design are shown in table 9.2.

Table 9.2   Comparison of Costs for Two Sampling Designs

	DESIGN	
Costs	*Simple Random Sampling*	*Simple Two-Stage Cluster Sampling*
listing costs in person-hours	1.5 per development times 5 developments = 7.5	1.5 per development times 2 developments = 3.0
interviewing costs in person-hours	travel to 4 developments plus interviewing 10 households: 4(.5) + 10(.25) = 4.5	travel to 2 developments plus interviewing 10 households: 2(.5) + 10(.25) = 3.5
total field costs in person-hours	12.0	6.5

From the calculations in table 9.2 we see that, even for this small sample, the field costs involved in cluster sampling can be very much lower than the field costs of simple random sampling. The particular savings are in the listing and traveling costs.

9.3 A DISADVANTAGE OF CLUSTER SAMPLING: HIGH STANDARD ERRORS

Now that we have shown how economical cluster sampling can be and how feasible it often is, we must point out that the standard errors of estimates obtained from cluster sampling designs are often very high compared with those obtained from samples of the same number of listing units chosen by other sampling designs. The reason for this situation is that listing units within the same cluster are often homogeneous with respect to many characteristics. For example, households on the same block are often quite similar with respect to socioeconomic status, ethnicity, and other variables. Because of homogeneity among listing units within the same cluster, selection of more than one household within the same cluster, as is done in cluster sampling, is in a sense redundant. And the effect of this redundancy becomes evident in the high standard errors of estimates that are so often seen in cluster sampling.

High standard errors will result if there is homogeneity within clusters

    If we were to choose between cluster sampling and some alternative design solely on the basis of cost or feasibility, cluster sampling would inevitably be the sampling design of choice. On the other hand, if we were to choose a design solely on the basis of the reliability of estimates, then cluster sampling would never be the design of choice. Generally in choosing between cluster sampling and alternatives, we use criteria that incorporate both reliability and cost. In fact, we generally choose the sampling design that gives the lowest possible standard error at a specified cost—or, conversely, we choose the sampling design that yields, at the lowest cost, estimates having specified standard errors.

9.4 HOW CLUSTER SAMPLING IS TREATED IN THIS BOOK

Following the overview of cluster sampling given in this chapter, we develop specific cluster sampling designs in the next three chapters by going from very simple to very complex designs. The simplest type of cluster sampling is single-stage cluster sampling where clusters are selected by simple random sampling, and this type of cluster sampling is discussed in the next chapter (Chapter 10). The following two chapters (chapters 11 and 12) both deal with two-stage cluster sampling. In two-stage cluster sampling, estimates of population characteristics and estimates of the standard errors of those statistics used to estimate population characteristics are relatively easy to obtain if each cluster in the population has the same number of listing units. Two-stage cluster sampling in this situation is treated in chapter 11. Two-stage cluster sampling at its most complex occurs when each cluster in the population does not have the same number of listing units. Unfortunately, this happens in many practical situations, and we feel that it should be covered in this book in spite of the fact that it entails the use of formulas that are more involved than those that appear in the rest of the book. We develop this type of cluster sampling in chapter 12.

The development in the next three chapters proceeds from simple to complex

    Our treatment of cluster sampling is very similar to our treatment of the other designs. In particular, we discuss how samples are taken, how estimates are obtained, the nature of the sampling distributions of these estimates, and the methods of estimating the standard errors of these estimates.

SUMMARY

In this chapter we presented an overview of cluster sampling. We introduced the concept of a cluster of enumeration or listing units, and we defined cluster sampling as any sampling design that uses a sampling frame consisting of clusters of listing units. Some examples of clusters were given and some characteristics of cluster sampling were discussed, such as its sequential, stepwise nature and the fact that the listing units need to be listed only from sample clusters rather than from all clusters. We pointed out the advantages of cluster sampling—namely, feasibility and economy—as well as its major disadvantage, namely, the high standard errors of estimates. However, because of the potential for taking more observations for the same budget than are possible with other designs, it is often possible to reduce the standard errors to the point where cluster sampling is the method of choice.

10
Simple One-Stage Cluster Sampling

We begin our development of some of the commonly used cluster sampling designs with a discussion of simple one-stage cluster sampling. As we mentioned in chapter 9, **simple one-stage cluster sampling** is a sampling plan in which clusters are chosen by simple random sampling, and within each cluster all listing units are selected.

Simple one-stage cluster sampling is frequently used in situations in which the cost of obtaining every listing unit within a cluster is no higher or only slightly higher than the cost of obtaining a sample of listing units. Let us consider, for example, a sample survey in which hospitals are clusters and patients hospitalized with a certain diagnosis are listing units. If the information needed for the survey can be obtained from computer printouts that summarize the experience of each patient, and if these are either already available or can be furnished relatively easily by the hospital record librarian, it might be cheaper and more convenient to select every patient having the specified diagnosis than to select a sample of these patients. On the other hand, if the data needed from each patient must be extracted from information on the original hospital records (which is often a costly and time-consuming process), then it might be more economical to select a sample of these patients rather than to take all of them.

As we will see later in this chapter, the estimation procedures associated with simple one-stage cluster sampling are virtually identical to those associated with simple random sampling if we consider the cluster itself to be the

Cost is often a major factor in the decision to use cluster sampling

Table 10.1 Number of Persons over 65 Years of Age and Number over 65 Years Needing Services of Visiting Nurse for Five Housing Developments

	DEVELOPMENT 1			DEVELOPMENT 2			DEVELOPMENT 3			DEVELOPMENT 4			DEVELOPMENT 5	
House-hold	No. of Persons over 65	No. over 65 Needing Nurse	House-hold	No. of Persons over 65	No. over 65 Needing Nurse	House-hold	No. of Persons over 65	No. over 65 Needing Nurse	House-hold	No. of Persons over 65	No. over 65 Needing Nurse	House-hold	No. of Persons over 65	No. over 65 Needing Nurse
1	3	1	1	2	1	1	3	0	1	3	0	1	1	1
2	1	0	2	1	0	2	2	1	2	1	0	2	1	0
3	1	1	3	2	0	3	2	1	3	3	0	3	3	1
4	1	1	4	1	1	4	3	1	4	1	0	4	2	1
5	1	1	5	1	0	5	2	1	5	2	0	5	2	0
6	1	1	6	1	0	6	2	0	6	2	0	6	1	1
7	1	1	7	2	1	7	1	0	7	1	0	7	3	0
8	1	0	8	1	1	8	1	1	8	3	1	8	1	0
9	3	1	9	3	1	9	3	0	9	1	1	9	1	2
10	3	2	10	1	1	10	3	1	10	1	0	10	3	1
11	3	2	11	1	0	11	2	1	11	1	0	11	2	1
12	1	0	12	2	1	12	3	1	12	3	1	12	3	0
13	1	1	13	1	0	13	1	2	13	3	0	13	1	1
14	1	0	14	3	1	14	1	0	14	1	0	14	1	0
15	1	1	15	1	0	15	2	1	15	1	0	15	2	1
16	3	1	16	3	2	16	1	0	16	1	0	16	2	0
17	1	2	17	1	0	17	3	0	17	1	1	17	1	1
18	3	1	18	2	0	18	1	1	18	1	0	18	1	0
19	1	1	19	1	1	19	2	0	19	1	0	19	2	1
20	1	1	20	3	0	20	1	2	20	1	0	20	1	1
Total	32	19		33	11		39	14		32	4		34	12

effective listing unit. We will elaborate on this concept later in the chapter. A disadvantage of this type of sampling, however, is that the sampling errors associated with estimates obtained from simple one-stage cluster sampling are generally much higher than those obtained from a simple random sample of the same number of listing units, especially when listing units within clusters are homogeneous with respect to the variable being measured. Suppose, for example, that we are attempting to estimate the proportion of all families below the poverty level in a community from a simple one-stage cluster sample in which city blocks are clusters and households are listing units. Since the households within any city block are likely to contain families of very similar income, the inclusion in the sample of every household on a selected block is a wasteful way of allocating the sample listing units and is likely to yield estimates having high sampling errors.

10.1 HOW TO TAKE A SIMPLE ONE-STAGE CLUSTER SAMPLE

We take a one-stage cluster sample by first listing all clusters in the population and then taking, in the usual manner, a simple random sample of clusters. Within each of the clusters selected in the sample, we then include all listing units.

For example, let us suppose that the total number of persons over 65 and the number of persons over 65 requiring the services of a visiting nurse are as given in table 10.1 for the households in the five housing developments discussed in chapter 9. We will use these data to illustrate how cluster sampling is performed.

Suppose that we wish to take a simple one-stage cluster sample of two housing developments from the five housing developments in table 10.1. We would choose two random numbers between 1 and 5 and then interview every household in the two housing developments chosen in the sample. Suppose that the random numbers chosen were 2 and 5. Then all households in developments 2 and 5 would be interviewed and the relevant data would be collected.

10.2 ESTIMATION OF POPULATION CHARACTERISTICS

Once the sample of clusters is selected, the required data are collected from every listing unit within the chosen clusters. The forms used to collect these data would, of course, depend on the type of information needed and the manner in which the data are to be collected (e.g., mail, personal interview, telephone, extraction from records, etc.). Then the estimates of population characteristics are calculated by using the data that have been collected.

Let us investigate the estimation procedures by considering an example.

ILLUSTRATIVE EXAMPLE

Suppose that from the sample of two housing developments discussed above, we wish to estimate the following population characteristics:

1. the total number of persons over 65 years of age in the five housing projects

2. the total number of persons over 65 years of age requiring the services of a visiting nurse

3. the proportion of all persons over 65 years of age requiring the services of a visiting nurse

4. the mean number of persons over 65 years of age per housing development

5. the proportion of all households having at least one individual over 65 years of age who requires the services of a visiting nurse

To obtain these estimates, the form shown in figure 10.1 might be suitable for collecting the data by personal interview.

Figure 10.1   Form for Collecting Data from Sample Households in Housing Developments

Housing Development: *Kingwood Manor Apartments*

Sample Development No: *2*

Household Number: *10*

Name of Household Head: *Jones, John*

List All Persons in Household Beginning with Respondent:

		Does this person require the services of a visiting nurse? (Answer only for persons over 65 years of age.)	
Person	Age	Yes	No
1. Lydia Jones	67		X
2. John Jones	68	X	
3. Samantha Jones	75	X	
4. Edgar Jones	60		
5.			
6.			

If housing developments 2 and 5 are those selected in the sample, then the form shown in figure 10.1 illustrates data that may have been collected from household 10 in development 5 (sample development 2). Note that there are three individuals over 65 years of age in this household and that two of them require the services of a visiting nurse. There would be 20 such forms collected from this housing development and also from housing development 2 (sample development 1).

From these household forms summary information for each sample development is tabulated in a format similar to that shown in table 10.2. We then obtain the desired estimates as follows from the summary data shown in the table.

Table 10.2   Summary Data for the Two Clusters Selected in the Sample

Sample Development	No. of Households	No. of Persons over 65	No. over 65 Needing Nurse	No. of Households with at Least One Person over 65 Needing Nurse
1 (housing development 2)	20	33	11	10
2 (housing development 5)	20	34	12	11
Total	40	67	23	21

To find the estimated total number of persons over 65 years of age, we first compute the average number of persons over 65 per sample cluster. Then the estimated total number of persons over 65 years in the population is obtained by multiplying this cluster average by the total number of clusters in the population. That is,

$$\text{cluster average} = \tfrac{67}{2} = 33.5$$

$$\text{estimated population total of persons over } 65 = 5(33.5) = 167.5$$

Alternatively, the sample total may be inflated by the ratio of total clusters in the population to total sample clusters (i.e., $\tfrac{5}{2}$). Then the estimated population total of persons over 65 is $(\tfrac{5}{2})(67) = 167.5$.

To find the estimated total number of persons over 65 years needing the services of a visiting nurse, we inflate the sample total by $\tfrac{5}{2}$, as we did above:

$$\text{estimated total over 65 needing nurse} = (\tfrac{5}{2})(23) = 57.5$$

To find the proportion of all persons over 65 years of age requiring the services of a visiting nurse, we take the ratio of the appropriate sample totals:

$$\text{estimated proportion of all persons over 65 needing nurse} = \tfrac{23}{67} = .3433$$

To find the estimated mean number of persons over 65 years of age per housing development, we divide the total number of persons over 65 years in the sample by the total number of housing developments in the sample:

$$\text{estimated mean number over 65 per development} = \tfrac{67}{2} = 33.5$$

To find the estimated proportion of all households having at least one individual over 65 years who requires the services of a visiting nurse, we divide the total number of households in the sample having at least one individual over 65 who requires the services of a visiting nurse by the number of households in the sample:

$$\text{estimated proportion of households with 1 or more over 65 needing nurse} = \tfrac{21}{40} = .525$$

The estimates shown above include estimated population totals, ratios, and means.

In cluster sampling the mean level of a characteristic $\mathcal{X}$ per cluster is generally denoted by $\bar{X}$, as distinguished from the expression $\bar{\bar{X}}$, which is used to denote the mean level of $\mathcal{X}$ per listing unit. To generalize, let us use the notation shown in box 10.1.

Using the notation of box 10.1, we list, in box 10.2, the formulas used to compute estimated population characteristics and estimated standard errors of these estimated population characteristics. Note that the subscript "clu" is

---

Box 10.1 Notation Used in Simple One-Stage Cluster Sampling

General Notation

M = number of clusters in the population

m = number of clusters in the sample

x_{ij} = level of characteristic $\mathcal{X}$ for sample listing unit j in sample cluster i

y_{ij} = level of characteristic $\mathcal{Y}$ for sample listing unit j in sample cluster i

N_i = number of listing units in sample cluster i

$x_i = \displaystyle\sum_{j=1}^{N_i} x_{ij}$ = aggregate of characteristic $\mathcal{X}$ for the ith sample cluster

$y_i = \displaystyle\sum_{j=1}^{N_i} y_{ij}$ = aggregate of characteristic $\mathcal{Y}$ for the ith sample cluster

$x = \displaystyle\sum_{i=1}^{m} x_i$ = sample total for characteristic $\mathcal{X}$

Box 10.1 (*continued*)

General Notation

$y = \sum\limits_{i=1}^{m} y_i$ = sample total for characteristic $\mathcal{Y}$

N = total number of listing units in population

$\bar{N} = \dfrac{N}{M}$ = average number of listing units per cluster in population

Population Characteristics

X_{ij} = level of characteristic $\mathcal{X}$ for population listing unit j in population cluster i

Y_{ij} = level of characteristic $\mathcal{Y}$ for population listing unit j in population cluster i

$X_i = \sum\limits_{j=1}^{N_i} X_{ij}$ = aggregate of characteristic $\mathcal{X}$ for ith population cluster

$Y_i = \sum\limits_{j=1}^{N_i} Y_{ij}$ = aggregate of characteristic $\mathcal{Y}$ for ith population cluster

$X = \sum\limits_{i=1}^{M} \sum\limits_{j=1}^{N_i} X_{ij}$ = population total for characteristic $\mathcal{X}$

$\bar{X} = \dfrac{X}{M}$ = mean level of $\mathcal{X}$ per cluster

$\bar{\bar{X}} = \dfrac{X}{N}$ = mean level of $\mathcal{X}$ per listing unit

$\sigma_{1x}^2 = \dfrac{\sum\limits_{i=1}^{M} (X_i - \bar{X})^2}{M}$ = variance of distribution of $\mathcal{X}$ over all clusters

$\sigma_{1y}^2 = \dfrac{\sum\limits_{i=1}^{M} (Y_i - \bar{Y})^2}{M}$ = variance of distribution of $\mathcal{Y}$ over all clusters

$\sigma_{1xy} = \dfrac{\sum\limits_{i=1}^{M} (X_i - \bar{X})(Y_i - \bar{Y})}{M}$ = covariance of $\mathcal{X}$ and $\mathcal{Y}$ over all clusters

Box 10.2 Estimated Population Characteristics and Estimated Standard Errors for Simple One-Stage Cluster Sampling

Total, **X**

$$x'_{clu} = \left(\frac{M}{m}\right)(x) \quad \widehat{SE}(x'_{clu}) = \left(\frac{M}{\sqrt{m}}\right)(\hat{\sigma}_{1x})\left(\frac{M-m}{M-1}\right)^{1/2}$$

Mean Per Cluster, $\bar{X}$

$$\bar{x}_{clu} = \frac{x}{m} \quad \widehat{SE}(\bar{x}_{clu}) = \left(\frac{1}{\sqrt{m}}\right)(\hat{\sigma}_{1x})\left(\frac{M-m}{M-1}\right)^{1/2}$$

Mean Per Listing Unit, $\bar{\bar{X}}$

$$\bar{\bar{x}}_{clu} = \frac{x}{m\bar{N}} \quad \widehat{SE}(\bar{\bar{x}}_{clu}) = \left(\frac{1}{\sqrt{m\bar{N}}}\right)(\hat{\sigma}_{1x})\left(\frac{M-m}{M-1}\right)^{1/2}$$

Ratio, **R = X/Y**

$$r_{clu} = \frac{x}{y}$$

$$\widehat{SE}(r_{clu}) = (r_{clu})\left\{\frac{[\widehat{SE}(\bar{x}_{clu})]^2}{\bar{x}_{clu}^2} + \frac{[\widehat{SE}(\bar{y}_{clu})]^2}{\bar{y}_{clu}^2}\right.$$

$$\left. - \left(\frac{2}{m}\right)\left(\frac{M-m}{M}\right)\left(\frac{1}{\bar{x}_{clu}\bar{y}_{clu}}\right)\left[\frac{\sum_{i=1}^{m}(x_i - \bar{x}_{clu})(y_i - \bar{y}_{clu})}{m-1}\right]\right\}$$

where $\hat{\sigma}_{1x}$ is defined as

$$\hat{\sigma}_{1x} = \left[\frac{\sum_{i=1}^{m}(x_i - \bar{x}_{clu})^2}{m-1}\right]^{1/2}\left(\frac{M-1}{M}\right)^{1/2}$$

and $\hat{\sigma}_{1y}$ is defined in a similar fashion. All other notation is defined in box 10.1.

used to indicate that the estimate is obtained by cluster sampling. For example, the expression x'_{clu} indicates an estimated population total obtained by cluster sampling.

Examining the expressions for estimates given in box 10.2, we see their close resemblance to the expressions for equivalent estimates under simple random sampling developed in chapter 3. Since in simple one-stage cluster sampling every listing unit within every sample cluster is selected in the sample, the sampling variability among listing units within clusters is not a factor in determining the sampling variability of estimates under this sampling plan. Effectively, then, cluster totals are the building blocks on which the estimation formulas in box 10.2 are built. Use of these formulas for the data in table 10.2 is illustrated next.

Cluster totals are the building blocks for estimation

ILLUSTRATIVE EXAMPLE

Let us consider again the data in table 10.2. Then we have

$$m = 2 \text{ housing developments in sample}$$

$$M = 5 \text{ housing developments in population}$$

$$N = 100 \text{ households in population}$$

$$N_1 = N_2 = 20 \text{ households per development} = \bar{N}$$

Calculations using the formulas of box 10.2

For x'_{clu}

First we consider the estimation of the mean number of persons over 65 years of age per housing development requiring the services of a visiting nurse. The computations for $\bar{x}_{clu}$ are

$$x_1 = 11, \qquad x_2 = 12, \qquad x = 23$$

$$\bar{x}_{clu} = \frac{23}{2} = 11.5$$

The computations for $\widehat{SE}(\bar{x}_{clu})$ are

$$\frac{\sum\limits_{i=1}^{m} (x_i - \bar{x}_{clu})^2}{m - 1} = \frac{(11 - 11.5)^2 + (12 - 11.5)^2}{2 - 1} = .5$$

$$\hat{\sigma}_{1x} = \left[\frac{\sum\limits_{i=1}^{m} (x_i - \bar{x}_{clu})^2}{m - 1} \right]^{1/2} \left(\frac{M - 1}{M} \right)^{1/2}$$

$$= (.5)^{1/2} \left(\frac{5 - 1}{5} \right)^{1/2} = .6325$$

$$\widehat{SE}(\bar{x}_{clu}) = \left(\frac{1}{\sqrt{m}} \right) (\hat{\sigma}_{1x}) \left(\frac{M - m}{M - 1} \right)^{1/2} = \left(\frac{1}{\sqrt{2}} \right) (.6325) \left(\frac{5 - 2}{5 - 1} \right)^{1/2} = .3873$$

A 95% confidence interval for $\bar{X}$ is

$$\bar{x}_{clu} - (1.96)[\widehat{SE}(\bar{x}_{clu})] \leq \bar{X} \leq \bar{x}_{clu} + (1.96)[\widehat{SE}(\bar{x}_{clu})]$$

$$11.5 - (1.96)(.3873) \leq \bar{X} \leq 11.5 + (1.96)(.3873)$$

$$10.74 \leq \bar{X} \leq 12.26$$

For x'clu

Now we consider the estimation of the total number of persons over 65 years of age requiring the services of a visiting nurse. The computation of x'_{clu} is

$$x'_{clu} = \left(\frac{M}{m}\right)(x) = \left(\frac{5}{2}\right)(23) = 57.5$$

The computation of $\widehat{SE}(x'_{clu})$ is

$$\widehat{SE}(x'_{clu}) = \left(\frac{M}{\sqrt{m}}\right)(\hat{\sigma}_{1x})\left(\frac{M-m}{M-1}\right)^{1/2} = \left(\frac{5}{\sqrt{2}}\right)(.6325)\left(\frac{5-2}{5-1}\right)^{1/2} = 1.94$$

A 95% confidence interval for X is

$$x'_{clu} - (1.96)[\widehat{SE}(x'_{clu})] \leq X \leq x'_{clu} + (1.96)[\widehat{SE}(x'_{clu})]$$

$$57.5 - (1.96)(1.94) \leq X \leq 57.5 + (1.96)(1.94)$$

$$53.7 \leq X \leq 61.3$$

For x̄̄clu

Now we consider the estimation of the mean number of persons over 65 years of age requiring the services of a visiting nurse per household. The computation of $\bar{\bar{x}}_{clu}$ is

$$\bar{\bar{x}}_{clu} = \frac{x}{m\bar{N}} = \frac{23}{(2)(20)} = .5750$$

The computation of $\widehat{SE}(\bar{\bar{x}}_{clu})$ is

$$\widehat{SE}(\bar{\bar{x}}_{clu}) = \left(\frac{1}{\sqrt{m}\,\bar{N}}\right)(\hat{\sigma}_{1x})\left(\frac{M-m}{M-1}\right)^{1/2}$$

$$= \left(\frac{1}{\sqrt{2}(20)}\right)(.6325)\left(\frac{5-2}{5-1}\right)^{1/2} = .0194$$

A 95% confidence interval for $\bar{\bar{X}}$ is

$$\bar{\bar{x}}_{clu} - (1.96)[\widehat{SE}(\bar{\bar{x}}_{clu})] \leq \bar{\bar{X}} \leq \bar{\bar{x}}_{clu} + (1.96)[\widehat{SE}(\bar{\bar{x}}_{clu})]$$

$$.5750 - (1.96)(.0194) \leq \bar{\bar{X}} \leq .5750 + (1.96)(.0194)$$

$$.5370 \leq \bar{\bar{X}} \leq .6130$$

For ȳclu

Now we consider the estimation of the mean number of persons over 65 years of age per housing development. The computations for $\bar{y}_{clu}$ are

$$y_1 = 33, \qquad y_2 = 34, \qquad y = 67$$

$$\bar{y}_{clu} = \frac{y}{m} = \frac{67}{2} = 33.5$$

The computations for $\widehat{SE}(\bar{y}_{clu})$ are

$$\frac{\sum\limits_{i=1}^{m}(y_i - \bar{y}_{clu})^2}{m - 1} = \frac{(33 - 33.5)^2 + (34 - 33.5)^2}{2 - 1} = .5$$

$$\hat{\sigma}_{1y} = \left[\frac{\sum\limits_{i=1}^{m}(y_i - \bar{y}_{clu})^2}{m - 1}\right]^{1/2}\left(\frac{M - 1}{M}\right)^{1/2}$$

$$= (.5)^{1/2}\left(\frac{5 - 1}{5}\right)^{1/2} = .6325$$

$$\widehat{SE}(\bar{y}_{clu}) = \left(\frac{\hat{\sigma}_{1y}}{\sqrt{m}}\right)\left(\frac{M - m}{M - 1}\right)^{1/2} = \left(\frac{.6325}{\sqrt{2}}\right)\left(\frac{5 - 2}{5 - 1}\right)^{1/2} = .3873$$

A 95% confidence interval for $\bar{Y}$ is

$$\bar{y}_{clu} - (1.96)[\widehat{SE}(\bar{y}_{clu})] \le \bar{Y} \le \bar{y}_{clu} + (1.96)[\widehat{SE}(\bar{y}_{clu})]$$

$$33.5 - (1.96)(.3873) \le \bar{Y} \le 33.5 + (1.96)(.3873)$$

$$32.7 \le \bar{Y} \le 34.3$$

Finally, we consider the estimation of the proportion of persons over 65 years of age requiring the services of a visiting nurse. The computation of r_{clu} is   ***For r_{clu}***

$$r_{clu} = \frac{x}{y} = \frac{23}{67} = .3433$$

The computations for $\widehat{SE}(r_{clu})$ are

$$\frac{\sum\limits_{i=1}^{m}(x_i - \bar{x}_{clu})(y_i - \bar{y}_{clu})}{m - 1} = \frac{(11 - 11.5)(33 - 33.5) + (12 - 11.5)(34 - 33.5)}{2 - 1} = .5$$

$$\widehat{SE}(r_{clu}) = (r_{clu})\left\{\frac{[\widehat{SE}(\bar{x}_{clu})]^2}{\bar{x}_{clu}^2} + \frac{[\widehat{SE}(\bar{y}_{clu})]^2}{\bar{y}_{clu}^2}\right.$$

$$- \left(\frac{2}{m}\right)\left(\frac{M - m}{M}\right)\left(\frac{1}{\bar{x}_{clu}\bar{y}_{clu}}\right)$$

$$\left.\times \left[\frac{\sum\limits_{i=1}^{m}(x_i - \bar{x}_{clu})(y_i - \bar{y}_{clu})}{m - 1}\right]\right\}^{1/2}$$

$$= (.3433)\left\{\frac{(.3873)^2}{(11.5)^2} + \frac{(.3873)^2}{(33.5)^2}\right.$$

$$\left.- \left(\frac{2}{2}\right)\left(\frac{5 - 2}{5}\right)\left[\frac{1}{(11.5)(33.5)}\right](.5)\right\}^{1/2}$$

$$= .0076$$

A 95% confidence interval for R is

$$r_{clu} - (1.96)[\widehat{SE}(r_{clu})] \leq R \leq r_{clu} + (1.96)[\widehat{SE}(r_{clu})]$$
$$.3433 - (1.96)(.0076) \leq R \leq .3433 + (1.96)(.0076)$$
$$.3284 \leq R \leq .3582$$

Ratio estimates are most useful in cluster sampling

In cluster sampling the clusters themselves are often constructs used to provide an efficient sampling plan, and it is often not of primary importance to estimate characteristics on a per-cluster basis. In order to obtain estimates on a per-element basis from a cluster sample, ratio estimates must be used. For example, in order to estimate the proportion of all persons requiring the services of a visiting nurse, a ratio estimate is necessary since the number of persons in the sample is subject to sampling variability. Thus ratio estimates are very important in cluster sampling.

10.3 SAMPLING DISTRIBUTIONS OF ESTIMATES

Let us first look at an example of the sampling distributions of estimates.

ILLUSTRATIVE EXAMPLE

In the example above in which a simple one-stage cluster sample of two housing developments is selected from a population of five developments, there are ten possible samples, each having the same chance of being selected. The sampling distributions of three estimates—the total number of persons over 65 years of age requiring the services of a

Table 10.3   Sampling Distribution of Three Estimates

Clusters in Sample	x'_{clu}	y'_{clu}	r_{clu}	Clusters in Sample	x'_{clu}	y'_{clu}	r_{clu}
1,2	75	162.5	.462	2,4	37.5	162.5	.231
1,3	82.5	177.5	.465	2,5	57.5	167.5	.343
1,4	57.6	160	.359	3,4	45	177.5	.254
1,5	77.5	165	.470	3,5	65	182.5	.356
2,3	62.5	180	.347	4,5	40	165	.242

visiting nurse (x'_{clu}), the total number of persons over 65 years of age (y'_{clu}), and the proportion of persons over 65 years of age requiring the services of a visiting nurse (r_{clu})—are shown in table 10.3.

The means and standard errors of x'_{clu}, y'_{clu}, and r_{clu} obtained by enumeration over all samples are shown in table 10.4, along with the true population values (X, Y, and R).

Table 10.4   Means and Standard Errors of Estimates

Estimate	Mean of Estimate	Standard Error of Estimate	Population Value
x'_{clu}	$E(x'_{clu}) = 60$	$SE(x'_{clu}) = 14.87$	$X = 60$
y'_{clu}	$E(y'_{clu}) - 170$	$SE(y'_{clu}) = 7.98$	$Y = 170$
r_{clu}	$E(r_{clu}) = .35287$	$SE(r_{clu}) = .087$	$R = .35294$

Note that in this example $E(x'_{clu}) = X$ and $E(y'_{clu}) = Y$, and this is true in general about totals estimated from simple single-stage cluster sampling. Note also that while the ratio estimate r_{clu} is not an unbiased estimate of the population ratio R, the magnitude of the bias is small.   **_Estimated totals are unbiased_**

Expressions for the theoretical standard errors of estimated totals, means, and ratios are shown in box 10.3 for simple one-stage cluster sampling in terms of the population parameters. The expressions X_i and $\bar{X}$ appearing in box 10.3 were defined in box 10.1 and are as follows:

$$X_i = \sum_{j=1}^{N_i} X_{ij}$$

where

$X_{ij} =$ the level of characteristic $\mathscr{X}$ for the jth listing unit in cluster i

$$\bar{X} = \frac{\sum_{i=1}^{M} X_i}{M}$$

In other words, the X_i are cluster totals and $\bar{X}$ is the mean level of $\mathscr{X}$ per cluster. As in earlier chapters these entities are capitalized when we are discussing population characteristics and are lowercased when we are discussing sample characteristics.

Box 10.3 Theoretical Standard Errors for Estimates Under Simple Single-Stage Cluster Sampling

Total, x'_{clu}

$$\text{SE}(x'_{clu}) = \left(\frac{M}{\sqrt{m}}\right)\left[\frac{\sum\limits_{i=1}^{M}(X_i - \bar{X})^2}{M}\right]^{1/2}\left(\frac{M - m}{M - 1}\right)^{1/2}$$

Mean Per Cluster, $\bar{x}_{clu}$

$$\text{SE}(\bar{x}_{clu}) = \left(\frac{1}{\sqrt{m}}\right)\left[\frac{\sum\limits_{i=1}^{M}(X_i - \bar{X})^2}{M}\right]^{1/2}\left(\frac{M - m}{M - 1}\right)^{1/2}$$

Mean Per Enumeration Unit, $\bar{\bar{x}}_{clu}$

$$\text{SE}(\bar{\bar{x}}_{clu}) = \left(\frac{1}{\sqrt{m\bar{N}}}\right)\left[\frac{\sum\limits_{i=1}^{M}(X_i - \bar{X})^2}{M}\right]^{1/2}\left(\frac{M - m}{M - 1}\right)^{1/2}$$

Ratio, r_{clu}

$$\text{SE}(r_{clu}) \approx \left(\frac{R}{\sqrt{m}}\right)\left(\frac{M - m}{M - 1}\right)^{1/2}\left[\frac{\sum\limits_{i=1}^{M}(X_i - \bar{X})^2}{M\bar{X}^2} + \frac{\sum\limits_{i=1}^{M}(Y_i - \bar{Y})^2}{M\bar{Y}^2}\right.$$

$$\left. - \frac{2\sum\limits_{i=1}^{M}(X_i - \bar{X})(Y_i - \bar{Y})}{M\bar{X}\bar{Y}}\right]^{1/2}$$

The notation used here is defined in box 10.1. The population estimates are defined in box 10.2.

The use of these formulas for the population of five housing developments given in table 10.1 is illustrated next.

ILLUSTRATIVE EXAMPLE

For the population given in table 10.1, we have

$$M = 5, \quad Y_1 = 32, \quad Y_2 = 33, \quad Y_3 = 39, \quad Y_4 = 32, \quad Y_5 = 34$$

Calculations using the formulas in box 10.3

$$\bar{Y} = 34, \quad \sigma_{1y}^2 = \frac{\sum_{i=1}^{M}(Y_i - \bar{Y})^2}{M} = 6.8$$

$$X_1 = 19, \quad X_2 = 11, \quad X_3 = 14, \quad X_4 = 4, \quad X_5 = 12$$

$$\bar{X} = 12, \quad \sigma_{1x}^2 = \frac{\sum_{i=1}^{M}(X_i - \bar{X})^2}{M} = 23.6$$

$$\sigma_{1xy} = \frac{\sum_{i=1}^{M}(X_i - \bar{X})(Y_i - \bar{Y})}{M} = 2.6, \quad R = \frac{12}{34} = .353$$

Then for samples of $m = 2$ clusters, we have

$$\text{SE}(y'_{\text{clu}}) = \left(\frac{5}{\sqrt{2}}\right)(6.8)^{1/2}\left(\frac{5-2}{5-1}\right)^{1/2} = 7.98$$

$$\text{SE}(x'_{\text{clu}}) = \left(\frac{5}{\sqrt{2}}\right)(23.6)^{1/2}\left(\frac{5-2}{5-1}\right)^{1/2} = 14.87$$

$$\text{SE}(\bar{x}_{\text{clu}}) = \left(\frac{1}{\sqrt{2}}\right)(23.6)^{1/2}\left(\frac{5-2}{5-1}\right)^{1/2} = 2.97$$

$$\text{SE}(\bar{\bar{x}}_{\text{clu}}) = \left(\frac{1}{\sqrt{40}}\right)(23.6)^{1/2}\left(\frac{5-2}{5-1}\right)^{1/2} = .665$$

$$\text{SE}(r_{\text{clu}}) = \left(\frac{.353}{\sqrt{2}}\right)\left(\frac{5-2}{5-1}\right)^{1/2}\left[\frac{23.6}{(12)^2} + \frac{6.8}{(34)^2} - \frac{2(2.6)}{(12)(34)}\right]^{1/2} = .0857$$

Note in the example that $\text{SE}(x'_{\text{clu}})$ and $\text{SE}(y'_{\text{clu}})$ as computed from the formulas in box 10.3 are exactly equal to what was obtained earlier by complete enumeration of all samples (table 10.4). This is true in general for estimated totals and means obtained from simple cluster sampling. The formula for the standard error of r_{clu}, however, is only an approximation.

The expression $\sum_{i=1}^{M}(X_i - \bar{X})^2/M$ that appears in the formulas in box 10.3 is really the variance of the distribution of the cluster totals X_i. This expression, denoted by σ_{1x}^2, is often referred to as a **first-stage variance** and is descriptive

**Box 10.4 Exact and Approximate Sample Sizes
Required Under Simple One-Stage Cluster Sampling**

| | EXACT | APPROXIMATE |

Total

$$m = \frac{z_{1-\alpha/2}^2 M V_{1x}^2}{z_{1-\alpha/2}^2 V_{1x}^2 + (M-1)\varepsilon^2} \qquad m \approx \frac{z_{1-\alpha/2}^2 V_{1x}^2}{\varepsilon^2}$$

Mean Per Cluster

$$m = \frac{z_{1-\alpha/2}^2 M V_{1x}^2}{z_{1-\alpha/2}^2 V_{1x}^2 + (M-1)\varepsilon^2} \qquad m \approx \frac{z_{1-\alpha/2}^2 V_{1x}^2}{\varepsilon^2}$$

Mean Per Listing Unit

$$m = \frac{z_{1-\alpha/2}^2 M V_{1x}^2}{z_{1-\alpha/2}^2 V_{1x}^2 + (M-1)\varepsilon^2} \qquad m \approx \frac{z_{1-\alpha/2}^2 V_{1x}^2}{\varepsilon^2}$$

Ratio

$$m = \frac{z_{1-\alpha/2}^2 M V_{1R}^2}{z_{1-\alpha/2}^2 V_{1R}^2 + (M-1)\varepsilon^2} \qquad m \approx \frac{z_{1-\alpha/2}^2 V_{1R}^2}{\varepsilon^2}$$

where

$$V_{1x}^2 = \frac{\sigma_{1x}^2}{\bar{X}^2}$$

$$V_{1R}^2 = \left[\frac{\sigma_{1x}^2}{\bar{X}^2} + \frac{\sigma_{1y}^2}{\bar{Y}^2} - (2)\left(\frac{\sigma_{1xy}}{\bar{X}\bar{Y}}\right)\right]\Big/ R^2$$

$$\sigma_{1xy} = \frac{\sum_{i=1}^{M}(X_i - \bar{X})(Y_i - \bar{Y})}{M}$$

M is the number of clusters in the population, $z_{1-\alpha/2}$ is the reliability coefficient for $100(1-\alpha)\%$ confidence, and ε represents the specifications set on our estimate in terms of the maximum relative difference allowed between it and the unknown population parameter.

of the variation among clusters with respect to the distribution of total levels of characteristic $\mathscr{X}$. In other words, we define, for any characteristic $\mathscr{X}$,

$$\sigma_{1x}^2 = \frac{\sum\limits_{i=1}^{M}(X_i - \bar{X})^2}{M} \qquad (10.1)$$

If we examine the formulas in box 10.3, substituting relation (10.1) in the appropriate places, we see that these expressions are exactly the same as the expressions for the standard errors of the analogous estimates in simple random sampling, with the exception that m replaces n, M replaces N, and σ_{1x}^2 replaces σ_x^2. This result is not surprising since simple one-stage cluster sampling is exactly the same as simple random sampling with the aggregate of all listing units in the cluster serving as an effective enumeration unit.

Note the similarity of simple one-stage cluster sampling formulas to the expressions for simple random sampling

The estimated standard errors of estimated means, totals, and ratios shown in box 10.2 are obtained from the theoretical standard errors of these estimates shown in box 10.3 by substitution of $\hat{\sigma}_{1x}^2$ for σ_{1x}^2 in the appropriate places, where $\hat{\sigma}_{1x}^2$ is an estimate from the data of σ_{1x}^2, given by

$$\hat{\sigma}_{1x}^2 = \left[\frac{\sum\limits_{i=1}^{m}(x_i - \bar{x}_{\text{clu}})^2}{m-1}\right]\left(\frac{M-1}{M}\right)$$

as defined in box 10.2.

10.4 HOW LARGE A SAMPLE IS NEEDED?

Suppose that we intend to use a simple one-stage cluster sample design and wish to be virtually certain of obtaining estimates that differ in relative terms from the true values of the unknown parameters by no more than ε (where ε is as defined in chapter 3, p. 55). Then the required number m of sample clusters is as given in box 10.4.

Let us look at a calculation that uses one of these formulas.

ILLUSTRATIVE EXAMPLE

In the example based on the data in table 10.1, suppose that we wish to be virtually certain (i.e., $z = 3$) of estimating the total number Y of persons over 65 years residing in the five housing developments to within 10% of the true value. With $\sigma_{1y}^2 = 6.8$, $M = 5$, $\varepsilon = .10$, and $\bar{Y} = 34$, we have

$$V_{1y}^2 = \frac{\sigma_{1y}^2}{\bar{Y}^2} = \frac{6.8}{34^2} = .0059$$

and from box 10.4

$$m = \frac{Z_{1-\alpha/2}^2 MV_{1y}^2}{Z_{1-\alpha/2}^2 V_{1y}^2 + (M-1)\varepsilon^2} = \frac{(9)(5)(.0059)}{9(.0059) + 4(.10)^2} = 2.85$$

Rounding up, we have $m = 3$. Thus we would need a simple one-stage cluster sample of 3 clusters to meet these specifications.

To determine sample size, we must know or estimate σ_{1x}^2 and $\bar{X}^2$

In order to determine the sample size that meets the specifications required for the reliability of the estimate, it is necessary to know the value of V_{1x}^2, which is the ratio of σ_{1x}^2, the variance of the distribution of cluster totals, to $\bar{X}^2$, the square of the mean level of characteristic $\mathcal{X}$ per cluster. These quantities are population parameters that in general would be unknown and would have to be either estimated from preliminary studies or else guessed by means of intuition or past experience.

10.5 RELIABILITY OF ESTIMATES AND COSTS INVOLVED

One of the major advantages of simple one-stage cluster sampling is that the cost of obtaining a sample of listing units by this method is often lower than that of obtaining a sample of the same number of listing units by other methods. In this section we illustrate, using the example based on the population shown in table 10.1, the comparatively low field costs involved in simple one-stage cluster sampling as well as the comparatively high standard errors that are characteristic of this method. Finally, we introduce the concept of comparing sampling designs on the basis of the standard errors of estimates that can be obtained at preassigned field costs.

Low field costs are associated with cluster sampling

ILLUSTRATIVE EXAMPLE

Let us consider again the population of five housing developments shown in table 10.1. In chapter 9 we specified the following costs associated with field operations of traveling, listing, and interviewing for a survey of these housing developments:

travel to developments: .5 person-hour per development

listing of households: 3 person-minutes per household (or .05 person-hour)

interviewing: 15 minutes per household (or .25 person-hour)

Using the cost components discussed above, let us consider what the field costs would be of taking a simple one-stage cluster sample of two housing developments.

The construction of the sampling frame requires 3 person-hours. This total is the sum of the time needed to travel to the sample housing developments, which is

$$(2 \text{ sample developments}) \times (.5 \text{ person-hour per development})$$
$$= 1.0 \text{ person-hour}$$

Field costs for cluster sample

and the time needed to list households, which is

$$(40 \text{ households}) \times (.05 \text{ person-hour per household}) = 2.0 \text{ person-hours}$$

The collection of data requires 11 person-hours. This total is the sum of the time needed to travel to the housing developments, which is

$$(2 \text{ developments}) \times (.5 \text{ person-hour per development}) = 1 \text{ person-hour}$$

and the time needed to interview the sample households, which is

$$(40 \text{ households}) \times (.25 \text{ person-hour per household}) = 10 \text{ person-hours}$$

Then we have

$$\text{total field costs} = 3 + 11 = 14 \text{ person-hours}$$

Thus the field costs involved in a simple one-stage cluster sample of two housing developments are 14 person-hours. In the example following box 10.3 we calculated the standard error of x'_{clu}, the estimated number of persons over 65 years of age requiring the services of a visiting nurse, as 14.87.

The simple one-stage cluster sample of two housing developments yielded 40 sample households. Let us now see what the field costs would be for a simple random sample of 40 households. In chapter 9 we calculated that the costs of constructing the sampling frame would be 7.5 person-hours for a simple random sample design. Since a simple random sample of 40 households would almost certainly include at least one household from each development, the field costs for data collection are as listed below:

Field costs for simple random sample

$$\text{travel:} \quad (5 \text{ developments}) \times (.5 \text{ person-hour per development})$$
$$= 2.5 \text{ person-hours}$$
$$\text{interviewing:} \quad (40 \text{ households}) \times (.25 \text{ person-hour per household})$$
$$= 10 \text{ person-hours}$$

Thus the total data collection costs are $10 + 2.5 = 12.5$ person-hours, and the total field costs are $7.5 + 12.5 = 20.0$ person-hours.

The standard error of the estimated total x' of persons over 65 years of age requiring the services of a visiting nurse from a simple random sample of 40 households is given by

$$SE(x') = \left(\frac{N}{\sqrt{n}}\right)(\sigma_x)\left(\frac{N-n}{N-1}\right)^{1/2}$$

where $N = 100$, $n = 40$, and $\sigma_x = .6164$ (from the data in table 10.1), which gives

$$SE(x') = 7.59$$

The standard errors of x' and x'_{clu} are shown in table 10.5 along with the field costs of obtaining these estimates.

Table 10.5   Standard Errors and Field Costs

Sample Design	Total Households Sampled	Field Costs in Person-Hours	Standard Error of Estimated Total
simple random sampling	40	20.00	7.59
simple one-stage sampling of 2 clusters	40	14.00	14.87

From the table we see that the simple one-stage cluster sample yields an estimate having a larger standard error than that of the simple random sample. However, the field costs of the simple random sample are greater than those of the simple cluster sample.

Comparison of the two designs for the same field costs

Perhaps a better way to compare the two designs is to examine the standard error of the estimated totals at equivalent field costs. For example, at a field cost of 14.00 person-hours, a simple random sample of approximately 16 households could be taken. The standard error of an estimated total from such a simple random sample would be

$$\text{SE}(x') = \left(\frac{100}{\sqrt{16}}\right)(.6164)\left(\frac{100 - 16}{100 - 1}\right)^{1/2} = 14.19$$

Thus at an equivalent cost of 14.00 person-hours, a simple random sample of approximately 16 households can be taken. At the same cost a simple one-stage cluster sample of 40 households can be taken. The simple random sample of 16 households will yield an estimate of the total persons over 65 years requiring the services of a visiting nurse which has a slightly lower standard error than the analogous estimate obtained at the same cost from the simple one-stage cluster sample of 40 households. In contrast to what was found in this example, it is not uncommon for cluster sampling to provide more precise estimates of a population parameter than simple random sampling if the budget available to carry out either type of survey is the same.

10.6 CHOOSING A SAMPLING DESIGN BASED ON COST AND RELIABILITY

There are essentially two widely used strategies for choosing among several possible sample designs. The first strategy consists of the four steps shown below (for simplicity, we will assume that only one estimate is to be taken into consideration in choosing the sample design).

1. Determine the relative error ε required for the estimate.
2. For each sample design under consideration, determine the sample size required to obtain, with specified confidence, an estimate that meets the specifications listed in step 1.
3. For each sample design estimate the field costs involved in obtaining the sample size given in step 2.
4. Choose the sample design that yields the lowest field costs, as calculated in step 3. In other words, this strategy chooses from among the competing designs the sample design that meets the required specifications at the lowest field costs.

One strategy for choosing a sample design

    Let us see how this strategy could be used by looking at an example.

ILLUSTRATIVE EXAMPLE

Let us again use the data in table 10.1. Suppose that we wish to decide between a simple one-stage cluster sample and a simple random sample, and that we wish to be virtually certain of estimating Y, the total number of persons over 65 years of age residing in the five housing developments, to within 10% of the true value (i.e., $\varepsilon = .10$). In section 10.4 we showed that a sample of three clusters was necessary to meet this specification if we were to use simple one-stage cluster sampling. Using the cost components introduced in section 10.5, we can compute the field costs for this sample design as follows.

    For the construction of the sampling frame we have the time to travel to the sample housing developments, which is

$$\text{(3 sample developments)} \times \text{(.5 person-hour per development)}$$
$$= 1.5 \text{ person-hours}$$

Field costs for cluster sample

and the time to list households, which is

$$\text{(60 households)} \times \text{(.05 person-hour per household)} = 3.0 \text{ person-hours}$$

Thus the construction of the sampling frame requires 4.5 person-hours.

    For the collection of data we have the time to travel to the housing developments, which is

$$\text{(3 developments)} \times \text{(.5 person-hour per development)} = 1.5 \text{ person-hours}$$

and the time to interview sample households, which is

$$\text{(60 households)} \times \text{(.25 person-hour per household)} = 15 \text{ person-hours}$$

So collection of data requires 16.5 person-hours.

Thus for a simple one-stage cluster sample that meets the specifications, we have

total field costs = 21 person-hours

Let us now determine the necessary sample size and field costs for a simple random sample that would meet the same specifications. From box 3.4 (with $N = 100$, $\varepsilon = .10$, $\sigma_y^2 = .71$, $z = 3$, and $\bar{\bar{Y}} = 1.7^*$), we would require a sample of 69 households. The field costs of this sample design are computed as follows.

For the construction of the sampling frame we have the time to travel to the sample housing developments, which is

Field costs for simple random sample

(5 sample developments) × (.5 person-hour per development)

= 2.5 person-hours

and the time to list households, which is

(100 households) × (.05 person-hour per household) = 5.0 person-hours

Thus the construction of the sampling frame requires 7.5 person-hours.

For the collection of data we have the time to travel to the housing developments[†] which is

(5 developments) × (.5 person-hour per development) = 2.5 person-hours

and the time to interview sample households, which is

(69 households) × (.25 person-hour per household) = 17.25 person-hours

So collection of data requires 19.75 person-hours.

Thus for a simple random sample we have

total field costs = 27.25 person-hours

The two designs are summarized in table 10.6.

---

* The computations for $\bar{\bar{Y}}$ and σ_y^2 are as follows:

$$\bar{\bar{Y}} = \frac{\sum_{i=1}^{M} \sum_{j=1}^{N_i} Y_{ij}}{N} = \frac{170}{100} = 1.7$$

Note that $\bar{\bar{Y}}$ has the same interpretation as did the expression $\bar{Y}$ in chapter 3.

$$\sigma_y^2 = \frac{\sum_{i=1}^{M} \sum_{j=1}^{N_i} (Y_{ij} - \bar{\bar{Y}})^2}{N} = \frac{(3 - 1.7)^2 + \cdots + (1 - 1.7)^2}{100} = .71$$

Note that in the notation of chapter 3 this is equivalent to $\sum_{i=1}^{N} (Y_i - \bar{Y})^2 / N$.

† A sample of 69 households would almost certainly involve at least one household from each of the five developments.

Table 10.6 Summary of Two Sampling Designs

	Simple One-Stage Cluster Sampling	Simple Random Sampling
Specification for Reliability of Estimate	$\varepsilon = .10$	$\varepsilon = .10$
Number of Households in Sample	60	69
Field Costs (in person-hours)		
Construction of Sampling Frame	4.5	7.5
Collection of Data	16.5	19.75
Total Field Costs	21	27.25

Thus from table 10.6 we see that of the two designs simple one-stage cluster sampling would be the choice, because the desired level of reliability could be achieved at lower cost then with simple random sampling.

A second strategy that is widely used in choosing among alternative sampling designs is to first determine the sample design that produces estimates having the lowest variance at the field costs that have been specified. This is done by first computing the sample size that can be taken within the specified fields costs and then calculating the variance of the estimate for that particular sample size. *A second strategy for choosing a sample design*

In order for this strategy to be used easily, it helps to have an equation relating sample size to field costs. Such an equation is called a **cost function** and is a very useful tool that enables an investigator to choose from among competing sample designs the one that will produce the lowest variance at a specified cost. We show below how such a simple cost function might be obtained.

Let us examine in a slightly different way the field costs involved in each of the two sample designs we have been discussing. For the simple random sampling design the cost of constructing the sample frame is independent of the number of enumeration units selected in the sample since each enumeration unit must be listed prior to selection of the sample. Also, the travel costs associated with the interviewing are, to a large extent, independent of the number of enumeration units selected. The other costs might be considered as depending on the number of enumeration units selected. Thus a reasonable estimate of field costs for a simple random sampling design might be given by the expression *Cost function for simple random sampling*

$$C = C_0 + C_1 n \qquad (10.2)$$

where C_0 is the cost component associated with construction of the sampling frame plus travel costs that are not dependent on sample size and C_1 is the interviewing cost per enumeration unit. For the example discussed earlier we have values of C_0 and C_1 given by

$$C_0 = 10.00 \text{ person-hours} \quad \text{and} \quad C_1 = .25 \text{ person-hour}$$

Thus as indicated earlier, a simple random sample of 69 households would have a field cost of

$$C = 10.00 + 69(.25) = 27.25 \text{ person-hours}$$

Cost function for simple cluster sampling

The field costs involved in simple cluster sampling have a different form. Since the frame construction costs as well as the travel costs depend on the number of clusters selected, the field costs involved in a simple one-stage cluster sample can be described by the following equation:

$$C = C'_1 m + C'_2 m \bar{N} \tag{10.3}$$

The cost component C'_1 associated with clusters includes the cost of traveling to each sample cluster, once for listing (.5 person-hour) and once for data collection (.5 person-hour). The cost component C'_2 includes the cost of listing and interviewing each sample household (.05 person-hour per household + .25 person-hour per household, or .30 person-hour per sample household). Thus in our example we have

$$C'_1 = 1.00 \quad \text{and} \quad C'_2 = .30$$

So as shown earlier, a simple one-stage cluster sample of 3 clusters would have a field cost of

$$C = 1.00(3) + (.30)(3)(20) = 21 \text{ person-hours}$$

The cost functions discussed above are rough approximations to the true field costs and are useful in arriving at order-of-magnitude costs and in choosing between alternative sample designs. Such cost functions will be used when we discuss cost efficiency in later chapters.

Now let us look at an illustration of this second strategy, using the same example as before.

ILLUSTRATIVE EXAMPLE

Let us suppose that we have a budget that allocates 20 person-hours to field costs and that we wish to choose between simple random sampling and simple cluster sampling.

From relation (10.2) with $C = 20$, $C_0 = 10.00$, and $C_1 = .25$, we can take a simple random sample of $n = 40$ households, which would yield an estimated total having a variance (from box 3.1) given by

$$\text{Var}(y') = \left(\frac{N^2}{n}\right)(\sigma_y^2)\left(\frac{N-n}{N-1}\right) = \left(\frac{100^2}{40}\right)(.71)\left(\frac{100-40}{100-1}\right) = 107.57$$

From relation (10.3) with $C_1' = 1.00$ and $C_2' = .30$, a simple cluster sample at field costs of 20 person-hours would allow 2.85 clusters to be sampled. We round this down to two clusters so as not to exceed the available budget. Our estimated total, then, would have the following variance [from box 10.3 and equation (10.1)]:

$$\text{Var}(y'_{\text{clu}}) = \left(\frac{M^2}{m}\right)(\sigma_{1y}^2)\left(\frac{M-m}{M-1}\right) = \left(\frac{5^2}{2}\right)(6.8)\left(\frac{5-2}{5-1}\right) = 63.75$$

Thus if a budget of 20 person-hours is allocated to the field costs of the survey, simple one-stage cluster sampling would be the sample design of choice over simple random sampling, since it will produce an estimated total having the lower variance.

The discussion in this section has been oversimplified in order to illustrate the concepts involved in taking costs into consideration when we choose between one or more sample designs. In our discussion we made our choice on the basis of one estimate, namely, the estimated total number of persons over 65 years of age in the five housing developments. In real situations many estimates would be involved in the survey, and the sample design of choice would be the one that performs best in the sense discussed in this section when all the estimates are taken into consideration. The cost functions used in this discussion were simple linear functions of enumeration units or clusters. Although these simplified functions are often useful in practice, more complex functions are sometimes needed to describe costs in a realistic way. Excellent discussions of cost functions are given in the books by Hansen, Hurwitz, and Madow (2) and by Jessen (3).

In practice, many estimates would be considered in choosing a sample design

SUMMARY

In this chapter we discussed the basic concepts of simple one-stage cluster sampling for situations in which each cluster in the population contains the same number of enumeration units or listing units. Simple one-stage cluster sampling involves taking a simple random sample of clusters and including in the sample every listing unit within each sample cluster. We developed methods for estimating means, totals, and ratios under simple one-stage cluster sampling, and we discussed the sampling distributions of these estimates. In addition, we presented methods for estimating the standard errors of these estimates from the data in the sample.

We discussed determination of the sample size required to meet specifications set for the reliability of estimates obtained under simple cluster sampling, and the formulas developed were shown to be very similar to those developed earlier for simple random sampling, with the cluster totals serving as the effective observations. We presented strategies for choosing between alternative sample designs taking costs into consideration. Finally, we discussed the concepts of cost components and cost functions.

EXERCISES

1. Suppose that the elementary schools in a city are grouped into 30 school districts, with each school district containing four schools. Suppose that a simple one-stage cluster sample of three school districts is taken for purposes of estimating the number of schoolchildren in the city who are color-blind (as measured by a standard test) and that the accompanying data are obtained from this sample. Estimate and obtain a 95% confidence interval for the total number of color-blind children and for the proportion of all children who are color-blind.

Sample School District	School	No. of Children	No. of Color-blind Children
1	1	130	2
	2	150	3
	3	160	3
	4	120	5
2	1	110	2
	2	120	4
	3	100	0
	4	120	1
3	1	89	4
	2	130	2
	3	100	0
	4	150	2

2. A sample of patients is to be taken from the patient records of a large psychiatric outpatient clinic for purposes of estimating the total number of patients who were given Valium as part of their therapeutic regimen. The records are organized in file drawers, each containing 20 patient records, and there are 40 such file drawers.

(a) Suppose that we wish to use simple random sampling of patient records. How large a sample is needed if we wish to be virtually certain of estimating the total number of persons given Valium to within 10% of its true value and if we anticipate that approximately 20% of all patients were given Valium?

(b) What would be the field costs involved in taking the sample specified in part (a)? Make some assumptions about the cost components in determining these field costs.

(c) What sample size is needed if the design is to be a simple one-stage cluster sample?

(d) What would be the field costs for a simple one-stage cluster sample? Again, make some assumptions about the cost components in determining these field costs.

(e) Which of the two alternative sample designs would you use? Why?

3. A simple one-stage cluster sample was taken of ten hospitals in a midwestern state from a population of 33 hospitals that have received state funds to upgrade the emergency medical services in that state. Within each of the hospitals selected in the sample, the records of all patients hospitalized in calendar year 1978 for trauma conditions (i.e., accidents, poisonings, violence, burns, etc.) were examined. The number of patients hospitalized for trauma conditions and the number discharged dead are shown in the accompanying table for each hospital in the sample.

Hospital	Total Number of Patients Hospitalized for Trauma Conditions	Total Number Discharged Dead Among All Patients Hospitalized with Trauma Conditions
1	560	4
2	190	4
3	260	2
4	370	4
5	190	4
6	130	0
7	170	9
8	170	2
9	60	0
10	110	1

(a) For this sample, what are the clusters, what are the listing units, and what are the elementary units?

(b) Estimate and give a 95% confidence interval for the total number of persons hospitalized for trauma conditions among the 33 hospitals.

(c) Estimate and give a 95% confidence interval for the total number of patients discharged dead among all persons hospitalized for trauma conditions.

(d) Estimate and give a 95% confidence interval for the proportion of persons discharged dead among all persons hospitalized with trauma conditions.

4. The number of beds in each of the ten hospitals sampled in exercise 3 is shown in the accompanying table. The remaining 23 hospitals not appearing in the sample have a total of 3687 beds. Use this information to obtain improved estimates and confidence intervals for the following:

(a) the total number of persons hospitalized with trauma conditions.

(b) the total number of persons discharged dead among all persons hospitalized with trauma conditions

Hospital	1	2	3	4	5	6	7	8	9	10
No. of Beds	824	312	329	648	358	252	256	263	138	150

BIBLIOGRAPHY

The following publications contain more detailed discussions of cluster sampling.

1. COCHRAN, W. G. *Sampling techniques*. 3d ed. New York: Wiley, 1977.

2. HANSEN, M. H.; HURWITZ, W. N.; and MADOW, W. G. *Sample survey methods and theory*. Vol. 1. New York: Wiley, 1953.

3. JESSEN, R. J. *Statistical survey techniques*. New York: Wiley, 1978.

4. KISH, L. *Survey sampling*. New York: Wiley: 1965.

5. SCHEAFFER, R. L.; MENDENHALL, W.; and OTT, L. *Elementary survey sampling*. 2d ed. N. Scituate, MA: Duxbury Press, 1979.

6. SUDMAN, S. *Applied sampling*. New York: Academic Press, 1976.

11

Simple Two-Stage Cluster Sampling

In the previous chapter we discussed simple one-stage cluster sampling, which involves taking a simple random sample of clusters and then sampling every enumeration or listing unit within each sample cluster. In some situations it is more efficient to sample in more than one stage. For example, when the listing units within clusters are very homogeneous with respect to the variables being measured, there is a large amount of redundancy in sampling every listing unit within a sample cluster. In such situations it is often better to take a sample of listing units within selected clusters rather than to select all of them. In other words, it is often best to draw the sample in two stages, with the first stage being a sample of clusters and the second stage being a sample of listing units within each sample cluster.

If listing units within clusters are homogeneous, it may be better to take a sample (rather than all) of them

In this chapter and in the next we will discuss two-stage cluster sampling designs. The sampling designs considered in this chapter involve **simple two-stage cluster sampling** as defined in chapter 9. These are designs in which clusters are selected at the first stage by simple random sampling, listing units are selected at the second stage by simple random sampling within each cluster selected at the first stage of sampling, and the fraction of listing units selected at the second stage is the same for each sample cluster.

The sample of listing units is the second stage

In this chapter we consider the case in which the number of listing units is the same among clusters

If the number of listing units is not the same within each cluster, then it is not always possible for the sampling fraction of listing units to be exactly the same within sample cluster. For example, if one city block contains ten households and another contains five households, it would not be possible to take a 50% sample of households from each of these two blocks. In chapter 12 we treat the more complex situation in which the number of listing units varies among clusters.

199

There are many situations in which each cluster has the same number of listing units. Some examples are listed in the following paragraphs.

Weeks in the calendar year may serve as clusters in certain situations, with days serving as listing units. In such instances each cluster (week) would have the same number of listing units (days).

Examples of clusters with the same number of listing units

Health records are sometimes organized on computer tapes in reels, with each reel containing the same number of records. Hence in a cluster sampling design using reels as clusters and individual records as listing units, each cluster (reel) would have the same number of listing units (records).

In quality control sampling, individual units of a product are often organized into batches, with each batch serving as a cluster and the individual units serving as listing units.

11.1 HOW TO TAKE A SIMPLE TWO-STAGE CLUSTER SAMPLE

We will use a practical example to illustrate how a simple two-stage cluster sample may be taken.

ILLUSTRATIVE EXAMPLE

In this example we will use the data shown in table 11.1. Let us suppose that a local health department administers five community health centers and that each community health

Table 11.1   Number of Patients Seen by Nurse Practitioners and Number Referred to a Physician for Five Community Health Centers

Health Center	Nurse Practitioner	Number of Patients Seen, $\mathscr{X}$	Number of Patients Referred to Physician, $\mathscr{Y}$
1	1	58	5
	2	44	6
	3	18	6
2	1	42	3
	2	53	19
	3	10	2
3	1	13	12
	2	18	6
	3	37	10
4	1	16	5
	2	32	14
	3	10	4
5	1	25	17
	2	23	9
	3	23	14

center uses three nurse practitioners for primary care. Suppose further that it is desired to take a sample of three clinics and within each clinic to take a subsample of two of the nurse practitioners employed there. Each nurse in the sample will be requested to keep a log of the patients seen during a particular week and the number of these patients referred to a physician.

First we take a simple random sample of three centers

To take a simple two-stage cluster sample of three community health centers and two nurse practitioners from each health center sampled, we first number the health centers from 1 to 5 and then choose three random numbers between 1 and 5 (e.g., 1, 2, and 4). Next, within each of these three sample centers we identify each nurse practitioner by a number, and then we take two random numbers. The nurse practitioners corresponding to these numbers are then selected in the sample (e.g., nurse practitioners 2 and 3 from community health center 1, nurse practitioners 1 and 3 from health center 2, and nurse practitioners 1 and 2 from health center 4).

Within each center we take a simple random sample of two practitioners

11.2 ESTIMATION OF POPULATION CHARACTERISTICS

Once the sample of clusters and listing units is selected, the required data are collected from every listing unit selected in the sample. The forms that are used to collect these data would, as discussed in chapter 10, depend on the nature of the data and on the manner in which the data are collected. Then estimates of population characteristics are calculated by using the data that have been collected.

Let us investigate the estimation procedures by considering an example.

ILLUSTRATIVE EXAMPLE

Suppose that from our sample of three community health centers and two nurse practitioners within each of the selected community health centers, we wish to estimate the following population characteristics:

1. the total number of patients seen by nurse practitioners in the five community health centers

2. the total number of patients referred by nurse practitioners to physicians in the five community health centers

3. the proportion among all persons seen by nurse practitioners that is referred to a physician

4. the mean number of persons seen by nurse practitioners per community health center

5. the mean number of patients seen per nurse practitioner

The data might be collected by obtaining, from the records of each nurse practitioner selected in the sample, the total number of patients seen and the total number referred to physicians. Suppose that these data are as summarized in table 11.2. We then obtain the desired estimates as follows from the summary data shown in table 11.2.

To find the estimated total number of patients seen by nurse practitioners in the five community health centers, we first compute the total number of patients seen by all nurse

Table 11.2   Summary Data for the Three Clusters Selected in the Sample

Health Center	Nurse Practitioner	Number of Patients Seen, $\mathcal{X}$	Number of Patients Referred to Physician, $\mathcal{Y}$
1	2	44	6
	3	18	6
2	1	42	3
	3	10	2
4	1	16	5
	2	32	14
Total		162	36

practitioners in the sample. Then we divide that total by the overall sampling fraction. That is,

total patients seen $= 162$

overall sampling fraction $= (\frac{3}{5}$ of all centers$) \times (\frac{2}{3}$ of all nurses$) = \frac{6}{15}$

estimated population total of persons seen by nurses $= \dfrac{162}{\frac{6}{15}} = 405$

To find the estimated total number of patients referred by nurse practitioners to physicians in the five community health centers, we use computations similar to the previous computations.

total patients referred to physician $= 36$

overall sampling fraction $= \frac{6}{15}$

estimated total number of patients referred to physician $= \dfrac{36}{\frac{6}{15}} = 90$

To find the estimated proportion referred to physicians among all patients seen by nurse practitioners, we compute the ratio of the two estimated totals computed above. That is,

estimated proportion referred to physician $= \dfrac{90}{405} = .2222$

To find the estimated mean number of patients seen by nurse practitioners per community health center, we divide the estimated total number of patients seen by nurse practitioners in all community health centers by the number of community health centers. That is,

estimated mean number of patients seen by nurses per center $= \dfrac{405}{5} = 81$

To find the estimated mean number of patients seen per nurse practitioner, we divide the estimated total number of patients seen by nurse practitioners in all community health centers by the total number of nurse practitioners. That is,

estimated mean number of patients seen per nurse $= \dfrac{405}{15} = 27$

The notation used in simple two-stage cluster sampling from clusters having equal numbers of listing units is very similar to the notation used for simple one-stage cluster sampling. This notation is shown next in box 11.1.

Box 11.1 Notation Used in Simple Two-Stage Cluster Sampling

M = number of clusters in the population

m = number of clusters in the sample

x_{ij} = level of characteristic $\mathcal{X}$ for sample listing unit j in sample cluster i

y_{ij} = level of characteristic $\mathcal{Y}$ for sample listing unit j in sample cluster i

$\bar{n}$ = number of listing units sampled from each cluster

$n = \bar{n}m$ = total number of listing units in the sample

$$x_i = \sum_{j=1}^{\bar{n}} x_{ij} = \text{sample total of characteristic } \mathcal{X} \text{ for } i\text{th sample cluster}$$

$$y_i = \sum_{j=1}^{\bar{n}} y_{ij} = \text{sample total of characteristic } \mathcal{Y} \text{ for } i\text{th sample cluster}$$

$$x = \sum_{i=1}^{m} x_i = \text{sample total for characteristic } \mathcal{X}$$

$$y = \sum_{i=1}^{m} y_i = \text{sample total for characteristic } \mathcal{Y}$$

$$\bar{N} = \frac{N}{M} = \text{average number of listing units per cluster in population}$$

$N = \bar{N}M$ = total number of listing units in population

$$f_1 = \frac{m}{M} = \text{first-stage sampling fraction}$$

$$f_2 = \frac{\bar{n}}{\bar{N}} = \text{second-stage sampling fraction}$$

$f = f_1 f_2$ = overall sampling fraction

$$\bar{x} = \frac{x}{m}$$

$$\bar{y} = \frac{y}{m}$$

Using the notation of box 11.1, we list, in box 11.2, the algebraic formulas used to compute estimated population characteristics and estimated standard errors of these estimated population characteristics.

Box 11.2 Estimated Population Characteristics and Estimated Standard Errors for Simple Two-Stage Cluster Sampling

Total, X

$$x'_{clu} = \frac{x}{f} \qquad \widehat{SE}(x'_{clu}) = \left(\frac{M}{\sqrt{m}f_2}\right)\left[\frac{\sum\limits_{i=1}^{m}(x_i - \bar{x})^2}{m - 1}\right]^{1/2}\left(\frac{N - n}{N}\right)^{1/2}$$

Mean Per Cluster, $\bar{X}$

$$\bar{x}_{clu} = \frac{x'_{clu}}{M} \qquad \widehat{SE}(\bar{x}_{clu}) = \left(\frac{1}{\sqrt{m}f_2}\right)\left[\frac{\sum\limits_{i=1}^{m}(x_i - \bar{x})^2}{m - 1}\right]^{1/2}\left(\frac{N - n}{N}\right)^{1/2}$$

Mean Per Listing Unit, $\bar{\bar{X}}$

$$\bar{\bar{x}}_{clu} = \frac{x'_{clu}}{N} \qquad \widehat{SE}(\bar{\bar{x}}_{clu}) = \left(\frac{1}{\bar{N}\sqrt{m}f_2}\right)\left[\frac{\sum\limits_{i=1}^{m}(x_i - \bar{x})^2}{m - 1}\right]^{1/2}\left(\frac{N - n}{N}\right)^{1/2}$$

Ratio, R

$$r_{clu} = \frac{y}{x}$$

$$\widehat{SE}(r_{clu}) = r_{clu}\left\{\left[\frac{\widehat{SE}(\bar{y}_{clu})}{\bar{y}_{clu}}\right]^2 + \left[\frac{\widehat{SE}(\bar{x}_{clu})}{\bar{x}_{clu}}\right]^2\right.$$

$$\left. - \left(\frac{2}{f_2^2}\right)\left(\frac{N - n}{N}\right)\left[\frac{\sum\limits_{i=1}^{m}(x_i - \bar{x})(y_i - \bar{y})}{(m - 1)m\bar{x}_{clu}\bar{y}_{clu}}\right]\right\}^{1/2}$$

The notation used in these formulas is defined in box 11.1.

The expressions given in box 11.2 for estimating standard errors of estimates from these simple two-stage cluster sampling designs are known as **ultimate cluster estimates** and are based on manipulation of the totals x_i over the listing units selected in each sample cluster. Note that the mean $\bar{x}$ appearing in these formulas is not the same as $\bar{x}_{clu}$, the estimated mean per cluster. In fact, $\bar{x}_{clu} = (\bar{N}/\bar{n})(\bar{x})$.

Use of these formulas with the data given in table 11.2 is illustrated in the next example.

ILLUSTRATIVE EXAMPLE

To use the estimation procedures shown in box 11.2, let us consider the data shown in table 11.2. We have the following information:

$m = 3$ community health centers in the sample

$M = 5$ community health centers in the population

$\bar{n} = 2$ nurse practitioners sampled from each health center selected

$\bar{N} = 3$ nurse practitioners employed at each health center

$$f_1 = \frac{m}{M} = \frac{3}{5} = .6 = \text{first-stage sampling fraction}$$

$$f_2 = \frac{\bar{n}}{\bar{N}} = \frac{2}{3} = .67 = \text{second-stage sampling fraction}$$

$$f = f_1 f_2 = \left(\frac{3}{5}\right)\left(\frac{2}{3}\right) = .4 = \text{overall sampling fraction}$$

$n = 6$ nurse practitioners in sample

$N = 15$ nurse practitioners in population

First we consider the estimation of y'_{clu}, the total number of patients referred to a physician among those seen by the nurse practitioners in the five centers. The computations for y'_{clu} are

Calculations using formulas of box 11.2

$$y_1 = 12, \quad y_2 = 5, \quad y_3 = 19, \quad y = 36$$

$$y'_{clu} = \frac{36}{.4} = 90$$

The computations for $\widehat{SE}(y'_{clu})$ are

$$\bar{y} = \frac{12 + 5 + 19}{3} = 12$$

$$\frac{\sum_{i=1}^{m} (y_i - \bar{y})^2}{m - 1} = \frac{(12 - 12)^2 + (5 - 12)^2 + (19 - 12)^2}{3 - 1} = 49$$

$$\widehat{SE}(y'_{clu}) = \left[\frac{5}{\sqrt{3(.67)}}\right](49)^{1/2}\left(\frac{15 - 6}{15}\right)^{1/2} = 23.48$$

A 95% confidence interval for Y is

$$y'_{clu} - (1.96)[\widehat{SE}(y'_{clu})] \leq Y \leq y'_{clu} + (1.96)[\widehat{SE}(y'_{clu})]$$
$$90 - (1.96)(23.48) \leq Y \leq 90 + (1.96)(23.48)$$
$$43.98 \leq Y \leq 136.02$$

Now we consider the estimation of $\bar{y}_{clu}$, the mean number of patients per health center referred to a physician by a nurse practitioner. The computation of $\bar{y}_{clu}$ is

$$\bar{y}_{clu} = \frac{90}{5} = 18$$

The computation of $\widehat{SE}(\bar{y}_{clu})$ is

$$\widehat{SE}(\bar{y}_{clu}) = \left[\frac{1}{\sqrt{3(.67)}}\right](49)^{1/2}\left(\frac{15 - 6}{15}\right)^{1/2} = 4.70$$

A 95% confidence interval for $\bar{Y}$ is

$$\bar{y}_{clu} - (1.96)[\widehat{SE}(\bar{y}_{clu})] \leq \bar{Y} \leq \bar{y}_{clu} + (1.96)[\widehat{SE}(\bar{y}_{clu})]$$
$$18 - (1.96)(4.70) \leq \bar{Y} \leq 18 + (1.96)(4.70)$$
$$8.78 \leq \bar{Y} \leq 27.21$$

Now we consider the estimation of $\bar{\bar{y}}_{clu}$, the mean number of patients per nurse practitioner referred to a physician. The computation of $\bar{\bar{y}}_{clu}$ is

$$\bar{\bar{y}}_{clu} = \frac{90}{15} = 6$$

The computation of $\widehat{SE}(\bar{\bar{y}}_{clu})$ is

$$\widehat{SE}(\bar{\bar{y}}_{clu}) = \left[\frac{1}{3\sqrt{3(.67)}}\right](49)^{1/2}\left(\frac{15 - 6}{15}\right)^{1/2} = 1.57$$

A 95% confidence interval for $\bar{\bar{Y}}$ is

$$\bar{\bar{y}}_{clu} - (1.96)[\widehat{SE}(\bar{\bar{y}}_{clu})] \le \bar{\bar{Y}} \le \bar{\bar{y}}_{clu} + (1.96)[\widehat{SE}(\bar{\bar{y}}_{clu})]$$
$$6 - (1.96)(1.57) \le \bar{\bar{Y}} \le 6 + (1.96)(1.57)$$
$$2.92 \le \bar{\bar{Y}} \le 9.08$$

Finally, we consider the estimation of r_{clu}, the proportion of all patients referred to a physician among those seen by nurse practitioners. The computations for r_{clu} are

$$y = 36 \qquad x_1 = 62 \qquad x_2 = 52 \qquad x_3 = 48 \qquad x = 162$$

$$r_{clu} = \frac{36}{162} = .2222$$

The computations for $\widehat{SE}(r_{clu})$ are

$$\bar{x} = \frac{62 + 52 + 48}{3} = 54$$

$$\frac{\sum_{i=1}^{m}(x_i - \bar{x})^2}{m - 1} = \frac{(62 - 54)^2 + (52 - 54)^2 + (48 - 54)^2}{3 - 1} = 52$$

$$x'_{clu} = \frac{162}{.4} = 405 \qquad \bar{x}_{clu} = \frac{405}{5} = 81$$

$$\widehat{SE}(\bar{x}_{clu}) = \left[\frac{1}{\sqrt{3(.67)}}\right](52)^{1/2}\left(\frac{15 - 6}{15}\right)^{1/2} = 4.84$$

$$\sum_{i=1}^{m}(x_i - \bar{x})(y_i - \bar{y}) = (62 - 54)(12 - 12) + (52 - 54)(5 - 12)$$

$$+ (48 - 54)(19 - 12) = -28$$

$$\widehat{SE}(r_{clu}) = (.2222)\left\{\left[\left(\frac{4.70}{18}\right)^2 + \left(\frac{4.84}{81}\right)^2\right.\right.$$

$$\left.\left. - \left[\frac{2}{(.67)^2}\right]\left(\frac{15 - 6}{15}\right)\left[\frac{-28}{(3 - 1)(3)(81)(18)}\right]\right\}^{1/2}$$

$$= .1808$$

A 95% confidence interval for R is

$$r_{clu} - (1.96)[\widehat{SE}(r_{clu})] \le R \le r_{clu} + (1.96)[\widehat{SE}(r_{clu})]$$
$$.2222 - (1.96)(.1808) \le R \le .2222 + (1.96)(.1808)$$
$$0 \le R \le .5765$$

11.3 SAMPLING DISTRIBUTIONS OF ESTIMATES

Total number of possible samples

Let us consider a simple two-stage cluster sample in which m clusters are chosen at the first stage from the M clusters in the population, and within each sample cluster $\bar{n}$ listing units are sampled from the $\bar{N}$ listing units in the cluster. The total number of possible samples is given by

$$\binom{M}{m}\binom{\bar{N}}{\bar{n}}^{m}$$

For example, refer to the data in table 11.1. If we wish to take a simple two-stage cluster sample of two health centers from the five in the population as the first-stage sample, and two nurse practitioners from the three available within each sample health center as the second-stage sample, we can select

$$\binom{5}{2}\binom{3}{2}^{2} = 10 \times 3^2 = 90 \text{ possible samples}$$

From each of these 90 samples, we can estimate population characteristics such as totals, means, and ratios.

The estimated means are unbiased estimates

In this section we discuss properties of the sampling distributions of the estimated population characteristics. In particular, the means, $E(x'_{\text{clu}})$, $E(\bar{x}_{\text{clu}})$, and $E(\bar{\bar{x}}_{\text{clu}})$, of the sampling distributions of estimated totals x'_{clu}, means per cluster $\bar{x}_{\text{clu}}$, and means per listing unit $\bar{\bar{x}}_{\text{clu}}$ are equal to the corresponding population parameters $(X, \bar{X}, \text{and } \bar{\bar{X}})$, as defined in box 10.1. In other words, these are unbiased estimates. Estimated ratios r_{clu}, on the other hand, are not unbiased, but as discussed earlier for other sample designs, their biases are generally small for reasonably large sample sizes. The theoretical standard errors of these estimates are given next in box 11.3.

Thus we see that the sampling variance of estimated means and totals from simple two-stage cluster sampling consist of two terms, one depending on the value of σ^2_{1x}, the variance among clusters of the distribution of cluster totals X_i, and the other depending on σ^2_{2x}, a term representing the variance among listing units with respect to the level of the characteristic $\mathcal{X}$ for the listing units. These terms are known as **first-stage** and **second-stage components,** respectively. If every cluster is included in the sample—or, in other words, if $m = M$—then the first-stage components in the expressions shown in box 11.3 drop out since the factor $(M - m)/(M - 1)$ becomes zero. This makes sense intuitively, because if every cluster is included in the sample, then sampling variability due to differences among the clusters should not be a factor in the sampling distribution of estimates. The resulting estimates are then identical to those for stratified sampling. Similarly, if within each sample cluster, every listing unit is included in the sample—or, in other words, if $\bar{n} = \bar{N}$—then the second-stage components in the expressions shown in box 11.3 drop out since the factor $(\bar{N} - \bar{n})/(\bar{N} - 1)$

Box 11.3 Standard Errors for Population Estimates Under Simple Two-Stage Cluster Sampling

Total, x'_{clu}

$$\mathrm{SE}(x'_{\mathrm{clu}}) = \left[\left(\frac{M^2}{m} \right)(\sigma^2_{1x})\left(\frac{M - m}{M - 1} \right) + \left(\frac{N^2}{n} \right)(\sigma^2_{2x})\left(\frac{\bar{N} - \bar{n}}{\bar{N} - 1} \right) \right]^{1/2}$$

Mean Per Cluster, $\bar{\mathrm{x}}_{clu}$

$$\mathrm{SE}(\bar{x}_{\mathrm{clu}}) = \left[\left(\frac{\sigma^2_{1x}}{m} \right)\left(\frac{M - m}{M - 1} \right) + \left(\frac{\bar{N}^2}{n} \right)(\sigma^2_{2x})\left(\frac{\bar{N} - \bar{n}}{\bar{N} - 1} \right) \right]^{1/2}$$

Mean Per Element, $\bar{\bar{\mathrm{x}}}_{clu}$

$$\mathrm{SE}(\bar{\bar{x}}_{\mathrm{clu}}) = \left[\left(\frac{1}{\bar{N}^2} \right)\left(\frac{\sigma^2_{1x}}{m} \right)\left(\frac{M - m}{M - 1} \right) + \left(\frac{\sigma^2_{2x}}{n} \right)\left(\frac{\bar{N} - \bar{n}}{\bar{N} - 1} \right) \right]^{1/2}$$

Ratio, r_{clu}

$$\mathrm{SE}(r_{\mathrm{clu}}) \approx (R)\left[\left(\frac{\sigma^2_{1R}}{m\bar{X}^2} \right)\left(\frac{M - m}{M - 1} \right) + \left(\frac{\sigma^2_{2R}}{m\bar{n}\bar{\bar{X}}^2} \right)\left(\frac{\bar{N} - \bar{n}}{\bar{N} - 1} \right) \right]^{1/2}$$

The expression σ^2_{1x} appearing in these formulas is the variance among cluster totals, defined in chapter 10, equation (10.1), as

$$\sigma^2_{1x} = \frac{\sum\limits_{i=1}^{M} (X_i - \bar{X})^2}{M}$$

The expression σ^2_{2x} appearing in these expressions is given by

$$\sigma^2_{2x} = \frac{\sum\limits_{i=1}^{M} \sum\limits_{j=1}^{\bar{N}} (X_{ij} - \bar{\bar{X}}_i)^2}{N} \tag{11.1}$$

where $\bar{\bar{X}}_i$ is the mean level of characteristic $\mathscr{X}$ per listing unit for those listing units in cluster i, as given by

$$\bar{\bar{X}}_i = \frac{\sum\limits_{j=1}^{\bar{N}} X_{ij}}{\bar{N}}$$

The formula for the approximate standard error of an estimated ratio r_{clu} is an approximation that is valid whenever the coefficient of variation, $V(\bar{y}_{\mathrm{clu}})$, of the denominator of the ratio is less than .05. The

---

Box 11.3 (*continued*)

parameters σ_{1R}^2 and σ_{2R}^2 appearing in the expression for SE(r_{clu}) are given by

$$\sigma_{1R}^2 = \sigma_{1y}^2 + R^2\sigma_{1x}^2 - 2R\sigma_{1xy} \qquad (11.2)$$

$$\sigma_{2R}^2 = \sigma_{2y}^2 + R^2\sigma_{2x}^2 - 2R\sigma_{2xy} \qquad (11.3)$$

where the expressions σ_{1xy} and σ_{2xy} are first- and second-stage covariances given by

$$\sigma_{1xy} = \frac{\sum\limits_{i=1}^{M}(X_i - \bar{X})(Y_i - \bar{Y})}{M} \qquad (11.4)$$

$$\sigma_{2xy} = \frac{\sum\limits_{i=1}^{M}\sum\limits_{j=1}^{\bar{N}}(X_{ij} - \bar{\bar{X}}_i)(Y_{ij} - \bar{\bar{Y}}_i)}{N} \qquad (11.5)$$

Other notation used in these formulas is defined in boxes 10.1 and 11.1.

---

reduces to zero and the variances of the estimates become identical to those for simple one-stage cluster sampling, shown in box 10.3. Again, this makes sense intuitively since within each sample cluster every listing unit is included. Hence there is no second stage of sampling and the process is in reality single-stage cluster sampling.

Now let us illustrate the use of the formulas of box 11.3 in an example.

ILLUSTRATIVE EXAMPLE

Calculations using formulas of box 11.3

Let us consider the population shown in table 11.1. Some preliminary calculations for this population are given in table 11.3; for all calculations we have

$$M = 5, \qquad \bar{N} = 3, \qquad N = 15$$

Based on the information in table 11.3 and the formulas in box 11.3, we can make the following calculations:

$$\sigma_{1x}^2 = \frac{2837.20}{5} = 567.44 \qquad \sigma_{1y}^2 = \frac{677.2}{5} = 135.44 \qquad \sigma_{1xy} = \frac{-830.80}{5} = -166.16$$

Table 11.3 Worksheet for Calculations Involving Cluster Totals

Cluster	X_i	Y_i	$(X_i - \bar{X})^2$	$(Y_i - \bar{Y})^2$	$(X_i - \bar{X})(Y_i - \bar{Y})$
1	120	17	1267.36	179.56	−477.04
2	105	24	424.36	40.96	−131.84
3	68	48	268.96	309.76	−288.64
4	58	23	696.96	54.76	195.36
5	71	40	179.56	92.16	−128.64
	$X = 422$	$Y = 152$	2837.20	677.20	−830.80
	$\bar{X} = 84.4$	$\bar{Y} = 30.4$			
	$\bar{\bar{X}} = 28.13$	$\bar{\bar{Y}} = 10.13$			

Now we consider the calculations for the listing units. Some preliminary calculations are shown in table 11.4.

Table 11.4 Worksheet for Calculations Involving Listing Units

Cluster	j	X_{ij}	$\bar{X}_i$	$(X_{ij} - \bar{X}_i)^2$	Y_{ij}	$\bar{Y}_i$	$(Y_{ij} - \bar{Y}_i)^2$	$(X_{ij} - \bar{X}_i)(Y_{ij} - \bar{Y}_i)$
1	1	58		324	5		.45	−12.07
	2	44	40	16	6	5.67	.11	1.32
	3	18		484	6		.11	−7.26
2	1	42		49	3		25	−35
	2	53	35	324	19	8	121	198
	3	10		625	2		36	150
3	1	13		93.51	12		16	38.68
	2	18	22.67	21.81	6	16	100	46.70
	3	37		205.35	30		196	200.62
4	1	16		11.09	5		7.13	8.89
	2	32	19.33	160.53	14	7.67	40.07	80.20
	3	10		87.05	4		13.47	34.24
5	1	25		1.77	17		13.47	4.88
	2	23	23.67	0.45	9	13.33	18.75	2.90
	3	23		0.45	14		.45	−.45
				2404.01			588.01	711.65

Using the information in table 11.4, we have the following calculations:

$$\sigma_{2x}^2 = \frac{2404.01}{15} = 160.27 \qquad \sigma_{2y}^2 = \frac{588.01}{15} = 39.20 \qquad \sigma_{2xy} = \frac{711.65}{15} = 47.44$$

Using the formula given in box 11.3, we can calculate the theoretical standard error $SE(x'_{clu})$ of x'_{clu}, the total number of patients seen by the 15 nurse practitioners as estimated from the two-stage cluster sample of two centers and two nurses within each sample center.

$$SE(x'_{clu}) = \left[\left(\frac{5^2}{2}\right)(567.44)\left(\frac{5-2}{5-1}\right) + \left(\frac{15^2}{4}\right)(160.27)\left(\frac{3-2}{3-1}\right) \right]^{1/2} = 99.13$$

Similarly, the theoretical standard errors of $\bar{x}_{clu}$, $\bar{\bar{x}}_{clu}$, y'_{clu}, $\bar{y}_{clu}$, and $\bar{\bar{y}}_{clu}$ can be obtained by substituting the parameters calculated in tables 11.3 and 11.4 into the appropriate expressions given in box 11.3.

11.4 HOW LARGE A SAMPLE IS NEEDED?

$\bar{n}$ *determined on bases of costs and sizes of first- and second-stage variances*

In simple two-stage cluster sampling, as we will see in a later section, the desired number $\bar{n}$ of listing units to be selected at the second stage from each cluster sampled at the first stage is determined on the basis of costs and on the basis of the relative sizes of the first- and second-stage variance components (e.g., σ_{1x}^2, σ_{2x}^2). Once the number $\bar{n}$ has been fixed, we might then wish to determine the total number m of clusters to be selected at the first stage of sampling in order to be $100(1 - \alpha)\%$ confident of obtaining estimates that differ by no more than ε from the true value of the population characteristic being estimated. The formulas used to calculate the **number m of clusters sampled** that would satisfy these specifications are given below.

For estimated **totals** (x'_{clu}) or **means** $(\bar{x}_{clu}, \bar{\bar{x}}_{clu})$,

m *is number of clusters sampled*

$$m = \frac{\left(\dfrac{\sigma_{1x}^2}{\bar{X}^2}\right)\left(\dfrac{M}{M-1}\right) + \left(\dfrac{1}{\bar{n}}\right)\left(\dfrac{\sigma_{2x}^2}{\bar{\bar{X}}^2}\right)\left(\dfrac{\bar{N}-\bar{n}}{\bar{N}-1}\right)}{\dfrac{\varepsilon^2}{z_{1-\alpha/2}^2} + \dfrac{\sigma_{1x}^2}{\bar{X}^2(M-1)}} \qquad (11.6)$$

and for estimated **ratios** $(r_{clu} = x/y)$,

$$m = \frac{\left(\dfrac{\sigma_{1R}^2}{\bar{X}^2}\right)\left(\dfrac{M}{M-1}\right) + \left(\dfrac{1}{\bar{n}}\right)\left(\dfrac{\sigma_{2R}^2}{(\bar{\bar{X}})^2}\right)\left(\dfrac{\bar{N}-\bar{n}}{\bar{N}-1}\right)}{\dfrac{\varepsilon^2}{z_{1-\alpha/2}^2} + \dfrac{\sigma_{1R}^2}{\bar{X}^2(M-1)}} \qquad (11.7)$$

ILLUSTRATIVE EXAMPLE

Let us suppose that from the population of nurse practitioners shown in table 11.1, we wish to take a two-stage cluster sample with two practitioners chosen at the second stage from each health center selected at the first stage. Let us suppose that we wish to be 95%

confident of obtaining an estimate x'_{clu}, the total number of patients seen by nurse practitioners, that is within 30% of the true value and an estimate r_{clu}, the proportion of these patients referred to a physician, that is also within 30% of the true value. From earlier computations we have

$$\sigma_{1x}^2 = 567.44 \qquad \sigma_{2x}^2 = 160.27 \qquad \bar{X} = 84.4$$

$$\bar{\bar{X}} = 28.13 \qquad M = 5 \qquad \bar{N} = 3$$

Since $\bar{n} = 2$ and $\varepsilon = .3$, we have from relation (11.6)

$$m = \frac{\left[\dfrac{567.44}{(84.4)^2}\right]\left(\dfrac{5}{5-1}\right) + \left(\dfrac{1}{2}\right)\left[\dfrac{160.27}{(28.13)^2}\right]\left(\dfrac{3-2}{3-1}\right)}{\dfrac{(.3)^2}{(1.96)^2} + \dfrac{567.44}{(84.4)^2(5-1)}} = 3.47$$

That is, four clusters must be selected.

Using information determined in the previous example, we have

$$R = \frac{Y}{X} = \frac{152}{422} = .3602$$

$$\sigma_{1R}^2 = \sigma_{1y}^2 + R^2\sigma_{1x}^2 - 2R\sigma_{1xy}$$

$$= 135.44 + (.3602)^2(567.44) - 2(.3602)(-166.16) = 328.76$$

$$\sigma_{2R}^2 = \sigma_{2y}^2 + R^2\sigma_{2x}^2 - 2R\sigma_{2xy}$$

$$= 39.20 + (.3602)^2(160.27) - 2(.3602)(47.44) = 25.82$$

Then from relation (11.7), we have

$$m = \frac{\left[\dfrac{328.76}{(84.4)^2}\right]\left(\dfrac{5}{5-1}\right) + \left(\dfrac{1}{2}\right)\left[\dfrac{25.82}{(28.13)^2}\right]\left(\dfrac{3-2}{3-1}\right)}{\dfrac{(.3)^2}{(1.96)^2} + \dfrac{328.76}{(84.4)^2(5-1)}} = 1.88$$

That is, two clusters must be selected.

Thus we would need a first-stage sample of four health centers in order to be 95% confident that the estimated total number of persons seen by nurse practitioners (x'_{clu}) meets the stated specifications. However, we would need a sample of only two health centers in order to be 95% confident that the estimated proportion referred to a physician (r_{clu}) meets the stated specifications. Therefore, we would take a sample of four health centers if we wish both of these estimates to meet the given specifications.

In practice, the parameters σ_{1x}^2, σ_{2x}^2, and so forth, which are needed for determination of the required number m of sample clusters, are rarely known and must be either estimated from available data or guessed from experience or intuition.

11.5 CHOOSING THE OPTIMAL CLUSTER SIZE $\bar{n}$ CONSIDERING COSTS

We must consider both m and $\bar{n}$

Suppose that we wish to choose, from among several sample designs, that design which meets, at the lowest cost, the specifications set on the reliability of the estimates, and suppose that we wish to investigate simple two-stage cluster sampling as a possible design. Simple two-stage cluster sampling, however, is a class of designs characterized by a first-stage number m of clusters and a second-stage number $\bar{n}$ of listing units. The problem, then, is to investigate which combination of m and $\bar{n}$ would meet the required specifications at the lowest cost. Let us explore this problem through an example.

ILLUSTRATIVE EXAMPLE

Let us use the population of five housing projects shown in table 10.1 (p. 172). We have already discussed the cost components associated with this example for simple random sampling, stratified random sampling, and simple one-stage cluster sampling. In particular, we showed that for simple one-stage cluster sampling, the approximate field costs C are determined by the following function [equation (10.3)]:

$$C = C'_1 m + C'_2 m \bar{N}$$

The **field costs** for a two-stage simple cluster sample can be approximated by a similar function of the form

Cost function for simple two-stage cluster sampling

$$C = C^*_1 m + C^*_2 m \bar{n} \qquad (11.8)$$

where C^*_1 is composed of the cost of traveling to each sample cluster for the purpose of listing the $\bar{N}$ sampling units, the cost of listing and selecting a sample of $\bar{n}$ of the $\bar{N}$ sampling units from each list, and the cost of traveling back to the cluster to do the interviewing. C^*_2 is the cost of interviewing each of the sampling units selected.

In the example considered in chapter 10, it cost .5 person-hour to travel to each of the sample clusters. Suppose it costs 1 person-hour to list the 20 sampling units in the selected clusters and to then select a random sample of these sampling units, and it costs .5 person-hour to return to the cluster for the purpose of interviewing. Hence $C^*_1 = .5 + 1.00 + .5 = 2.00$. Also, as in the example of chapter 10, the cost of interviewing each of the sampled households is .25 person-hour. Hence $C^*_2 = .25$. The cost function (11.8) then becomes

$$C = 2.00m + .25m\bar{n}$$

Note that the expression $m\bar{N}$ appearing in the second term of relation (10.3) is the total number of listing units included in the sample for the simple one-stage cluster sampling design. Likewise, the expression $m\bar{n}$ appearing in the second term of relation (11.8) is the number of listing units included in the sample for the simple two-stage cluster sampling design. Thus the cost functions. (10.3) and (11.8) are very similar.

Suppose that we wish to estimate the total number of persons in the five housing developments and we wish to be virtually certain that this estimate will be within 25% of the true value. Let us examine, using relation (11.6), the number of clusters m required to meet this specification for various second-stage cluster sizes $\bar{n}$. Then we will use relation (11.8) to determine the field costs for each of these designs. Those designs that satisfy the specification are listed in table 11.5.

Calculations for estimating total

Table 11.5   Designs Satisfying Specification on Total

Number of Listing Units Taken in Second State, n̄	*Number of Clusters m Needed to Meet Specification ε = .25*	*Field Cost (in person-hours), C = 2.0m + .25mn̄*
6	5	17.5
7	4	15.0
8	4	16.0
9	3	12.75
10	3	13.5
11	3	14.25
12	2	10.0
13	2	10.5
14	2	11.0
15	2	11.5
16	2	12.0
17	2	12.5
18	2	13.0
19	1	6.75
20	1	7.0

To illustrate how some of the computations in table 11.5 are made, let us consider a simple two-stage cluster sampling design with the number of households to be sampled set equal to 5 (i.e., $\bar{n} = 5$). From table 10.1 we can calculate the following:

$$\sigma_{1y}^2 = 6.8 \qquad \bar{Y} = 34 \qquad \sigma_{2y}^2 = .693$$
$$\bar{\bar{Y}} = 1.7 \qquad M = 5 \qquad \bar{N} = 20$$

Then from relation (11.6) we have

$$m = \frac{\left[\dfrac{6.8}{(34)^2}\right]\left(\dfrac{5}{5-1}\right) + \left(\dfrac{1}{5}\right)\left[\dfrac{.693}{(1.7)^2}\right]\left(\dfrac{20-5}{20-1}\right)}{\dfrac{(.25)^2}{9} + \dfrac{6.8}{(34)^2(5-1)}} = 5.23$$

That is, six clusters must be selected. Thus it would take a sample of six clusters to meet the specification. Since there are only five clusters in the population, it would be impossible for the specification to be met if $\bar{n} = 5$.

Let us now set $\bar{n} = 6$. From relation (11.6) we have

$$m = \frac{\left[\dfrac{6.8}{(34)^2}\right]\left(\dfrac{5}{5-1}\right) + \left(\dfrac{1}{6}\right)\left[\dfrac{.693}{(1.7)^2}\right]\left(\dfrac{20-6}{20-1}\right)}{\dfrac{(.25)^2}{9} + \dfrac{6.8}{(34)^2(5-1)}} = 4.37$$

That is, five clusters must be selected. Thus a sample of $m = 5$ clusters (i.e., every cluster in the population) would meet the specification if $\bar{n} = 6$. The field costs of such a sample design are

$$C = (2.0)(5) + (.25)(5)(6) = 17.5 \text{ person-hours}$$

Among all the simple cluster sample designs listed in table 11.5 that satisfy the specifications, the design characterized by a first-stage sample of $m = 1$ cluster followed by a second-stage sample $\bar{n} = 19$ listing units would do so at the lowest field cost (i.e., 6.75 person-hours) and hence would be the design of choice.

Calculations for estimating ratio

If we wished to estimate a ratio—for example, the proportion R of all persons requiring the services of a visiting nurse—we would go through the same process except that we would use relation (11.7) rather than relation (11.6). If we set $\varepsilon = .25$ again, the two-stage cluster designs listed in table 11.6 would satisfy this specification on the estimated ratio.

Table 11.6   Designs Satisfying Specification on Ratio

Number of Listing Units Taken in Second State, $\bar{n}$	Number of Clusters m Needed to Meet Specification $\varepsilon = .25$	Field Cost (in person-hours), $C = 2.0m + .25m\bar{n}$
12	5	25
13	5	26.25
14	5	27.50
15	5	28.75
16	5	30
17	5	31.25
18	5	32.5
19	5	35
20	5	35

From the data in table 10.1 we can calculate the following values in order to determine the costs given in table 11.6: $X = 60$, $Y = 170$, $R = .35294$, $\sigma_{1x}^2 = 23.6$, $\sigma_{1y}^2 = 6.8$, $\sigma_{1xy} = 2.6$, $\sigma_{2y}^2 = .693$, $\sigma_{2x}^2 = .321$, $\sigma_{2xy} = .1435$, $\sigma_{1R}^2 = 22.61$, $\sigma_{2R}^2 = .3060$.

Examining table 11.6, we see that a two-stage cluster sample with all five housing developments sampled at the first stage and 12 households sampled from each housing development at the second stage would be the design that would satisfy, at the lowest field costs, the specification set for estimation of the proportion R of persons requiring the services of a visiting nurse.

11.6 SOME SHORTCUT FORMULAS FOR DETERMINING THE OPTIMAL NUMBER $\bar{n}$

In the previous section we chose the values of $\bar{n}$ and m that would meet the specifications at the lowest possible field costs as follows: We enumerated all possible combinations of m and $\bar{n}$, eliminating those combinations that would not meet the specifications [by use of relations (11.6) or (11.7)]. Then from among those designs remaining we chose the one that would meet the specifications at the lowest possible cost. This process can be very tedious, especially if M and $\bar{N}$ are large numbers.

There is a shortcut formula that can be used for choosing the optimal value of $\bar{n}$. It is useful if the field costs can be approximated by a function of the form $C_1^* m + C_2^* m\bar{n}$ and if the number of clusters M in the population is large in comparison with the number of clusters chosen in the sample. This formula (valid for estimating means or totals) is

$$\bar{n} = \sqrt{\left(\frac{C_1^*}{C_2^*}\right)\left(\frac{1 - \delta_x}{\delta_x}\right)}$$ (11.9) ***Shortcut formula (means or totals)***

where C_1^* and C_2^* are the cost components introduced earlier and δ_x is the **intraclass correlation coefficient** defined previously in our discussion of systematic sampling [equation (4.5)]. It can be expressed in the form

$$\delta_x = \frac{(1/\bar{N})\sigma_{1x}^2 - \sigma_x^2}{(\bar{N} - 1)\sigma_x^2}$$ (11.10)

which is algebraically identical to expression (4.5) provided that the number of listing units N_i are the same for each cluster.

Once the optimal cluster size $\bar{n}$ is obtained from relation (11.9), the number m of clusters to be selected at the first stage is then obtained from relation (11.6).

For estimation of ratios, relations (11.9) and (11.10) are modified as follows:

$$\bar{n} = \sqrt{\left(\frac{C_1^*}{C_2^*}\right)\left(\frac{1 - \delta_R}{\delta_R}\right)}$$ (11.11) ***Shortcut formula (ratios)***

where

$$\delta_R = \frac{(1/\bar{N})\sigma_{1R}^2 - \sigma_R^2}{(\bar{N} - 1)\sigma_R^2}$$ (11.12)

To illustrate these concepts, let us consider the following example.

ILLUSTRATIVE EXAMPLE

Suppose that a survey is to be taken in a general hospital for purposes of estimating the total amount of money billed to Medicare during a particular quarter (13 weeks). A cluster sample is to be taken by taking a simple random sample of weeks followed by a simple random sample of days within each selected week. For each day chosen in the sample, the amount billed to Medicare is obtained by a review of all items billed during that day. The data for the entire quarter (not known, of course, in advance of the survey) are shown, by days, in table 11.7.

With weeks as clusters, days as listing units, and X as the amount billed to Medicare on a particular day, we have the following calculations:

$$\sigma_x^2 = \frac{\sum_{i=1}^{13} \sum_{j=1}^{7} (X_{ij} - \bar{\bar{X}})^2}{91} = 1{,}304.58 \qquad \sigma_{1x}^2 = \frac{\sum_{i=1}^{13} (X_i - \bar{X})^2}{13} = 26{,}624.44$$

$$\bar{\bar{X}} = 110.45 \qquad \bar{X} = 773.15 \qquad \sigma_{2x}^2 = 761.22$$

$$M = 13 \qquad \bar{N} = 7 \qquad N = 91$$

$$\delta_x = \frac{(1/7)(26{,}624.44) - 1{,}304.58}{(7 - 1)(1{,}304.58)} = .3192$$

Let us now consider the field costs that might be involved in collecting the data. For each day selected in the sample it would be necessary to obtain data pertaining to the amount billed on that day to Medicare for each patient hospitalized. This could take a considerable amount of record retrieval and abstracting. Let us assume that there are an average of five patients per day in the hospital who are covered by Medicare and that for each patient .5 hour of time is required for retrieval and abstracting on the part of a research associate who is paid $4.00 per hour. In addition, let us assume that for each patient it costs approximately $3.00 to code the data, prepare it for the computer, and process it. Then the total cost C_2^* per listing unit (day) selected in the sample is given by

$$C_2^* = (5 \text{ patients per day}) \times (2.00 + 3.00) \text{ per patient} = \$25 \text{ per day}$$

Let us suppose that patient cost records are organized on computer tape by week and that for each week chosen in the sample the *entire week's* records must be listed by computer in order for the daily costs to be identified and that this costs $50 in computer time. Let us assume that other costs associated with the clusters (weeks) are negligible, so that the cost component C_1^* is given by

$$C_1^* = \$50 \text{ per sample week}$$

Since $\delta \approx .32$ for these data, we have the optimal cluster size $\bar{n}$ given by

$$\bar{n} = \sqrt{\left(\frac{50}{25}\right)\left(\frac{.68}{.32}\right)} \approx 2$$

Table 11.7 Amount of Money Billed to Medicare by Day and Week

| | AMOUNT BILLED ($\times \$10$) | | | | | | | | |
Week	Sunday	Monday	Tuesday	Wednesday	Thursday	Friday	Saturday	X_i	$\sum(X_{ij} - \bar{X}_i)^2$
1	121	88	138	69	85	59	63	623	5418
2	152	105	179	127	145	116	165	989	4273.43
3	134	62	44	128	92	127	141	728	8882
4	94	123	81	109	110	101	34	652	5134.86
5	210	182	120	120	154	98	178	1062	9907.43
6	104	100	70	115	142	139	131	801	3929.71
7	80	43	59	50	20	69	64	385	2312
8	123	59	140	146	149	109	111	837	5847.71
9	137	168	84	120	123	87	121	840	4988
10	110	132	104	65	97	98	84	690	2619.71
11	158	114	93	147	91	125	132	860	3890.86
12	79	156	142	154	133	74	83	821	8219.43
13	97	96	110	83	89	146	142	763	3848

Then from relation (11.6) with $M = 13, \bar{n} = 2, \sigma_{1x}^2 = 26{,}624.44, \sigma_{2x}^2 = 761.22, \bar{\bar{X}} = 110.45,$ $\bar{X} = 773.15$, and $\bar{N} = 7$, if we wish to be virtually certain of estimating the total amount of money billed to Medicare during the quarter to within 25% of the true value (i.e., $\varepsilon = .25$), we have

$$m = \frac{\left[\dfrac{26{,}624.44}{(773.15)^2}\right]\left(\dfrac{13}{13 - 1}\right) + \left(\dfrac{1}{2}\right)\left[\dfrac{761.22}{(110.45)^2}\right]\left(\dfrac{7 - 2}{7 - 1}\right)}{\dfrac{(.25)^2}{9} + \dfrac{26{,}624.44}{(773.15)^2(13 - 1)}} = 6.97$$

Hence seven clusters must be selected.

Thus with a two-stage cluster sample of $m = 7$ weeks and $\bar{n} = 2$ days, the specifications can be met at minimal cost in relation to other two-stage cluster designs. This can be verified by examining the costs of other cluster designs meeting these specifications, as shown in table 11.8.

Table 11.8   Designs Satisfying Specification on Total

Number of Listing Units in Sample, $\bar{n}$	Number of Clusters, m Needed to Meet Specification $\varepsilon = .25$	Field Costs, $C = 50m + 25m\bar{n}$
1	10	750
2	7	700
3	7	875
4	6	900
5	6	1050
6	6	1200
7	6	1350

δ_x is useful in two procedures

The intraclass correlation coefficient δ_x is a parameter that is very important in sampling theory. It is useful, as shown above, in determining the optimal number of listing units that should be selected at the second stage of cluster sampling. It is also useful in relating the standard error of an estimated mean or total from a two-stage cluster sample to one that would have been obtained from a simple random sample of the same number n of listing units. If the number M of clusters in the population is large in comparison to the number selected at the first stage of sampling, then the following relations are true:

Formulas relating standard errors and δ_x

$$\text{SE}(x'_{\text{clu}}) = \left(\frac{N\sigma_x}{\sqrt{n}}\right)\sqrt{1 + \delta_x(\bar{n} - 1)} \qquad (11.13)$$

$$\text{SE}(\bar{x}_{\text{clu}}) = \left(\frac{N\sigma_x}{\sqrt{M}\sqrt{n}}\right)\sqrt{1 + \delta_x(\bar{n} - 1)} \qquad (11.14)$$

$$\text{SE}(\bar{\bar{x}}_{\text{clu}}) = \left(\frac{\sigma_x}{\sqrt{n}}\right)\sqrt{1 + \delta_x(\bar{n} - 1)} \qquad (11.15)$$

These relations are important because they show that the standard errors of estimated means and totals obtained from cluster samples are approximately $\sqrt{1 + \delta_x(\bar{n} - 1)}$ times as large as those obtained from a simple random sample of the same number n of listing units. This factor, $\sqrt{1 + \delta_x(\bar{n} - 1)}$, is known as the **design effect** and depends on the intraclass correlation coefficient δ_x as well as the number $\bar{n}$ of listing units selected in the sample.

It can be seen by some algebraic manipulation of relation (11.10) that the intraclass correlation coefficient δ_x is a number lying between $-1/(\bar{N} - 1)$ and $+1$. It is essentially a measure of the homogeneity of listing units within clusters with respect to levels of the characteristic $\mathcal{X}$ being measured. If listing units within clusters tend to be similar in this respect, the value of δ_x will tend to be high and the design effect $\sqrt{1 + \delta_x(\bar{n} - 1)}$ would be potentially high if $\bar{n}$ were large. This makes sense intuitively, because a high value of δ_x implies that taking a large number of listing units within a sample cluster would be a wasteful procedure, since the listing units within clusters are similar with respect to levels of the characteristic $\mathcal{X}$ being measured.

δ_x essentially measures homogeneity of listing units

Knowledge of the value of δ_x for different types of clusters and different variables is extremely useful in planning surveys, and more detailed discussion of this is available in more advanced books on sampling (1, 2).

11.7 SYSTEMATIC SAMPLING AS CLUSTER SAMPLING

A systematic sample of one in M listing units beginning with a random start, as described in chapter 4, is in reality a single-stage cluster sample in which only one PSU is sampled. This is evident if we consider the listing units (numbered as they appear on the list) as being grouped into the following M clusters:

CLUSTER	LISTING UNITS
1	$1, 1 + M, 1 + 2M, 1 + 3M, \ldots$
2	$2, 2 + M, 2 + 2M, 2 + 3M, \ldots$
3	$3, 3 + M, 3 + 2M, 3 + 3M, \ldots$
$\vdots$	$\vdots$
$M - 1$	$M - 1, 2M - 1, 3M - 1, 4M - 1, \ldots$
M	$M, 2M, 3M, 4M, \ldots$

For simplicity, let us assume that the number N of listing units is exactly divisible by M so that each of the clusters listed above contains $\bar{N} = N/M$ listing units. Then if the random number chosen to start the systematic sampling is one, the sample will consist of every listing unit in cluster 1—that is, listing units, 1, $1 + M$, $1 + 2M$, $1 + (\bar{N} - 1)M$. Likewise, if the random number is 2, the sample will consist of all listing units in cluster 2; and so on. Thus the theory of systematic sampling with a random start is a special case of single-stage cluster sampling with $m = 1$ and $\bar{n} = \bar{N}$.

SUMMARY

In this chapter we developed the basic concepts of simple two-stage cluster sampling for situations in which each cluster in the population contains the same number of enumeration units or listing units. Simple two-stage cluster sampling involves first taking a simple random sample of clusters and then within each of these selected clusters taking a simple random sample of $\bar{n}$ listing units. We developed methods for estimating means, totals, and ratios under simple two-stage cluster sampling, and we discussed the sampling distributions of these estimates. In addition, we developed methods for estimating, from the data obtained in the sample, the standard errors of these estimates.

We discussed the determination of the sample size required to meet specifications set for the reliability of estimates. Strategies were developed for choosing the optimal number $\bar{n}$ of listing units to be selected at the second stage taking costs into consideration. We introduced the intraclass correlation coefficient as an index of the homogeneity among listing units within sample clusters with respect to a characteristic $\mathscr{X}$ being measured. This index is an important determinant of the optimal number of listing units $\bar{n}$ that should be sampled at the second stage as well as a determinant of the standard errors of estimates obtained from two-stage cluster sampling. We also introduced the concept of the design effect and discussed it briefly. Finally, we showed that systematic sampling is, in reality, simple one-stage cluster sampling with one cluster selected from the population.

EXERCISES

1. Suppose that Chicago is divided into 75 community areas and that each community area contains 20 retail pharmacies. Suppose that you wish to estimate the average prices charged for some standard prescription drugs by taking a simple random sample of eight community areas followed by a simple random sample of four pharmacies within each of the eight community areas selected.

   (a) Prepare a simple cost function for estimating the overall survey cost including the field costs. Specify each of the cost components.

   (b) How would the total cost indicated above be affected if 16 community areas and two pharmacies per community area were selected?

(c) Suppose it is guessed that the standard deviation σ among all stores in Chicago with respect to the price of a certain drug is $0.75 and that the average cost of this drug in Chicago is $5.00. Using the cost function you specified in part (a), determine the optimum value of $\bar{n}$ if the intraclass correlation coefficient is equal to .35. What then would be the coefficient of variation of the estimate if six PSUs were used?

2. (a) Suppose that the elementary schools in a city were grouped into 30 school districts with each school district containing ten schools. Suppose that a simple random sample of three school districts was taken and that within each sample school district a simple random sample of four schools was taken for purposes of estimating the number of school-children in the city that are color-blind (as measured by a standard test). The data shown in the accompanying table were obtained from this sample. Estimate and obtain a 95% confidence interval for the total number of color-blind schoolchildren in the city.

(b) Estimate and obtain a 95% confidence interval for the proportion of schoolchildren in the city who are color-blind.

Sample School District	Sample School	Number of Children	Number of Color-blind Children
1	1	130	2
	2	150	3
	3	160	3
	4	120	5
2	1	110	2
	2	120	4
	3	100	0
	4	120	1
3	1	89	4
	2	130	2
	3	100	0
	4	150	2

3. A simple random sample requires 400 listing units in order for estimated means and totals to meet specifications of precision. If all PSUs have the same number $\bar{N}$ of listing units, how large a simple cluster sample with cluster size $\bar{n}$ equal to 4 would be needed to achieve the same precision when the intraclass correlation coefficient is equal to .6?

4. Suppose that during the peak season the number of visitors to a state park and the number of injuries occurring among these visitors are as given in the accompanying table by week and day. (The park is closed on Fridays.)

	NUMBER OF VISITORS						NUMBER OF INJURIES					
Week	Su	M	Tu	W	Th	Sa	Su	M	Tu	W	Th	Sa
1	200	150	130	140	150	190	2	3	1	4	3	8
2	120	105	111	103	111	130	1	0	0	1	0	3
3	310	200	180	130	125	208	4	0	1	0	1	3
4	200	107	101	98	103	137	3	0	2	0	1	8
5	170	160	130	121	107	114	3	0	0	1	0	5
6	250	237	209	212	231	180	2	0	0	0	0	1
7	380	378	325	330	306	331	4	3	0	8	0	2
8	495	400	315	302	350	395	4	0	3	2	2	4
9	206	200	108	95	107	190	1	2	3	0	1	4
10	308	300	293	206	200	300	0	0	1	2	0	3

Suppose that a simple two-stage cluster sample was taken with weeks as clusters, days as listing units, $m = 4$, and $\bar{n} = 3$. Suppose further that at the first stage of sampling, clusters 2, 6, 8, and 10 are selected. At the second stage of sampling, listing units 2, 3, and 5 are selected within cluster 2, listing units 1, 3, and 6 are selected within cluster 6, listing units 3, 4, and 6 are selected within cluster 8, and listing units 2, 4, and 5 are selected within cluster 10. From this sample estimate and obtain 95% confidence intervals for the following:
(a) the total number of visitors during the peak season
(b) the total number of injuries during the peak season
(c) the total number of injuries and visitors per week
(d) the total number of injuries and visitors per day
(e) the number of injuries per visitor

5. Suppose that a simple one-stage cluster sample was selected from the population shown in exercise 4 and that clusters 2 and 8 were selected. From this sample compute the 95% confidence intervals for the characteristics given in (a) through (e) of exercise 4. Compare the widths of these confidence intervals with those obtained from the two-stage sampling design.

6. From the population shown in exercise 4, compute the intraclass correlation coefficient for the number of visitors to the park.

7. Using the intraclass correlation coefficient calculated in exercise 6, and assuming $C_1^* = 2C_2^*$, what would be the optimal number of days to sample in a simple two-stage cluster sample with weeks as clusters?

BIBLIOGRAPHY

The following publications contain additional discussion and examples of simple two-stage cluster sampling.

1. COCHRAN, W. G. *Sampling techniques*. 3d ed. New York: Wiley, 1977.

2. HANSEN, M. H.; HURWITZ, W. N.; and MADOW, W. G. *Sample survey methods and theory*. Vols. 1 and 2. New York: Wiley, 1953.

3. SCHEAFFER, R. L.; MENDENHALL, W.; and OTT, L. *Elementary survey sampling*. 2d ed. N. Scituate, MA: Duxbury Press, 1979.

12

Cluster Sampling from Clusters Having Unequal Numbers of Listing Units

In some surveys clusters will not have equal numbers of listing units

In chapter 11 we developed methods for taking simple two-stage cluster samples from clusters having equal numbers of listing units. In other words, the number N_i of listing units was assumed to be the same (i.e., $N_i = \bar{N}$) for each cluster in the population. In most survey situations, however, the clusters do not contain equal numbers of listing units. For example, in household surveys the city block often serves as the cluster and the household as the listing unit. For most cities the number of households is not likely to be the same in each block. Similarly, in sample surveys of hospital records, hospitals often serve as clusters with admission or discharge records serving as listing units; and the number of discharges would probably not be the same for each hospital.

In our previous discussions of cluster sampling it was possible to talk about a uniform second-stage sampling fraction f_2, which would represent the fraction of listing units sampled at the second stage from each cluster selected at the first stage. If, however, the number N_i of listing units in each cluster varies among the clusters, then this concept is not meaningful. For example, if a community has 6 city blocks containing 20, 23, 25, 27, 28, and 35 households, it would not be possible to define a 40% sample of households in each block since a 40% sample of 23, 27, or 28 blocks is not an integer (e.g., 40% of 23 = 9.2). With this in mind, our treatment of cluster sampling must be modified in order to be meaningful in such situations.

12.1 HOW TO TAKE A TWO-STAGE CLUSTER SAMPLE FOR THIS DESIGN

Clusters are chosen by simple random sampling

As before, the clusters will be selected by labeling them from 1 to M and then taking m random numbers between 1 and M. Those clusters corresponding to the random numbers selected will be in the sample.

But before the listing units can be selected, there should be some operational rule for determining the number n_i of listing units to be selected from a cluster containing N_i listing units. For example, we may decide to select the same number $\bar{n}$ of listing units from each sample cluster. Alternatively, we may decide to select that number n_i that would make the ratio n_i/N_i as close as possible to some predetermined number f_2, which represents the desired second-stage sampling fraction. No matter what the operational rule is, the number of listing units N_i in the selected cluster should determine uniquely the number n_i to be selected at the second stage of sampling.

Next, a rule must be specified for determining the number of listing units to be selected

With this in mind, we would label the listing units within the ith cluster selected at the first stage from 1 to N_i and choose n_i different random numbers between 1 and N_i. Those listing units corresponding to the random numbers selected would appear in the sample.

Finally, listing units are chosen by simple random sampling

We illustrate the procedure in the following example.

ILLUSTRATIVE EXAMPLE

Let us consider an administrative area containing ten hospitals, with total 1977 admissions, total 1977 admissions with life-threatening conditions, and total 1977 admissions discharged dead as given in table 12.1.

Let us suppose that we wish to take a simple random sample of three hospitals and within each selected hospital take a sample of approximately 5% of all admission records for purposes of estimating the total number of patients discharged dead among all patients admitted to these ten hospitals. To do this, we first choose three random numbers between 1 and 10 (e.g., 1, 2, and 8). We then identify each admission within each sample hospital

Table 12.1   Total Admissions, Total Admissions with Life-threatening Conditions, and Total Admissions Discharged Dead from Ten Hospitals, 1977

Hospital	Total Admissions	Total with Life-threatening Conditions	Total Discharged Dead Among Those with Life-threatening Conditions
1	4,288	501	42
2	5,036	785	78
3	1,178	213	17
4	638	173	9
5	27,010	3,404	338
6	1,122	217	17
7	2,134	424	37
8	1,824	246	18
9	4,672	778	68
10	2,154	346	27

with a number from 1 to N_i and then choose by random numbers that number n_i of admissions that makes the ratio n_i/N_i closest to .05, the desired second-stage sampling fraction. For example, in hospital 1, $N_1 = 4288$, and $(.05)(4288) = 214.4$. Thus we would take $n_1 = 214$ admissions from hospital 1. In a similar manner, we would decide to select $n_2 = 252$ admissions from hospital 2 and $n_3 = 91$ admissions from hospital 8.

12.2 ESTIMATION OF POPULATION CHARACTERISTICS FROM SIMPLE TWO-STAGE CLUSTER SAMPLING

Estimated totals, means, and ratios from this type of cluster sampling, in which there are unequal numbers N_i of listing units in each cluster, are defined in the box that follows.

Box 12.1 Estimates of Population Characteristics Under Simple Two-Stage Cluster Sampling, Unequal Numbers of Listing Units

Total, x'_{clu}

$$x'_{clu} = \left(\frac{M}{m}\right)\left(\sum_{i=1}^{m} \frac{N_i}{n_i}\right)\left(\sum_{j=1}^{n_i} x_{ij}\right)$$

Mean Per Cluster, $\bar{x}_{clu}$

$$\bar{x}_{clu} = \left(\frac{1}{m}\right)\left(\sum_{i=1}^{m} \frac{N_i}{n_i}\right)\left(\sum_{j=1}^{n_i} x_{ij}\right)$$

Mean Per Listing, $\bar{\bar{x}}_{clu}$

$$\bar{\bar{x}}_{clu} = \frac{x'_{clu}}{N}$$

This formula is usable when the total number N of listing units is known in advance of the sampling.

Ratio, r_{clu}

$$r_{clu} = \frac{\bar{x}_{clu}}{\bar{y}_{clu}}$$

where N_i is the number of listing units in each cluster, n_i is the number of listing units sampled from each cluster, and other notation is as defined in box 11.1.

Note that if the number N_i of listing units is the same for each cluster (i.e., $N_i = \bar{N}$), and if the second-stage sampling fraction is the same for each sample cluster (i.e., $n_i = \bar{n}$), then the formulas for estimates shown in box 12.1 reduce to those shown in chapter 11.

12.3 ESTIMATION OF STANDARD ERRORS OF ESTIMATES

Estimating the standard errors of estimates obtained from sampling of clusters having unequal numbers of listing units is sometimes difficult when the clusters are chosen by simple random sampling. If, however, the second-stage sampling fractions, $f_2 = n_i/N_i$, are the same for each cluster, then the ultimate cluster variance estimates given in the previous chapter can be used with minor modifications. Appropriate formulas are shown in box 12.2; the notation is that defined in box 11.1.

Box 12.2 Estimated Standard Errors of Population Estimates for Simple Two-Stage Cluster Sampling, Unequal Numbers of Listing Units

Total, X

$$\widehat{SE}(x'_{clu}) = \left(\frac{M}{\sqrt{mf_2}}\right)\left[\frac{\sum\limits_{i=1}^{m}(x_i - \bar{x})^2}{m-1}\right]^{1/2}\left(\frac{N-n}{N}\right)^{1/2}$$

Mean Per Cluster, $\bar{X}$

$$\widehat{SE}(\bar{x}_{clu}) = \left(\frac{1}{\sqrt{mf_2}}\right)\left[\frac{\sum\limits_{i=1}^{m}(x_i - \bar{x})^2}{m-1}\right]^{1/2}\left(\frac{N-n}{N}\right)^{1/2}$$

Mean Per Listing Unit, $\bar{\bar{X}}$

$$\widehat{SE}(\bar{\bar{x}}_{clu}) = \left(\frac{M}{N\sqrt{mf_2}}\right)\left[\frac{\sum\limits_{i=1}^{m}(x_i - \bar{x})^2}{m-1}\right]^{1/2}\left(\frac{N-n}{N}\right)^{1/2}$$

Ratio, R

$$\widehat{SE}(r_{clu}) = (r_{clu})\left\{\left[\frac{\widehat{SE}(\bar{x}_{clu})}{\bar{x}_{clu}}\right]^2 + \left[\frac{\widehat{SE}(\bar{y}_{clu})}{\bar{y}_{clu}}\right]^2\right.$$

$$\left. - 2\left(\frac{N-n}{N-1}\right)\left(\frac{1}{f_2^2 m\bar{x}_{clu}\bar{y}_{clu}}\right)\left[\frac{\sum\limits_{i=1}^{m}(x_i - \bar{x})(y_i - \bar{y})}{m-1}\right]\right\}^{1/2}$$

The notation used here is defined in box 11.1.

To illustrate the use of these formulas, let us look at an example.

ILLUSTRATIVE EXAMPLE

Let us suppose that a simple random sample of three hospitals was taken from the population of ten hospitals shown in table 12.1 and that a subsample of 10% (to the nearest integer) was taken from the hospitals selected in the sample. Suppose that hospitals 1, 4, and 10 were selected and that the data shown in table 12.2 were obtained. We will use these data and the formulas given above to estimate population characteristics and standard errors.

Table 12.2   Summary Data for a Sample of Three Hospitals Selected
from the Ten Hospitals in Table 12.1

Hospital	Total Admissions, N_i	Total Admissions Sampled, n_i	Total Patients with Life-threatening Conditions, y_i	Total Patients Discharged Dead Among Those with Life-threatening Conditions, x_i
1	4288	429	47	5
4	638	64	78	7
10	2154	215	24	3
Total	7080	708	149	15

Calculations using formulas in boxes 12.1 and 12.2

First we consider estimation of the total number of persons discharged dead among those having life-threatening conditions. The computations for x'_{clu} are as follows:

$$x_1 = 5 \quad N_1 = 4288 \quad n_1 = 429 \quad \left(\frac{N_1}{n_1}\right)(x_1) = 49.98$$

$$x_2 = 7 \quad N_2 = 638 \quad n_2 = 64 \quad \left(\frac{N_2}{n_2}\right)(x_2) = 69.78$$

$$x_3 = 3 \quad N_3 = 2154 \quad n_3 = 215 \quad \left(\frac{N_3}{n_3}\right)(x_3) = 30.06$$

$$M = 10 \quad m = 3$$

$$x'_{\text{clu}} = \left(\frac{M}{m}\right)\left[\sum_{i=1}^{m}\left(\frac{N_i}{n_i}\right)(x_i)\right] = \left(\frac{10}{3}\right)(49.98 + 69.78 + 30.06) = 499.38$$

The computations for $\widehat{SE}(x'_{clu})$ are

$$\bar{x} = \frac{5 + 7 + 3}{3} = 5 \qquad f_2 = .10 \qquad N = 50,056 \qquad n = 708$$

$$\frac{\sum\limits_{i=1}^{m}(x_i - \bar{x})^2}{m - 1} = \frac{(5 - 5)^2 + (7 - 5)^2 + (3 - 5)^2}{3 - 1} = 4$$

$$\widehat{SE}(x'_{clu}) = \left[\frac{10}{\sqrt{3}(.10)}\right](4)^{1/2}\left(\frac{50,056 - 708}{50,056}\right)^{1/2} = 114.65$$

A 95% confidence interval for X is

$$x'_{clu} - (1.96)[\widehat{SE}(x'_{clu})] \le X \le x'_{clu} + (1.96)[\widehat{SE}(x'_{clu})]$$
$$499.38 - (1.96)(114.65) \le X \le 499.38 + (1.96)(114.65)$$
$$274.67 \le X \le 724.09$$

Next we consider estimation of the mean number of persons discharged dead per hospital among those having life-threatening conditions. The computation of $\bar{x}_{clu}$ is

$$\bar{x}_{clu} = \left(\frac{1}{m}\right)\left[\sum\limits_{i=1}^{m}\left(\frac{N_i}{n_i}\right)(x_i)\right] = \left(\frac{1}{3}\right)(49.98 + 69.78 + 30.06) = 49.94$$

The computation of $\widehat{SE}(\bar{x}_{clu})$ is

$$\widehat{SE}(\bar{x}_{clu}) = \left[\frac{1}{\sqrt{3}(.10)}\right](4)^{1/2}\left(\frac{50,056 - 708}{50,056}\right)^{1/2} = 11.47$$

A 95% confidence interval for $\bar{X}$ is

$$\bar{x}_{clu} - (1.96)[\widehat{SE}(\bar{x}_{clu})] \le \bar{X} \le \bar{x}_{clu} + (1.96)[\widehat{SE}(\bar{x}_{clu})]$$
$$49.94 - (1.96)(11.47) \le \bar{X} \le 49.94 + (1.96)(11.47)$$
$$27.46 \le \bar{X} \le 72.42$$

Next we consider estimation of the mean number of persons discharged dead per person admitted to the hospital. The computation of $\bar{\bar{x}}_{clu}$ is

$$\bar{\bar{x}}_{clu} = \frac{x'_{clu}}{N} = \frac{499.38}{50,056} = .0098$$

The computation of $\widehat{SE}(\bar{\bar{x}}_{clu})$ is

$$\widehat{SE}(\bar{\bar{x}}_{clu}) = \left[\frac{10}{(50,056)(\sqrt{3})(.10)}\right](4)^{1/2}\left(\frac{50,056 - 708}{50,056}\right)^{1/2} = .0023$$

A 95% confidence interval for $\bar{\bar{X}}$ is

$$\bar{\bar{x}}_{clu} - (1.96)[\widehat{SE}(\bar{\bar{x}}_{clu})] \leq \bar{\bar{X}} \leq \bar{\bar{x}}_{clu} + (1.96)[\widehat{SE}(\bar{\bar{x}}_{clu})]$$

$$.0098 - (1.96)(.0023) \leq \bar{\bar{X}} \leq .0098 + (1.96)(.0023)$$

$$.0053 \leq \bar{\bar{X}} \leq .0143$$

Finally, we consider estimation of the proportion discharged dead among those having life-threatening conditions. The computations for r_{clu} are

$$\bar{y}_{clu} = \left(\frac{1}{m}\right)\left[\sum_{i=1}^{m}\left(\frac{N_i}{n_i}\right)(y_i)\right] = \left(\frac{1}{3}\right)\left[\left(\frac{4288}{429}\right)(47) + \left(\frac{638}{64}\right)(78) + \left(\frac{2154}{215}\right)(24)\right]$$

$$= 495.93$$

$$r_{clu} = \frac{\bar{x}_{clu}}{\bar{y}_{clu}} = \frac{49.94}{495.93} = .1007$$

The computations for $\widehat{SE}(r_{clu})$ are

$$\bar{y} = \frac{47 + 78 + 24}{3} = 49.67$$

$$\frac{\sum_{i=1}^{m}(y_i - \bar{y})^2}{m - 1} = \frac{(47 - 49.67)^2 + (78 - 49.67)^2 + (24 - 49.67)^2}{3 - 1}$$

$$= 734.33$$

$$\sum_{i=1}^{m}(x_i - \bar{x})(y_i - \bar{y}) = 108$$

$$\widehat{SE}(\bar{y}_{clu}) = \left[\frac{1}{\sqrt{3(.10)}}\right](734.33)^{1/2}\left(\frac{50,056 - 708}{50,056}\right)^{1/2} = 155.34$$

$$\widehat{SE}(r_{clu}) = (.1007)\left\{\left(\frac{11.47}{49.94}\right)^2 + \left(\frac{155.34}{495.93}\right)^2 - (2)\left(\frac{50,056 - 708}{50,055}\right)\right.$$

$$\left. \times \left[\frac{1}{(.10)^2(3)(49.94)(495.93)}\right]\left(\frac{108}{3 - 1}\right)\right\}^{1/2}$$

$$= .0088$$

A 95% confidence interval for R is

$$r_{clu} - (1.96)[\widehat{SE}(r_{clu})] \leq R \leq r_{clu} + (1.96)[\widehat{SE}(r_{clu})]$$

$$.1007 - (1.96)(.0088) \leq R \leq .1007 + (1.96)(.0088)$$

$$.0835 \leq R \leq .1179$$

It should be emphasized that the expressions for the estimated standard errors of estimates are applicable only if the clusters are selected by simple random sampling and the sampling fraction of listing units taken at the second stage is the same for each cluster selected in the sample. Under this allocation every listing unit in the population has the same chance of being selected in the sample. In other words, the sample is **self-weighting,** as we discussed earlier in terms of stratified sampling. For sample designs that are not self-weighting, variance estimation becomes more complicated and is beyond the scope of this book.

The formulas in 12.2 are valid only when sample is self-weighting

12.4 SAMPLING DISTRIBUTIONS OF ESTIMATES IN SIMPLE TWO-STAGE CLUSTER SAMPLING

To illustrate the sampling distributions of estimates in simple two-stage cluster sampling from clusters having unequal numbers of listing units, let us look at an example.

ILLUSTRATIVE EXAMPLE

Suppose that we wish to estimate the total number X of patients discharged dead and the proportion R of all admissions discharged dead among the ten hospitals shown in table 12.1. (It will be assumed for this example that the only deaths are among those individuals having life-threatening conditions.) Suppose (for simplicity) that we will do this by a simple one-stage cluster sample of two hospitals. The sampling distributions of the estimated total discharged dead, x'_{clu}, the estimated total admissions, y'_{clu}, and the estimated proportion of all patients discharged dead, r_{clu}, are shown in table 12.3.

The mean, standard error, and coefficient of variation of the distribution of x'_{clu} and r_{clu}, obtained by enumeration over the 45 possible samples using the techniques of chapter 2, are as follows:

$$E(x'_{clu}) = 651 \qquad E(r_{clu}) = .0134$$
$$X = 651 \qquad R = .0130$$
$$SE(x'_{clu}) = 623.313 \qquad SE(r_{clu}) = .0017$$
$$V(x'_{clu}) = .9575 \qquad V(r_{clu}) = .1308$$

Note that the estimated total discharged dead, x'_{clu}, has a very large standard error and a coefficient of variation of over 95%, whereas the estimated proportion of patients discharged dead, r_{clu}, has both a low standard error and a low coefficient of variation. This high variability among estimated totals x'_{clu} is seen clearly in its frequency distribution over the 45 samples (table 12.4). Note that only two of the 45 samples yield values of x'_{clu} that fall into the interval 600–799, which contains the true total ($X = 651$). Note also that nine of the 45 samples yield values of x'_{clu} that grossly overestimate the true total.

Table 12.3   Sampling Distribution of x'_{clu}, y'_{clu}, and r_{clu}

Hospitals in Sample	y'_{clu}	x'_{clu}	r_{clu}	Hospitals in Sample	y'_{clu}	x'_{clu}	r_{clu}
1, 2	46,620	600	.0129	3, 10	16,660	220	.0132
1, 3	27,330	295	.0108	4, 5	138,240	1,735	.0126
1, 4	24,630	255	.0104	4, 6	8,800	130	.0148
1, 5	156,490	1,900	.0121	4, 7	13,860	230	.0166
1, 6	27,050	295	.0109	4, 8	12,310	135	.0110
1, 7	32,110	395	.0123	4, 9	26,550	385	.0145
1, 8	30,560	300	.0098	4, 10	13,960	180	.0129
1, 9	44,800	550	.0123	5, 6	140,660	1,775	.0126
1, 10	32,210	345	.0107	5, 7	145,720	1,875	.0129
2, 3	31,070	475	.0153	5, 8	144,170	1,780	.0123
2, 4	28,370	435	.0153	5, 9	158,410	2,030	.0128
2, 5	160,230	2,080	.0130	5, 10	145,820	1,825	.0125
2, 6	30,790	475	.0154	6, 7	16,280	270	.0166
2, 7	35,850	575	.0160	6, 8	14,730	175	.0119
2, 8	34,300	480	.0140	6, 9	28,970	425	.0147
2, 9	48,540	730	.0150	6, 10	16,380	220	.0134
2, 10	35,950	525	.0146	7, 8	19,790	275	.0139
3, 4	9,080	130	.0143	7, 9	34,030	525	.0154
3, 5	140,940	1,775	.0126	7, 10	21,440	320	.0149
3, 6	11,500	170	.0148	8, 9	32,480	430	.0132
3, 7	16,560	270	.0163	8, 10	19,890	225	.0113
3, 8	15,010	175	.0117	9, 10	34,130	475	.0139
3, 9	29,250	425	.0145				

The sampling distributions of x'_{clu} and r_{clu} are typical for this design

SE(x'_{clu}) is high since N_i is not considered in the estimation or sampling plan

The pattern shown in the distributions of x'_{clu} and r_{clu} in the example above is typical of what often happens when clusters having great variability with respect to the number of listing units are sampled by simple random sampling. Those clusters containing large numbers of listing units have no greater chance of being selected than those having small numbers of listing units. The estimation procedure does not take into consideration the number of listing units. In our example hospitals are the clusters and hospital admission records are the listing units. There is considerable variation among the ten hospitals with respect to numbers of admissions, with one hospital (hospital 5) admitting more patients than the combined total of the other nine hospitals. The number of patients discharged dead is highly correlated with the number of admissions and so it too varies tremendously from hospital to hospital, with hospital 5 accounting for more than 50% of the total fatalities in the ten hospitals. Since the number of admissions in a given hospital is not taken into consideration either in the sampling plan or in the estimation procedure, the distribution of estimated hospital deaths shows very high variability.

Table 12.4 Frequency Distribution of Estimated Total x'_{clu} over All Possible Samples of Two Hospitals

Estimated Total Number of Persons Discharged Dead, x'_{clu}	Frequency, f_i
0–199	7
200–399	15
400–599	12
600–799	2
800–999	0
1000–1199	0
1200–1399	0
1400–1599	0
1600–1799	4
1800–1999	3
2000–2199	2
Total	45

On the other hand, the *proportion* of patients discharged dead is roughly the same among each of the ten hospitals and shows little correlation with number of admissions. Thus, in contrast to the estimated total x'_{clu}, the estimated proportion of patients discharged dead has a relatively small standard error.

Later on in this chapter we will discuss methods of modifying the estimation procedure and/or the sampling design to yield estimated totals having lower standard errors when the number N_i of listing units varies greatly among the clusters and the level of the characteristic being estimated in the cluster is strongly related to the number of listing units in the cluster.

The theoretical standard errors of estimated totals, means, and ratios are given in the box that follows for cluster sampling in which clusters are chosen by simple random sampling and listing units are chosen within selected clusters also by simple random sampling.

These expressions reduce to those listed in box 11.3 when all N_i are equal (i.e., $N_i = \bar{N}$).

Examining the formula for the standard error of an estimated total, we see that it has a term depending on σ^2_{1x}, the variance among clusters with respect to the total level in the cluster of the characteristics being measured,

Box 12.3 Theoretical Standard Errors for Population Estimates for Simple Two-Stage Cluster Sampling, Unequal Numbers of Listing Units

Total, x'_{clu}

$$SE(x'_{clu}) = \left\{ \left(\frac{M^2}{m} \right) \left(\sigma^2_{1x} \right) \left(\frac{M - m}{M - 1} \right) \right.$$
$$\left. + \left(\frac{M}{m} \right) \left[\sum_{i=1}^{M} \left(\frac{N_i}{n_i} \right) \left(\frac{N_i - n_i}{N_i - 1} \right) \sum_{j=1}^{N_i} (X_{ij} - \bar{X}_i)^2 \right] \right\}^{1/2}$$

Mean Per Cluster, $\bar{x}_{clu}$

$$SE(\bar{x}_{clu}) = \left\{ \left(\frac{\sigma^2_{1x}}{m} \right) \left(\frac{M - m}{M - 1} \right) + \left(\frac{1}{Mm} \right) \right.$$
$$\left. \times \left[\sum_{i=1}^{M} \left(\frac{N_i}{n_i} \right) \left(\frac{N_i - n_i}{N_i - 1} \right) \sum_{j=1}^{N_i} (X_{ij} - \bar{\bar{X}}_i)^2 \right] \right\}^{1/2}$$

Mean Per Listing Unit, $\bar{\bar{x}}_{clu}$

$$SE(\bar{\bar{x}}_{clu}) = \left(\frac{1}{N} \right) \left\{ \left(\frac{M^2}{m} \right) (\sigma^2_{1x}) \left(\frac{M - m}{M - 1} \right) \right.$$
$$\left. + \left(\frac{M}{m} \right) \left[\sum_{i=1}^{M} \left(\frac{N_i}{n_i} \right) \left(\frac{N_i - n_i}{N_i - 1} \right) \sum_{j=1}^{N_i} (X_{ij} - \bar{\bar{X}}_i)^2 \right] \right\}^{1/2}$$

Ratio, r_{clu}

$$SE(r_{clu}) = (R) \left\{ \left(\frac{\sigma^2_{1R}}{m\bar{X}^2} \right) \left(\frac{M - m}{M - 1} \right) + \left(\frac{1}{m\bar{X}^2} \right) \sum_{i=1}^{M} \left(\frac{1}{N_i n_i} \right) \left(\frac{N_i - n_i}{N_i - 1} \right) \right.$$
$$\times \left[\sum_{j=1}^{N_i} (X_{ij} - \bar{\bar{X}}_i)^2 + R^2 \sum_{j=1}^{N_i} (Y_{ij} - \bar{\bar{Y}}_i)^2 \right.$$
$$\left. \left. - 2R \sum_{j=1}^{N_i} (X_{ij} - \bar{\bar{X}}_i)(Y_{ij} - \bar{\bar{Y}}_i) \right] \right\}^{1/2}$$

The notation used here is defined in boxes 11.1 and 11.3.

and a term depending on the variance among listing units within a given cluster with respect to the level of the characteristic. Again, when the cluster totals X_i are strongly correlated with the number N_i of listing units in the cluster, and when there is great diversity among clusters with respect to N_i, then σ_{1x}^2 might be very large and hence the standard error of the estimated total might be large (as we observed earlier).

The use of these formulas for the data of the ten hospitals shown in table 12.1 is illustrated in the next example.

ILLUSTRATIVE EXAMPLE

Suppose that we wish to estimate the total number of persons discharged dead and the proportion discharged dead among all those having life-threatening conditions. Suppose that we will estimate these based on a cluster sample of three hospitals chosen by simple random sampling and a 10% (to the nearest integer) simple random sample of admissions from each sample hospital. The following population characteristics are obtained directly from table 12.1: $N = 50,056$, $M = 10$, $m = 3$, $n_1 = 429$, $n_2 = 504$, $n_3 = 118$, $n_4 = 64$, $n_5 = 2,701$, $n_6 = 112$, $n_7 = 213$, $n_8 = 182$, $n_9 = 467$, and $n_{10} = 215$.

For the calculations involving the number discharged dead, we have

$$X_{ij} = \begin{cases} 1 & \text{if patient is discharged dead} \\ 0 & \text{otherwise} \end{cases}$$

$$X = 651, \qquad \bar{X} = 65.1, \qquad \bar{\bar{X}} = .013, \qquad \sigma_{1x}^2 = 8,741.69$$

Other calculations necessary are shown in table 12.5.
From table 12.5 we have

$$\sum_{i=1}^{M} \sum_{j=1}^{N_i} (X_{ij} - \bar{\bar{X}}_i)^2 = 642.37$$

and

$$\sum_{i=1}^{M} \left[\left(\frac{N_i}{n_i} \right) \left(\frac{N_i - n_i}{N_i - 1} \right) \sum_{j=1}^{N_i} (X_{ij} - \bar{\bar{X}}_i)^2 \right] = 5,783.2$$

Then we have

$$SE(x'_{clu}) = \left\{ \left(\frac{M^2}{m} \right) (\sigma_{1x}^2) \left(\frac{M - m}{M - 1} \right) + \left(\frac{M}{m} \right) \right.$$

$$\left. \times \left[\sum_{i=1}^{M} \left(\frac{N_i}{n_i} \right) \left(\frac{N_i - n_i}{N_i - 1} \right) \sum_{j=1}^{N_i} (X_{ij} - \bar{\bar{X}}_i)^2 \right] \right\}^{1/2}$$

$$= \left[\left(\frac{10^2}{3} \right) (8,741.69) \left(\frac{10 - 3}{10 - 1} \right) + \left(\frac{10}{3} \right) (5,783.20) \right]^{1/2} = 495.897$$

$$\sigma_{2x}^2 = \left(\frac{1}{N} \right) \sum_{i=1}^{M} \sum_{j=1}^{N_i} (X_{ij} - \bar{\bar{X}}_i)^2 = \frac{642.37}{50,056} = .01283$$

Table 12.5   Calculations Involving Number Discharged Dead

For the calculations in this example, it is helpful to tabulate intermediate computations, as we have done here

Cluster	Col. A $\left(\dfrac{N_i}{n_i}\right)\left(\dfrac{N_i - n_i}{N_i - 1}\right)$	Col. B $\sum\limits_{j=1}^{N_i} (X_{ij} - \bar{\bar{X}}_i)^2$	Col. A × Col. B
1	$\left(\dfrac{4{,}288}{429}\right)\left(\dfrac{4{,}288 - 429}{4{,}288 - 1}\right) = 8.997$	41.589	374.18
2	$\left(\dfrac{5{,}036}{504}\right)\left(\dfrac{5{,}036 - 504}{5{,}036 - 1}\right) = 8.994$	76.792	690.67
3	$\left(\dfrac{1{,}178}{118}\right)\left(\dfrac{1{,}178 - 118}{1{,}178 - 1}\right) = 8.991$	16.75	150.64
4	$\left(\dfrac{638}{64}\right)\left(\dfrac{638 - 64}{638 - 1}\right) = 8.983$	8.873	79.71
5	$\left(\dfrac{27{,}010}{2{,}701}\right)\left(\dfrac{27{,}010 - 2{,}701}{27{,}010 - 1}\right) = 9.000$	333.770	3,003.93
6	$\left(\dfrac{1{,}122}{112}\right)\left(\dfrac{1{,}122 - 112}{1{,}122 - 1}\right) = 9.026$	16.742	151.07
7	$\left(\dfrac{2{,}134}{213}\right)\left(\dfrac{2{,}134 - 213}{2{,}134 - 1}\right) = 9.023$	36.358	328.06
8	$\left(\dfrac{1{,}824}{182}\right)\left(\dfrac{1{,}824 - 182}{1{,}824 - 1}\right) = 9.027$	17.822	160.88
9	$\left(\dfrac{4{,}672}{467}\right)\left(\dfrac{4{,}672 - 467}{4{,}672 - 1}\right) = 9.006$	67.010	603.49
10	$\left(\dfrac{2{,}154}{215}\right)\left(\dfrac{2{,}154 - 215}{2{,}154 - 1}\right) = 9.023$	26.662	240.57
Total		642.37	5,783.2

For the calculations involving the number having life-threatening conditions, we have

$$Y_{ij} = \begin{cases} 1 & \text{if admission is life threatening} \\ 0 & \text{if it is not} \end{cases}$$

$$Y = 7{,}087 \qquad \bar{Y} = 708.7 \qquad \bar{\bar{Y}} = .14158 \qquad \sigma_{1y}^2 = 851{,}956.41$$

Other calculations necessary are shown in table 12.6.

From table 12.6 we have

$$\sum_{i=1}^{M}\sum_{j=1}^{N_i}(Y_{ij} - \bar{\bar{Y}}_i)^2 = 6{,}047.153 \qquad \text{and} \qquad \sum_{i=1}^{M}\left(\frac{N_i}{n_i}\right)\left(\frac{N_i - n_i}{N_i - 1}\right)\sum_{j=1}^{N_i}(Y_{ij} - \bar{\bar{Y}}_i)^2$$

$$= 54{,}445.10$$

Table 12.6   Calculations Involving Number with Life-threatening Conditions

Cluster i	Col. A $\left(\dfrac{N_i}{n_i}\right)\left(\dfrac{N_i - n_i}{N_i - 1}\right)$	Col. B $\sum\limits_{j=1}^{N_i} (Y_{ij} - \bar{\bar{Y}}_i)^2$	Col. A × Col. B
1	$\left(\dfrac{4{,}288}{429}\right)\left(\dfrac{4{,}288 - 429}{4{,}288 - 1}\right) = 8.997$	442.464	3,981.04
2	$\left(\dfrac{5{,}036}{504}\right)\left(\dfrac{5{,}036 - 504}{5{,}036 - 1}\right) = 8.994$	662.636	5,959.65
3	$\left(\dfrac{1{,}178}{118}\right)\left(\dfrac{1{,}178 - 118}{1{,}178 - 1}\right) = 8.991$	174.486	1,568.75
4	$\left(\dfrac{638}{64}\right)\left(\dfrac{638 - 64}{638 - 1}\right) = 8.983$	126.089	1,132.64
5	$\left(\dfrac{27{,}010}{2{,}701}\right)\left(\dfrac{27{,}010 - 2{,}701}{27{,}010 - 1}\right) = 9.000$	2,975.003	26,776.02
6	$\left(\dfrac{1{,}122}{112}\right)\left(\dfrac{1{,}122 - 112}{1{,}122 - 1}\right) = 9.026$	175.031	1,579.81
7	$\left(\dfrac{2{,}134}{213}\right)\left(\dfrac{2{,}134 - 213}{2{,}134 - 1}\right) = 9.023$	339.756	3,065.62
8	$\left(\dfrac{1{,}824}{182}\right)\left(\dfrac{1{,}824 - 182}{1{,}824 - 1}\right) = 9.027$	212.822	1,921.13
9	$\left(\dfrac{4{,}672}{467}\right)\left(\dfrac{4{,}672 - 467}{4{,}672 - 1}\right) = 9.006$	648.444	5,840.02
10	$\left(\dfrac{2{,}154}{215}\right)\left(\dfrac{2{,}154 - 215}{2{,}154 - 1}\right) = 9.023$	290.422	2,620.42
Total		6,047.53	54,445.10

Then we have

$$SE(y'_{clu}) = \left\{ \left(\frac{M^2}{m}\right)(\sigma_{1y}^2)\left(\frac{M - m}{M - 1}\right) + \left(\frac{M}{m}\right) \right.$$

$$\left. \times \left[\sum_{i=1}^{M} \left(\frac{N_i}{n_i}\right)\left(\frac{N_i - n_i}{N_i - 1}\right) \sum_{j=1}^{N_i} (Y_{ij} - \bar{\bar{Y}}_i)^2 \right] \right\}^{1/2}$$

$$= \left[\left(\frac{10^2}{3}\right)(851{,}956.41)\left(\frac{10 - 3}{10 - 1}\right) + \left(\frac{10}{3}\right)(54{,}445.10) \right]^{1/2} = 4{,}719.03$$

$$\sigma_{2y}^2 = \left(\frac{1}{N}\right) \sum_{i=1}^{M} \sum_{j=1}^{N_i} (Y_{ij} - \bar{\bar{Y}}_i)^2 = \frac{6{,}047.153}{50{,}056} = .12081$$

Table 12.7 Calculation Involving Proportion of Deaths Among Those with Life-threatening Conditions

Cluster i	Col. A $\sum_{j=1}^{N_i} (X_{ij} - \bar{X}_i)^2$	Col. B $R^2 \sum_{j=1}^{N_i} (Y_{ij} - \bar{Y}_i)^2$	Col. C $2R \sum_{j=1}^{N_i} (X_{ij} - \bar{X}_i)(Y_{ij} - \bar{Y}_i)$	$\left(\dfrac{1}{N_i n_i}\right)\left(\dfrac{N_i - n_i}{N_i - 1}\right)(Col.\,A + Col.\,B - Col.\,C)$
1	41.589	$(.09186)^2(442.464) = 3.734$	$2(.09186)(37.09) = 6.81$	$\left(\dfrac{1}{1{,}839{,}552}\right)(.900)(38.513) = .0000188$
2	76.792	$(.09186)^2(662.636) = 5.591$	$2(.09186)(65.84) = 12.10$	$\left(\dfrac{1}{2{,}538{,}144}\right)(.900)(70.283) = .0000249$
3	16.75	$(.09186)^2(174.486) = 1.472$	$2(.09186)(13.93) = 2.56$	$\left(\dfrac{1}{139{,}004}\right)(.901)(15.662) = .0001015$
4	8.873	$(.09186)^2(126.089) = 1.064$	$2(.09186)(6.56) = 1.21$	$\left(\dfrac{1}{40{,}832}\right)(.901)(8.727) = .00019257$
5	333.770	$(.09186)^2(2975.003) = 25.104$	$2(.09186)(295.40) = 54.27$	$\left(\dfrac{1}{72{,}954{,}010}\right)(.900)(304.604) = .00000$
6	16.742	$(.09186)^2(175.031) = 1.477$	$2(.09186)(13.71) = 2.52$	$\left(\dfrac{1}{125{,}664}\right)(.901)(15.699) = .0001126$
7	36.358	$(.09186)^2(339.756) = 2.867$	$2(.09186)(29.65) = 5.45$	$\left(\dfrac{1}{454{,}542}\right)(.901)(33.775) = .00006692$
8	17.822	$(.09186)^2(212.822) = 1.796$	$2(.09186)(15.57) = 2.86$	$\left(\dfrac{1}{331{,}968}\right)(.901)(16.758) = .00004547$
9	67.010	$(.09186)^2(648.444) = 5.472$	$2(.09186)(56.68) = 10.41$	$\left(\dfrac{1}{2{,}181{,}824}\right)(.900)(62.072) = .0000256$
10	26.662	$(.09186)^2(290.422) = 2.451$	$2(.09186)(22.66) = 4.16$	$\left(\dfrac{1}{463{,}110}\right)(.901)(24.953) = .00004853$
Total				.00064

For the calculations involving the proportion of deaths among those having life-threatening conditions, we have

$$R = \frac{X}{Y} = \frac{651}{7,087} = .09186$$

$$\sigma_{1xy} = \sum_{i=1}^{M} \frac{(x_i - \bar{X})(Y_i - \bar{Y})}{m} = \frac{\sum_{i=1}^{M} X_i Y_i - M\bar{X}\bar{Y}}{M}$$

$$= \frac{1,324,053 - (10)(65.1)(708.7)}{10} = 86,268.93$$

$$\sigma_{1R}^2 = \sigma_{1x}^2 + R^2\sigma_{1y}^2 - 2R\sigma_{1xy}$$
$$= 874.69 + (.09186)^2(851,956.41) - 2(.09186)(86,268.93) = 81.39$$

Other calculations necessary are shown in table 12.7.

Then from table 12.7 we have

$$SE(r_{\text{clu}}) = (R)\left\{\left(\frac{\sigma_{1R}^2}{m\bar{X}^2}\right)\left(\frac{M-m}{M-1}\right) + \left(\frac{1}{m\bar{\bar{X}}^2}\right)\sum_{i=1}^{M}\left(\frac{1}{N_i n_i}\right)\left(\frac{N_i - n_i}{N_i - 1}\right)\right.$$

$$\times \left[\sum_{j=1}^{N_i} (X_{ij} - \bar{\bar{X}}_i)^2 + R^2 \sum_{j=1}^{N_i} (Y_{ij} - \bar{\bar{Y}}_i)^2\right.$$

$$\left.\left. - 2R \sum_{j=1}^{N_i} (X_{ij} - \bar{\bar{X}}_i)(Y_{ij} - \bar{\bar{Y}}_i)\right]\right\}^{1/2}$$

$$= (.09186)\left\{\left[\frac{81.39}{3(65.1)^2}\right]\left(\frac{10-3}{10-1}\right) + \left[\frac{1}{3(.013)^2}\right](.00064)\right\}^{1/2} = .1034$$

$$\sigma_{2xy} = \frac{\sum_{i=1}^{M}\sum_{j=1}^{N_i}(X_{ij} - \bar{\bar{X}}_i)(Y_{ij} - \bar{\bar{Y}}_i)}{N} = \frac{557.09}{50,056} = .01113$$

In the example above in calculating the expressions $\sum_{j=1}^{N_i}[(X_{ij} - \bar{\bar{X}}_i) \times (Y_{ij} - \bar{\bar{Y}}_i)]$, we assumed that fatalities occurred only among those admitted to the hospital with life-threatening illnesses. Under this assumption, we have the relationship given by

$$\sum_{j=1}^{N_i}(X_{ij} - \bar{\bar{X}}_i)(Y_{ij} - \bar{\bar{Y}}_i) = N_i\bar{\bar{X}}_i(1 - \bar{\bar{Y}}_i)$$

It should also be noted that the tediousness of the calculations shown above is typical of those seen in two-stage cluster sampling designs where clusters are chosen by simple random sampling, listing units are also chosen by simple random sampling, approximately equal sampling fractions are taken in each selected cluster, and there are unequal numbers of listing units in each cluster.

12.5 HOW LARGE A SAMPLE DO WE NEED?

*We choose **m** after the sampling fractions have been decided on*

Suppose that we intend to take a two-stage cluster sample in which a simple random sample of clusters is taken at the first stage followed by a simple random sample of n_i listing units from the N_i listing units within each sample cluster. In other words, we are assuming that the second-stage sampling fractions have already been decided upon. We then wish to know how many clusters m are needed in our sample for us to be virtually certain that the relative differences between our estimates and the true values are no more than ε. Formulas for the **number m of clusters** needed to meet the specifications stated above are given below.

For estimated **totals** (x'_{clu}) or **means** ($\bar{x}_{clu}$, $\bar{\bar{x}}_{clu}$):

$$m = \frac{\left(\dfrac{\sigma_{1x}^2}{\bar{X}^2}\right)\left(\dfrac{M}{M-1}\right) + \left(\dfrac{M}{N^2\bar{\bar{X}}^2}\right)\left[\displaystyle\sum_{i=1}^{M}\left(\dfrac{N_i}{n_i}\right)\left(\dfrac{N_i - n_i}{N_i - 1}\right)\displaystyle\sum_{j=1}^{N_i}(X_{ij} - \bar{\bar{X}}_i)^2\right]}{\dfrac{\varepsilon^2}{z_{1-\alpha/2}^2} + \dfrac{\sigma_{1x}^2}{\bar{X}^2(M-1)}}$$

(12.1)

and for estimated **ratios** ($r_{clu} = \bar{x}_{clu}/\bar{y}_{clu}$):

$$m = \frac{\left\{\left(\dfrac{\sigma_{1R}^2}{\bar{X}^2}\right)\left(\dfrac{M}{N^2\bar{\bar{X}}^2}\right) + \left(\dfrac{M}{N^2\bar{\bar{X}}^2}\right)\displaystyle\sum_{i=1}^{M}\left(\dfrac{1}{n_i N_i}\right)\right.}{\left.\times\left[\displaystyle\sum_{j=1}^{N_i}(X_{ij} - \bar{\bar{X}}_i)^2 + R^2\displaystyle\sum_{j=1}^{N_i}(Y_{ij} - \bar{\bar{Y}}_i)^2 - 2R\displaystyle\sum_{j=1}^{N_i}(X_{ij} - \bar{\bar{X}}_i)(Y_{ij} - \bar{\bar{Y}}_i)\right]\right\}}{\dfrac{\varepsilon^2}{z_{1-\alpha/2}^2} + \dfrac{\sigma_{1R}^2}{\bar{X}^2(M-1)}}$$

(12.2)

ILLUSTRATIVE EXAMPLE

Let us suppose that we wish to be virtually certain of estimating the total number of persons discharged dead to within 30% of the true value and the proportion of deaths among persons admitted with life-threatening conditions to within 30% of its true value. Suppose that we take a second-stage sample of 20% (to the nearest integer) of all admissions from those hospitals selected at the first stage. Then from previous calculations, we have

$$\sigma_{1x}^2 = 8{,}741.69 \qquad \bar{X} = 65.1 \qquad \bar{\bar{X}} = .0130$$

$$\sum_{i=1}^{M}\left(\frac{N_i}{n_i}\right)\left(\frac{N_i - n_i}{N_i - 1}\right)\sum_{j=1}^{N_i}(X_{ij} - \bar{\bar{X}}_i)^2 = 5{,}783.32$$

$$\sum_{i=1}^{M} \left(\frac{1}{N_i n_i}\right)\left(\frac{N_i - n_i}{N_i - 1}\right)\left[\sum_{j=1}^{N_i} (X_{ij} - \bar{\bar{X}}_i)^2 + R^2 \sum_{j=1}^{N_i} (Y_{ij} - \bar{\bar{Y}}_i)^2\right.$$

$$\left. - 2R \sum_{j=1}^{N_i} (X_{ij} - \bar{\bar{X}}_i)(Y_{ij} - \bar{\bar{Y}}_i)\right] = .00064$$

$$\sigma_{1R}^2 = 81.39 \qquad N = 50{,}056 \qquad M = 10$$

Then from relation (12.1) with $\varepsilon = .30$, we have

$$m = \frac{\left[\frac{8{,}741.69}{(65.1)^2}\right]\left(\frac{10}{10 - 1}\right) + \left[\frac{10}{(50{,}056)^2(.0130)^2}\right](5{,}783.32)}{\dfrac{(.30)^2}{9} + \dfrac{8{,}741.69}{(65.1)^2(10 - 1)}} = 10.15 \approx 10.0$$

And from relation (12.2) with $\varepsilon = .30$, we have

$$m = \frac{\left[\frac{81.39}{(65.1)^2}\right]\left(\frac{10}{10 - 1}\right) + \left[\frac{10}{(50{,}056)^2(.0130)^2}\right](.00064)}{\dfrac{(.30)^2}{9} + \dfrac{81.39}{(65.1)^2(10 - 1)}} = 1.76 \approx 2$$

Thus we would need a sample of all ten hospitals to meet the specifications set for the estimated total discharged dead (X), whereas we would need only two clusters to meet the specifications set for the ratio of deaths to life-threatening illnesses (R).

12.6 CHOOSING THE OPTIMAL CLUSTER SIZE n̄ CONSIDERING COSTS

Let us again assume that the clusters will be taken by simple random sampling and that within each cluster the second-stage sampling fraction, n_i/N_i, will be the same (within the limitations of the N_i discussed earlier) for each cluster selected. Suppose we define the average cluster size $\bar{n}$ as

$$\bar{n} = \frac{\sum_{i=1}^{m} n_i}{m}$$

And suppose the **field costs** can be approximated by the function

$$C = C_1' m + C_2' m \bar{n}$$

Then the **optimal average cluster size** $\bar{n}$ that would yield estimated totals (x_{clu}') or means $(\bar{x}_{\text{clu}}, \bar{\bar{x}}_{\text{clu}})$ having the lowest standard errors among all other estimates obtained at the same field costs from two-stage cluster sampling with a constant second-stage sampling fraction is given by

For totals or means
$$\bar{n} = \left[\left(\frac{C'_1}{C'_2}\right)\left(\frac{1 - \delta_x}{\delta_x}\right)\right]^{1/2} \qquad (12.3)$$

where δ_x is a generalization of the intraclass correlation coefficient discussed earlier and is given by

$$\delta_x = \frac{[M/(M - 1)]\,(\sigma^2_{1x}) - \bar{N}\sigma^2_{2x}}{[M/(M - 1)]\,(\sigma^2_{1x}) + \bar{N}(\bar{N} - 1)\sigma^2_{2x}} \qquad (12.4)$$

and where

$$\bar{N} = \frac{\sum\limits_{i=1}^{M} N_i}{M}$$

$$\sigma^2_{2x} = \left(\frac{1}{N}\right) \sum\limits_{i=1}^{M} \left(\frac{N_i}{N_i - 1}\right) \sum\limits_{j=1}^{N_i} (X_{ij} - \bar{X}_i)^2 \qquad (12.5)$$

For estimation of ratios, $r_{clu} = \bar{x}_{clu}/\bar{y}_{clu}$, the optimal cluster size $\bar{n}$ is given by

For ratios
$$\bar{n} = \left[\left(\frac{C'_1}{C'_2}\right)\left(\frac{1 - \delta_R}{\delta_R}\right)\right]^{1/2} \qquad (12.6)$$

where

$$\delta_R = \frac{[M/(M - 1)](\sigma^2_{1R}) - \bar{N}\sigma^2_{2R}}{[M/(M - 1)](\sigma^2_{1R}) + \bar{N}(\bar{N} - 1)\sigma^2_{2R}} \qquad (12.7)$$

$$\sigma^2_{2R} = \frac{1}{N} \sum\limits_{i=1}^{M} \left(\frac{N_i}{N_i - 1}\right)\left[\sum\limits_{j=1}^{N_i} (X_{ij} - \bar{X}_i)^2 + R^2 \sum\limits_{j=1}^{N_i} (Y_{ij} - \bar{Y}_i)^2\right.$$

$$\left. - 2R \sum\limits_{j=1}^{N_i} (X_{ij} - \bar{X}_i)(Y_{ij} - \bar{Y}_i)\right] \qquad (12.8)$$

ILLUSTRATIVE EXAMPLE

To illustrate the use of these formulas, let us suppose that we wish to take a simple two-stage cluster sample from the population of ten hospitals shown in table 12.1 for purposes of estimating the total persons discharged dead (X) and the proportion discharged dead among those admitted with life-threatening illnesses (R). Suppose that it would cost approximately \$500 in administrative and travel costs for every hospital sampled and approximately \$5.00 per admission record. In other words, $C'_1 = 500$ and $C'_2 = 5$. From earlier calculations we have

$$\sigma^2_{1x} = 8{,}741.69 \qquad \sigma^2_{2x} = \frac{642.37}{50{,}056} = .01283 \qquad \bar{N} = 5{,}005.6$$

$$\delta_x = \frac{(\frac{10}{9})(8{,}741.69) - (5{,}005.6)(.01283)}{(\frac{10}{9})(8{,}741.69) + (5{,}005.6)(5{,}004.6)(.01382)} = .02914$$

Therefore,

$$\bar{n} = \left[\left(\frac{500}{5}\right)\left(\frac{1 - .02914}{.02914}\right)\right]^{1/2} = 57.73 \approx 58$$

Thus the optimal average cluster size for estimating the total number discharged dead is 58 admissions and the optimal second-stage sampling fraction would be $f_2 = 58/5005.6 = .011586$. Once the optimal second-stage sampling fraction has been determined, we would then use relation (12.1) to determine the number of clusters needed to meet the required specifications set on the estimate.

To illustrate the use of expression (12.6) for a ratio R, we have, from earlier calculations,

$$\sigma_{1R}^2 = 81.39$$

$$\sigma_{2R}^2 = \sigma_{2x}^2 + R^2\sigma_{2y}^2 - 2R\sigma_{2xy}$$

$$= .01283 + (.09186)^2(.12081) - 2(.09186)(.01113) = .01180$$

$$\delta_r = \frac{(\frac{10}{9})(81.39) - (5,005.6)(.01180)}{(\frac{10}{9})(81.39) + (5,005.6)(5,004.6)(.01180)} = .000106$$

Therefore,

$$\bar{n} = \left[\left(\frac{500}{5}\right)\left(\frac{1 - .000106}{.000106}\right)\right]^{1/2} = 971.234$$

Thus the optimal second-stage sampling fraction for estimating the ratio of persons discharged dead to persons admitted with life-threatening conditions is

$$f_2 = \frac{971.234}{5,005.6} = .194$$

We could then use relation (12.2) (with the n_i set equal to the f_2N_i) to determine the number of clusters that should be sampled in order for the specifications set on the estimate to be met.

It often happens (as it did in this example) that the optimal cluster sizes are not the same for each estimate needed. In practice, a compromise on the cluster size $\bar{n}$ is often made by some method such as taking the average optimal $\bar{n}$ over the most important estimates that are needed from the survey.

12.7 METHODS OF IMPROVING THE RELIABILITY OF ESTIMATED TOTALS

In our discussion of cluster sampling from clusters having unequal numbers of listing units, we pointed out the pitfalls that could arise in estimating totals if the clusters were sampled by simple random sampling. If there is great diversity

Reliability of estimated totals for cluster sampling could be quite low

among clusters in the number of listing units and if the total level in the cluster of the characteristic being measured is related to the number of listing units in the cluster, then the reliability of the resulting estimate could be very low. The reason for this is that σ_{1x}^2 in the formula for the standard error of an estimated total might be quite large. No matter how large the second-stage sampling fraction is, it would not affect this component.

Methods to improve reliability include the following:

1. ratio estimation

All this suggests that simple random sampling of clusters may not be a very good sampling scheme in such situations. One situation in which it could be used efficiently, however, arises when the total number N of listing units is known in advance of the sampling. We then can estimate the total by the expression $N(\bar{x}_{\text{clu}}/\bar{n}_{\text{clu}})$, where $\bar{n}_{\text{clu}}$ is the average number of listing units per cluster, $\bar{x}_{\text{clu}}$ is the average level of the characteristic per sample cluster, and N is the total number of listing units. This estimate would tend to have a lower standard error than the estimate x'_{clu} when the level of the characteristic in the cluster is highly related to the number of listing units in the cluster. It would have properties similar to those discussed in chapter 7 for totals estimated from a ratio.

2. stratification

When the number of listing units is known in advance of the sampling, the sampling plan can be altered in some way to produce estimated totals that have relatively low standard errors. One way to alter the sampling plan is to first group the clusters into two or more strata on the basis of their number N_i of listing units and then to sample the clusters independently within each stratum by simple random sampling. This procedure ensures that those clusters having large numbers of listing units are represented in the sample. For this type of sampling scheme methods of estimation developed earlier for stratified random sampling would be used together with methods developed for cluster sampling. In particular, we would use an estimation procedure appropriate for cluster sampling to estimate the total level of $\mathcal{X}$ within each stratum and then aggregate these estimated totals over all strata.

3. sampling with probability proportional to size of cluster

Another method commonly used to improve reliability of estimates is to sample the clusters with probability proportional to the number of listing units in the cluster. In this way clusters having large N_i have a greater chance of being included in the sample than clusters having small N_i. This sampling strategy is known as sampling with **probability proportional to size,** or **PPS sampling.** In PPS sampling the same number $\bar{n}$ of listing units (or some multiple of $\bar{n}$) is generally sampled from each cluster selected at the first stage. We illustrate the method in the next example.

ILLUSTRATIVE EXAMPLE

Let us consider the population of ten hospitals shown in table 12.1. Suppose that we wish to take a PPS sample of $n = 4\bar{n}$ listing units. We first list these clusters and cumulate the number of listing units, as shown in table 12.8.

Table 12.8   Procedure for PPS Sampling

Cluster	Number of Listing Units, N_i	Cumulative $\sum N_i$	Random Numbers	Random Number Chosen
1	4,288	4,288	00001–04288	04285
2	5,036	9,324	04289–09324	
3	1,178	10,502	09325–10502	
4	638	11,140	10503–11140	
5	27,010	38,150	11141–38150	11883; 35700; 36699
6	1,122	39,272	38151–39272	
7	2,134	41,406	39273–41406	
8	1,824	43,230	41407–43230	
9	4,672	47,902	43231–47902	
10	2,154	50,056	47903–50056	
Total	50,056			

As we see in the table, numbers 1–4288 are associated with cluster 1; numbers 4289–9324 are associated with cluster 2; numbers 9325–10502 are associated with cluster 3; and so on. We then take four random numbers between 1 and 50056 (e.g., 36699, 35700, 11883, 4285, corresponding to hospitals 5, 5, 5, and 1, respectively). For each of the m random numbers chosen, we take a simple random sample of $\bar{n}$ listing units from the cluster corresponding to the random number. For example, three independent simple random samples of $\bar{n}$ admission records would be taken from hospital 5 since it corresponds to three of the chosen random numbers, and one simple random sample of $\bar{n}$ listing units would be taken from hospital 1.

For PPS sampling the **estimated total,** which we will denote x'_{pps}, is given by

$$x'_{pps} = \left(\frac{N}{n}\right) \sum_{i=1}^{m} x_{i+} \qquad (12.9)$$

Formulas to use under PPS sampling

where x_{i+} is the total level of variable $\mathscr{X}$ obtained from the $\bar{n}$ listing units associated with the ith random number chosen, m is the number of random numbers selected, and $n = m\bar{n}$ is the total number of sample listing units.

It can be shown that x'_{pps}, as given by relation (12.9) under the sampling plan described above, has a **mean** $E(x'_{pps})$ given by

$$E(x'_{pps}) = X$$

the true population total (i.e., the estimate x'_{pps} is an unbiased estimate of the population total X), and a **standard error** $SE(x'_{pps})$ given by

$$SE(x'_{pps}) = \left\{ \left(\frac{N}{m}\right) \sum_{i=1}^{M} N_i(\bar{\bar{X}}_i - \bar{\bar{X}})^2 \right.$$

$$\left. + \left(\frac{N}{m}\right) \left[\frac{\sum_{i=1}^{M} \left(\frac{N_i - \bar{n}}{N_i - 1}\right) \sum_{j=1}^{N_i} (X_{ij} - \bar{\bar{X}}_i)^2}{\bar{n}} \right] \right\}^{1/2} \quad (12.10)$$

To illustrate that this method has, when used appropriately, a much smaller standard error than the estimate x'_{clu} obtained from simple random sampling of clusters, let us compare the two estimates based on a comparable total number n of listing units.

ILLUSTRATIVE EXAMPLE

We have already shown that the estimate x'_{clu} of the total number of persons discharged dead based on a first-stage sample of three hospitals from the ten hospitals shown in table 12.1 and a second-stage sampling fraction of 10% of admissions from the selected hospitals has a standard error $SE(x'_{clu}) = 495.9$. This corresponds to $m = 3$ and $\bar{n} = .1\bar{N} = .1(5,005.6) = 500.56 = 500$. Thus we would compare this sampling with a PPS sample of 1500 listing units with $\bar{n} = 500$.

From earlier calculations and from relation (12.10), we have

$$\sum_{i=1}^{M} N_i(\bar{\bar{X}}_i - \bar{\bar{X}})^2 = .1602$$

$$\frac{\sum_{i=1}^{M} \left(\frac{N_i - \bar{n}}{N_i - 1}\right) \sum_{j=1}^{N_i} (X_{ij} - \bar{\bar{X}}_i)^2}{\bar{n}} = \frac{575.52}{500} = 1.151$$

$$SE(x'_{pps}) = \left[\left(\frac{50,056}{3}\right)(.1602 + 1.151) \right]^{1/2} = 147.91$$

Intermediate calculations for this example are shown in table 12.9.

Thus we see in this instance that PPS sampling yields an estimated total that has a standard error which is 30% of the size of the standard error of the estimated total x'_{clu} obtained from ordinary cluster sampling of the same number of listing units.

One common variation of PPS sampling

There are many variations of PPS sampling commonly used in practice. In one variation, used when the N_i are not readily available in advance of the sampling, the clusters are chosen with probability proportional to some available variable that is related to the number of listing units and hence to the characteristic of interest. For example, the number of admissions in each hospital might not be known in advance but the number of beds might be known. We might then choose a sample of hospitals in such a way that the probability of a hospital appearing in the sample would be proportional to the number of beds in the hospital. An estimate of the total could then be constructed in a manner analogous to that for the estimate x'_{pps} discussed earlier, and this estimate would have properties very similar to x'_{pps}.

An **estimate of the standard error** $SE(x'_{pps})$ of an estimated total x'_{pps} obtained from PPS sampling can be constructed from the sample statistics as given below:

Table 12.9   Intermediate Calculations for Computing $SE(x'_{pps})$

Cluster	$\bar{\bar{X}}_i$	$(\bar{\bar{X}}_i - \bar{\bar{X}})^2$	N_i	$N_i(\bar{\bar{X}}_i - \bar{\bar{X}})^2$
1	$42/4288 = .0098$	$(-.0032)^2$	4,288	.0439
2	$78/5036 = .0155$	$(.0025)^2$	5,036	.0315
3	$17/1178 = .0144$	$(.0014)^2$	1,178	.0023
4	$9/638 = .0141$	$(.0011)^2$	638	.0008
5	$338/27,010 = .0141$	$(-.0005)^2$	27,010	.0068
6	$17/1122 = .0152$	$(.0022)^2$	1,122	.0054
7	$37/2134 = .0173$	$(.0043)^2$	2,134	.0395
8	$18/1824 = .0099$	$(-.0031)^2$	1,824	.0175
9	$68/4672 = .0146$	$(.0016)^2$	4,672	.0120
10	$27/2154 = .0125$	$(-.0005)^2$	2,154	.0005
				.1602

Cluster	Col. A $\dfrac{N_i - \bar{n}}{N_i - 1}$	Col. B $\sum\limits_{j=1}^{N_i} (X_{ij} - \bar{\bar{X}}_i)^2$	Col. A × Col. B
1	.8836	41.589	36.748
2	.9009	76.792	69.181
3	.5760	16.75	9.649
4	.2166	8.873	1.922
5	.9815	333.77	327.603
6	.5549	16.742	9.289
7	.7661	36.358	27.852
8	.7263	17.822	12.944
9	.8932	67.010	59.85
10	.7682	26.662	20.483
			575.52

$$\widehat{SE}(x'_{pps}) = \left\{ \left[\frac{1}{m(m-1)} \right] \sum_{i=1}^{m} \left(\frac{N x_i}{\bar{n}} - x'_{pps} \right)^2 \right\}^{1/2} \qquad (12.11)$$

This expression is very much like the ultimate cluster estimates of standard errors discussed earlier (box 11.2) for ordinary cluster sampling.

12.8 SOME COMMON USES OF CLUSTER SAMPLING WITH UNEQUAL NUMBERS OF LISTING UNITS

In these past four chapters we have developed the concepts and methods of cluster sampling. We conclude our treatment of cluster sampling with a discussion of some sampling designs that are frequently used in the health sciences.

Household Surveys

Two-stage cluster samples are often used

A sampling design that is widely used for surveys of urban areas [such as cities, towns, standard metropolitan statistical areas (SMSAs), etc.] is a two-stage cluster sample in which city blocks are clusters and households are listing units. City blocks are convenient for field use as clusters because they are generally well defined geographically and therefore easily identified. In addition, the U.S. Bureau of the Census publishes population and household counts of blocks for the urbanized portions of SMSAs. Thus for many urban areas it would be possible to sample the blocks by PPS sampling on the basis of the census data. The Census Bureau also has available maps of the blocks for those areas where block data are published.

The techniques of listing are very important

Once the blocks are sampled, the field team generally visits each selected block and lists the households. It is important that the field team be well instructed so that all households are listed and nonhouseholds such as institutions or business establishments are not included on the list. A good discussion of listing procedures is included in the textbooks by Sudman (3) and Kish (2). The listing of households is an important component of the sampling design since a household can be included in the sample only if it is on the list from which the sample is chosen. Proper techniques of listing, therefore, cannot be overemphasized.

Once the households on a selected block are listed, they can be sampled. The sampling can be done at the same time that the listing is done if the field team is equipped with random number tables and instructed on the use of these tables to pick simple random samples.

Listing units are not always selected by simple random sampling

So far the entire theory of cluster sampling discussed in this book has been based on the fact that the listing units are selected by simple random sampling. In practice, however, some other sampling procedure might be used to select the listing units. For example, the households on a block might be selected by systematic sampling. Alternatively, one of the four faces of the block might be chosen by use of random numbers and every household on that face might be included in the sample. As we discussed earlier, systematic sampling is an easier procedure to teach and perform in the field than is simple random sampling and so is more widely used. In calculating standard errors of estimates, however, those procedures appropriate for simple random sampling are generally used even when the households are chosen by systematic sampling or by some other procedure. In this situation it is accepted that the estimated standard errors of estimates are not affected very much by this deviance from simple random sampling.

Anyone contemplating a household survey should be thoroughly familiar with the basic issues of such a survey, such as identifying the blocks, listing the households, and choosing the sample of households. Household surveys are serious undertakings, and even a relatively modest one can require much in the way of time and resources.

Telephone Surveys

The use of telephone interviewing in sample surveys has increased greatly in recent years, primarily because field costs involved in personal visits to households are often prohibitive. If it is recognized that not all households have telephones, and if the totality of households having telephones is acceptable as a target population, then telephone interviewing should be considered as a possible alternative to personal household visits.

Telephone surveys are used when field costs of personal interviews become prohibitive

In telephone surveys households can be chosen in several ways for inclusion in the sample. The telephone directory of the target area can be used as the sampling frame. However, telephone directories contain neither unlisted numbers nor numbers assigned to households since the publication of the latest directory. Exclusion of these households may be a source of serious bias since households having unlisted numbers or new numbers might form a substantial percentage of households with telephones.

Telephone directories might be used as sampling frames

An alternative sampling frame for telephone surveys is a list of all possible four-digit numbers within existing telephone exchanges. A telephone number consists of ten digits. The first three digits designate the area code, the next three designate the telephone exchange, and the last four digits identify the particular phone listing. For example, to telephone the dean of the School of Health Sciences at the University of Massachusetts, you would first dial area code 413 (the area code for western Massachusetts), followed by the number 545 (the particular telephone exchange for all University of Massachusetts at Amherst numbers), followed by 1303 (the dean's office). The use of these digits as the sampling frame is known as **random digit dialing** and avoids the biases associated with telephone directories. Our ensuing discussion of random digit dialing is based primarily on methods reported by Waksberg (4).

Or random digit dialing might be used as an alternative to using telephone directories

A list of area codes and exchanges for the target area of a survey can be obtained from the local telephone company office. Thus within a given area code (e.g., 203) and exchange (e.g., 624), only the last four digits of a telephone number need to be chosen randomly. However, it turns out that a relatively large proportion (approximately 80%) of all telephone numbers within designated area codes and exchanges either are not used at all or else are assigned to

A disadvantage of random digit dialing

businesses, institutions, or other nonhouseholds. In other words, the process of taking random four-digit numbers within given area codes and exchanges would be wasteful, since we would expect to dial five telephone numbers for every household obtained.

An alternative procedure to overcome the disadvantage

Waksberg suggests an alternative procedure that increases the yield of numbers corresponding to households. In this procedure the telephone numbers are grouped into clusters defined by the first 8 (rather than the first 6) digits. For example, if the target population includes those households in area code 203, exchanges 624 and 823, the numbers are grouped into 200 clusters as follows, based on the first 8 digits:

203–624–00 to 203–624–99　(100 clusters)

203–823–00 to 203–823–99　(100 clusters)

The clusters are identified (e.g., 1 to 200 above) and sampled as follows: A random cluster is taken (e.g., 203–624–36) and a random number between 00 and 99 is taken (e.g., 73). The telephone number (e.g., 203–624–3673) is then dialed. If the number is a household, the cluster is retained and additional two-digit numbers are taken until a total of $\bar{n}$ residences (including the first one dialed) are reached. If the original number is not a residence, the cluster is rejected. This procedure is continued until a total of m clusters are sampled, which would result in a total of $m\bar{n}$ interviews.

Waksberg's procedure yields a great improvement in the ratio of households dialed to total numbers dialed because of the tendency of these clusters to contain either a very high proportion of households or else a very low proportion. The estimation procedure used is that of PPS sampling since the initial phone call made in the cluster determines whether the cluster is or is not included in the sample, and the probability of this initial phone call yielding a household depends on the proportion of the 100 numbers in the cluster that are associated with households. [If you are interested in further statistical and nonstatistical issues associated with this method, read the article by Waksberg (4). This article also includes a list of references on telephone surveys.]

More Complex Cluster Sampling

In this book we have limited our discussion to cluster sampling in which there are at most two stages of sampling. Most of the emphasis was placed on two-stage simple cluster sampling and on cluster sampling with probability proportional to size. For most projects involving the planning of a sample survey, the methods of cluster sampling considered thus far provide sufficient tools for developing a reasonably efficient sampling plan.

Examples of complex surveys

There are, however, projects that require sampling methods much more complex than what can be treated in this book. Typically these surveys cover a very large geographic area (such as a nation), require a very large staff and budget, and either require several years for completion or else are ongoing. Examples of such complex surveys are the Current Population Survey conducted by the U.S. Bureau of the Census, the Health Interview Survey conducted by the National Center for Health Statistics, and the large agricultural surveys conducted by the U.S. Department of Agriculture. Usually these surveys have the objective of providing general purpose information to be used by a variety of institutions and individuals. For example, the Current Population Survey provides up-to-date information on population size as well as information on such items as family and household structure, unemployment, and the size of the labor force. The Health Interview Survey provides information on morbidity, on disability due to chronic and acute disease, and on utilization of health care services.

Because of the importance of these surveys and the size of the projects, very elaborate procedures are used in obtaining the samples. Typically these surveys involve several stages of sampling. Before any sampling is done at all, primary sampling units are often grouped into strata on the basis of their similarities on variables thought to be related to the variables sought in the survey. The primary sampling units themselves are often fairly large areas such as counties or SMSAs.

In these surveys the sampling procedures are very elaborate

Not only is the sampling complex in such surveys, but the estimation procedures are also very complicated. Estimates often involve several stages of ratio adjustments, adjustments for nonresponse, and other devices used to reduce sampling and measurement error. Since the estimates are so complex, it is very difficult to obtain expressions for their variances. Often estimates of variances of estimated parameters are obtained by computing the estimates on the basis of part of the sample observations and examining the variability of the part-sample estimates.

And the estimation procedures are quite complicated

There are several publications that consider these complex sample surveys. For example, the textbooks by Hansen, Hurwitz, and Madow (1) and by Kish (2) give detailed treatment of complex sample surveys. Often the agency that is responsible for the survey publishes material on the sampling plan and estimation procedure used in the survey. For example, the National Center for Health Statistics has published monographs on the methodology used in the Health Interview Survey (5), the Health Examination Survey (7), and the Hospital Discharge Survey (6).

SUMMARY

In this chapter we developed methods for cluster sampling from clusters having unequal numbers of listing units. Estimation procedures were proposed for estimating totals, means, and ratios and for estimating the standard errors of these estimates. For specified second-stage sampling fractions we presented procedures for determining how many clusters should be sampled at the first stage in order to assure that the standard errors of the estimates be below the tolerances set for them. We discussed determination of the optimum second-stage sampling fraction on the basis of costs and intraclass correlation.

We suggested methods such as ratio estimation, stratification, and PPS sampling as procedures that are useful in reducing the standard error of estimated totals when there is great diversity among clusters with respect to the number N_i of listing units. Finally, we described several examples of the use of cluster sampling in practice.

EXERCISES

1. A sample of patient records is being planned in a city that has 25 local mental health centers. The objective of the survey is to estimate the total number of patients who were given Valium as part of their therapeutic regimen. The number of patients treated in each of the mental health centers is listed in the accompanying table. A 2% sample of patients is to be selected by choosing a sample of mental health centers and within each mental health center choosing a subsample of approximately 100 patients per sample center. Choose such a sample and justify the procedure that you use.

Health Center	No. of Patients	Health Center	No. of Patients	Health Center	No. of Patients
1	491	10	246	18	584
2	866	11	399	19	882
3	188	12	175	20	424
4	994	13	166	21	775
5	209	14	672	22	262
6	961	15	475	23	968
7	834	16	439	24	586
8	9820	17	392	25	809
9	348				

2. A household survey is to be conducted for estimating certain health status and utilization variables. The survey research laboratory contracted to perform the study has access to U.S. Census Bureau lists of households and can define clusters of 18 households from which a sample of households can be taken. From a study conducted on similar lists the intraclass correlation coefficients were estimated (see the accompanying table). It is estimated that the cost component associated with clusters is about one-fourth of that associated with listing units. On the basis of this information, choose between

the three different types of clusters, and determine the appropriate sample cluster size.

	Variable	Intraclass Correlation (δ_x) for Various Cluster Sizes		
		$N_i = 6$	$N_i = 9$	$N_i = 18$
number of bed-days in last 2 weeks		.022	.038	.011
number of hospital discharges in past 12 months		.057	.069	.077

3. A list of hospitals in a rural geographic region is shown in the accompanying table, by county. A sample survey is planned using a sampling design in which counties are clusters, hospitals are listing units, and one hospital is to be selected from each cluster. If it is assumed that the total expenses for a hospital are proportional to the number of admissions, how many counties should be selected in order to be 95% confident of estimating the total expenses per day among hospitals in that region to within 20% of the true value?

County	Hospital	No. of Beds	Average No. of Admissions per Day in 1979
1	1	72	4.8
2	1	87	8.4
	2	104	9.4
	3	34	2.0
3	1	99	5.1
4	1	48	4.4
5	1	99	6.2
6	1	131	9.1
	2	182	15.9
7	1	42	2.4
8	1	38	2.8
9	1	34	2.3
10	1	42	4.9
11	1	39	4.0
	2	59	4.1
12	1	76	5.2

County	Hospital	No. of Beds	Average No. of Admissions per Day in 1979
13	1	25	3.1
	2	80	5.3
14	1	50	4.9
15	1	88	7.1
16	1	50	4.4
17	1	63	5.1
18	1	45	3.9
19	1	75	8.5
20	1	17	3.8
	2	140	11.9
21	1	44	4.9
22	1	171	12.0
	2	85	4.6
23	1	48	3.8
	2	18	2.9
24	1	54	4.9
25	1	68	3.8
	2	68	5.5
26	1	44	3.5
27	1	32	1.0
	2	90	6.1
28	1	35	2.9
29	1	72	5.2
30	1	104	6.6
31	1	86	6.4
	2	91	6.4
	3	53	4.5
32	1	108	6.4
33	1	50	4.9
34	1	45	3.8
35	1	65	4.3
36	1	48	4.9
37	1	61	5.7

4. Suppose that a sample of five clusters is selected from the population shown in exercise 3 and that the clusters selected are 5, 8, 23, 30, and 36. Take a second-stage sample of one listing unit from each sample cluster and estimate from this sample the mean number of admissions per hospital bed.

BIBLIOGRAPHY

The following publications discuss household surveys.

1. HANSEN, M. H.; HURWITZ, W. N.; and MADOW, W. G. *Sample survey methods and theory.* Vol. 1. New York: Wiley, 1953.

2. KISH, L. *Survey sampling.* New York: Wiley, 1965.

3. SUDMAN, S. *Applied sampling.* New York: Academic Press, 1976.

The following publication gives practical details about telephone surveys.

4. WAKSBERG, J. Sampling methods for random digit dialing. *Journal of the American Statistical Association* (1978) 73:40–46.

The following publications discuss the methodology of actual surveys in the health professions.

5. National Center for Health Statistics. *Estimation and sampling variance in the health interview survey.* Vital and Health Statistics, Series 2, No. 38, PHS Publication No. 1000. Washington, DC: U.S. Government Printing Office, 1970.

6. National Center for Health Statistics. *Development of the design of the NCHS hospital discharge survey.* Vital and Health Statistics, Series 2, No. 39, PHS Publication No. 1000. Washington, DC: U.S. Government Printing Office, 1970.

7. National Center for Health Statistics. *Sample design and estimation procedures for a national health examination survey of children.* Vital and Health Statistics, Series 2, No. 43, PHS Publication No. 1000. Washington, DC: U.S. Government Printing Office, 1971.

13

Nonresponse and Missing Data in Sample Surveys

Nonresponse has become an increasing problem in recent years

Once a sample is selected, the field work begins and an attempt is made to collect the desired data from all listing units selected in the sample. Unfortunately, it is never possible to achieve complete success in obtaining the data from all sample units. In large-scale surveys it may take a considerable amount of resources to obtain a response rate even as high as 50% of all units originally selected in the sample. This is true even when the survey operation calls for revisiting households in which respondents were not at home at the time of the initial visits, for telephone follow-ups, or for second and third mailings in the case of mail surveys. A partial explanation for high nonresponse rates may be that since the number of sample surveys has proliferated greatly in recent years, there is a growing reluctance on the part of potential respondents to participate. This growing problem of nonresponse has attracted the attention of institutions, corporations, and agencies who either are in the business of conducting sample surveys or rely on sample surveys as decision-making tools. As a result, this topic has been the subject of much research over the past decade.

In this chapter we will first discuss, by use of a simple conceptual model, the impact of nonresponse on the accuracy of estimates obtained from sample surveys. We will then discuss some methods that might increase response rates and some statistical methods of handling missing data.

13.1 EFFECT OF NONRESPONSE ON ACCURACY OF ESTIMATES

The purpose of most sample surveys is to estimate with the greatest possible precision such population parameters as means, totals, and proportions. Each

258

of the sampling procedures described in this book can provide unbiased estimates of these parameters providing a response rate of 100% is attained. Clearly this will rarely be the case, and therefore resulting estimates will no longer be unbiased. In fact, as the nonresponse rate increases, the amount of bias will increase as well.

As the nonresponse rate increases, bias also increases

To examine this idea more formally, let us define the following entities:

Definition of notation

N = the total number of enumeration units in the population

N_1 = the total number of potential responding enumeration units in the population

N_2 = the total number of potential nonresponding enumeration units in the population (i.e., $N_2 = N - N_1$)

$\bar{X}_1$ = the mean level of a characteristic $\mathscr{X}$ among the N_1 potential responding enumeration units

$\bar{X}_2$ = the mean level of $\mathscr{X}$ among the N_2 potential nonresponding enumeration units

$\bar{X} = \dfrac{N_1\bar{X}_1 + N_2\bar{X}_2}{N}$ = the mean level of $\mathscr{X}$ among the total

population of N enumeration units

If we take a simple random sample of n enumeration units and if no attempt is made to obtain data from the potential nonresponders, we are effectively estimating the mean level of characteristic $\mathscr{X}$ for the subgroup of N_1 responding enumeration units rather than for the totality of N enumeration units in the population. From our discussion of estimates for subgroups from simple random sampling (chapter 3), we know that if our sample of n enumeration units (eu's) yields n_1 responding eu's, and if $\bar{x}$ denotes the mean level of $\mathscr{X}$ among these n_1 responding eu's, then the mean value of $\bar{x}$ is given by

In effect, we are estimating the mean of the subgroup of respondents

$$E(\bar{x}) = \bar{X}_1$$

and the bias of $\bar{x}$, denoted by $B(\bar{x})$, is given by

$$B(\bar{x}) = \bar{X}_1 - \bar{X} = \left(\frac{N_2}{N}\right)(\bar{X}_1 - \bar{X}_2) \qquad (13.1)$$

Upon examination of relation (13.1) we see that the bias due to nonresponse is independent of the number n_1 of units successfully sampled. Clearly it cannot be reduced by an increase in sample size, and other measures must be used to reduce this bias. One of these measures is to decrease the proportion N_2/N of potential nonrespondents, and this will be discussed in a later section. Thus the effect of nonresponse bias depends on the proportion of nonrespondents and the difference between the means of the potential nonrespondents and respondents. Unfortunately, the parameters $N_2, \bar{X}_1, \bar{X}_2$ are rarely known.

Bias in $\bar{x}$ does not depend on the number responding

Let us illustrate these ideas in an example.

ILLUSTRATIVE EXAMPLE

Suppose that a sample survey of 100 houholds obtained from simple random sampling is to be conducted in a rural area containing 2000 households for purposes of estimating the proportion of all households that do not have flush toilets. Suppose further than 20% (400) of the 2000 households would refuse to cooperate in the survey or else would not be reachable if selected in the sample (this, of course, would not be known in advance of the survey). Thus the 2000 households in the population consist of 400 potential nonresponding households and 1600 potential responding households. Suppose, finally, that 100 (or 25% of the 400 potential nonresponding households do not have flush toilets, whereas 160 (or 10%) of the 1600 potential respondents do not have flush toilets. Thus in the entire population of 2000 households, 260 (or 13%) of all households do not have flush toilets.

If, in the survey procedure, no attempt is made to obtain data from the potential nonresponding households, the distribution of estimated proportions not having flush toilets that could be obtained from the sample survey would center around .10 (the proportion not having flush toilets among the 1600 potential responders), whereas the target value is .13. In other words, the exclusion of the potential nonresponders would result in biased estimation.

In this example we have

$$N_1 = 1600, \quad \bar{X}_1 = .10, \quad N_2 = 400, \quad \bar{X}_2 = .25, \quad N = 2000$$

From relation (13.1) we have

$$B(\bar{x}) = \left(\frac{400}{2000}\right)(.10 - .25) = .03$$

13.2 METHODS OF INCREASING THE RESPONSE RATE IN SAMPLE SURVEYS

These methods are for household surveys

We can see from relation (13.1) that one of the ways in which the bias due to nonresponse can be decreased is by use of methodology that would result in reduction in the number of potential nonresponding enumeration units. In this section we list, for household surveys, some methods of decreasing the potential number of nonresponding households.

Increasing the Number of Households Contacted Successfully

In household surveys using direct interview, lack of contact will occur when nobody is home. Since in many households both parents work during the day and the children are at school, it is not likely that attempts to make contact with individuals in the household during the day will be successful. In the survey design provision should be made to revisit these households during the evening or, if the information can be obtained in a reasonably short time, to telephone the household during the evening.

Make provisions for contacting households in the evening

In mail surveys of households lack of contact may occur if the family no longer lives at the address from which the name was obtained and the mail is not forwardable. If the listing unit is the address rather than the particular family living there, a visit to the address might be necessary in order to obtain the name of its current resident. Since nearly one of every five American families moves every year, this type of problem is potentially large in mail surveys when the frame from which the name was obtained is not current. Another method of reducing this difficulty is to label the envelope "Mr. and Mrs. John Smith or current occupant."

Make provisions that allow for families that have moved

Increasing the Completion Rate on Mail Questionnaires

In mail questionnaires the response rate often can be increased by an attractive packaging of the questionnaire. The material sent to the household should contain a carefully worded covering letter explaining the purpose of the survey, identifying the organization responsible for the conduct of the survey, and stating that the information elicited from the respondent will be held in strict confidentiality and used in aggregate form for statistical purposes only. The statement of confidentiality is especially important if the information given by the respondent is potentially embarrassing or damaging.

Make the packaging attractive

The survey materials sent to the respondent should be of high quality and should be sent by first-class mail; the return envelope also should contain first-class postage. Agencies that conduct surveys have found, almost universally, that persons are more likely to respond to a mail questionnaire that has an attractive, professional appearance rather than to one that has a cheap and unattractive appearance. In addition, inordinately long questionnaires requiring 30 minutes or more for completion run a higher risk of refusal than do shorter questionnaires. (Mail surveys that incorporate in their design provisions for personal interviews of a subsample of nonrespondents are considered in section 13.3.)

Use high-quality materials and first-class postage

Decreasing the Number of Refusals in Face-to-face or Telephone Interviews

It is very easy for a designated respondent to refuse to complete a questionnaire sent by mail since the respondent has no direct contact with the organization conducting the survey. It is somewhat more difficult for the respondent to refuse a telephone interview since there is voice contact, and it is most difficult for the respondent to refuse a face-to-face interview since there is, in addition, eye-to-eye contact between respondent and interviewer.

Initiate a publicity campaign before starting the survey

In either telephone or face-to-face surveys (as well as in mail surveys), the nonresponse rates often can be reduced if an effective publicity campaign is initiated in advance of the survey. This, however, is not easily accomplished, especially in large metropolitan areas. For instance, the local media would probably be reluctant to use prime time or space to announce an up-coming survey of the frequency of utilization of branch libraries when OPEC has just announced a raise in oil prices and the local university's star basketball player has just decided to play professionally after his sophomore year.

Provide interviewer with proper credentials

Nonresponse rates might also be reduced, particularly in personal interviews, if the interviewer is provided with the proper credentials. This is especially true in large metropolitan areas where a fear of crime exists.

Using Endorsement

The response rate in household surveys might be increased if the survey is endorsed by an official agency or organization whose sphere of interest includes the subject matter of the survey. For example, a household health survey might benefit from the endorsement of a local medical society. In mail surveys the endorsement could be in the form of a covering letter sent with the survey material to the respondent. The covering letter should bear the logo of the endorsing agency and should be signed by a high official of the agency to have maximum impact.

Endorsement is particularly important in surveys of institutions, such as hospitals

Endorsement by an appropriate agency is especially important in surveys of institutions. For example, in a survey of hospitals the likelihood of success would increase if the project had a strong endorsement from the state hospital association. Sometimes an endorsement from the appropriate organization can be obtained more easily if the organization is included as a collaborator or as part of a steering committee for the study. One then gains the additional benefit of having the expertise and experience of the organization as part of the resources of the study.

Using Incentives

The reward given to a respondent for participating in a survey is called an *incentive*. Cash incentives, which are widely used in mail surveys but less widely used in personal interview or telephone surveys, have been found to be effective in increasing response rates. For example, response rates might be increased if the covering letter includes a shiny 25-cent piece or a brand new dollar bill. Incentives other than cash may also be used, but the problem of bias arises with nonmonetary incentives, because they may be more likely to attract special subgroups of the population than would money, which has a more universal appeal. In a controlled study the National Center for Health Statistics has shown

In mail surveys nonresponse rates may be reduced by including cash incentives with the covering letter

that a $10 honorarium promised to the designated sample persons if they would participate in a rather long physical examination and interview resulted in substantially higher response rate (3). An excellent discussion of the use of incentives is found in the book by Erdos on mail surveys (1).

13.3 MAIL SURVEYS COMBINED WITH INTERVIEWS OF NONRESPONDENTS

Mail surveys are generally less expensive than household surveys conducted by personal interview. However, it is often difficult to obtain a response rate from mail surveys that is high enough to meet specifications pertaining to the validity and reliability of the resulting estimates. If the initial response rate to the mailed questionnaire is low, the resulting estimates may be seriously biased. To overcome this problem, it is possible to use a two-stage sampling procedure in which the first stage is a mail survey and the second stage is a telephone and/or personal interview of a subsample of those who did not respond to the mail questionnaire. This procedure often can yield estimates having high reliability and can be done at reasonable cost. This type of sample design is described in the next example in some detail.

This design is a two-stage sampling procedure

ILLUSTRATIVE EXAMPLE

Suppose that in a community containing 300 physicians a questionnaire is sent to a simple random sample of 100 physicians; the questionnaire asks whether the physician accepts patients who cannot pay for their services either directly or indirectly. Of the 100 questionnaires sent out, let us suppose that 30 are returned. Let us suppose further that from the 70 physicians who did not respond to the mail questionnaire, a simple random sample of 20 is selected, that intensive effort is made by telephone and personal visit to obtain responses from these 20 physicians, and that 15 are successfully interviewed. Finally, let us suppose that the data shown in table 13.1 are obtained from the respondents.

Table 13.1   Data for Survey of Physicians

	Number	Number Responding "Yes"
Physicians Returning Mail Questionnaire	30	20
Physicians Responding to Telephone or Visit	15	3

To generalize, let us introduce the following notation as representing this situation:

Notation for this design

n = the number of enumeration units initially sampled by mail

N = the number of enumeration units in the population

n_1 = the number of enumeration units responding to the initial mailing

$n_2 = n - n_1$ = the number of enumeration units not responding to the initial mailing

n_2^* = the number of the n_2 nonresponding eu's selected for intensive effort (e.g., telephone or personal interview)

n_2' = the number of these n_2^* eu's for which responses are obtained successfully

$$\bar{x}_1 = \frac{\sum_{i=1}^{n_1} x_i}{n_1} = \text{the mean level of } \mathscr{X} \text{ among the } n_1 \text{ eu's successfully contacted at the first mailing}$$

$$\bar{x}_2 = \frac{\sum_{i=1}^{n_2'} x_i}{n_2'} = \text{the mean level of } \mathscr{X} \text{ among the } n_2' \text{ eu's successfully contacted through intensive effort}$$

Estimator of unknown population mean   An estimator, which we will denote by $\bar{x}_{\text{DUB}}$ (since it is based on a double sample), can be used to estimate the unknown population mean $\bar{X}$. This estimator is given by

$$\bar{x}_{\text{DUB}} = \frac{n_1\bar{x}_1 + n_2\bar{x}_2}{n} \qquad (13.2)$$

For this example we have

$$N = 300 \qquad n = 100 \qquad n_1 = 30 \qquad n_2 = 70 \qquad n_2^* = 20 \qquad n_2' = 15$$

$$\bar{x}_1 = \frac{20}{30} = .67 \qquad \bar{x}_2 = \frac{3}{15} = .20$$

and thus

$$\bar{x}_{\text{DUB}} = \frac{30(.67) + 70(.20)}{100} = .34$$

If the number n_2' of the initial nonresponding enumeration units successfully contacted through intensive effort is numerically close to n_2^*, the number actually chosen for intensive effort, then the estimator $\bar{x}_{\text{DUB}}$ is a nearly unbiased estimator of the unknown population mean $\bar{X}$.

The results of this example can be generalized to any appropriate survey.

Determination of Optimal Fraction of Initial Nonrespondents to Subsample for Intensive Effort

Suppose that we have decided on the two-stage sampling procedure consisting of an initial mail questionnaire followed by an intensive effort to obtain responses from a subsample of those enumeration units that do not respond to the initial mail questionnaire. An important decision to make is how large a sample, n_2^*, to take from the n_2 enumeration units not responding to the mail questionnaire. To make this decision, we propose a strategy originally developed by Hansen, Hurwitz, and Madow (2), which yields the optimum allocation for subsampling taking into consideration the field costs and the expected nonresponse rate.

First, let us discuss the unit costs associated with this sample design. Suppose the following **cost components** are defined:

C_0 = cost per mailing of the initial questionnaires

C_1 = cost per returned questionnaire of processing those questionnaires returned by mail

C_2 = cost per questionnaire of obtaining data from those initial nonresponding enumeration units designated for intensive effort and of processing the data once it is obtained

The cost component C_0 consists of the cost of materials used in the questionnaire (e.g., stamps, envelopes, etc.) plus labor required for preparation of these materials for mailing. The cost component C_1 consists of labor involved in editing and coding the data and other data preparation work plus data processing costs such as computer time and computer programming. The component C_2 is a combination of field costs and data preparation and processing costs.

C_0 and C_1 include costs involved with initial mail survey

C_2 includes costs involved in subsampling

An estimate of the **total field and processing costs** of the survey is given by

$$C = C_0 n + C_1 n_1 + C_2 n_2' \qquad (13.3)$$

Finally, if it is anticipated that a proportion P_1 of those initially sampled will respond to the initial mailing, then the **optimum number n_2^* that should be subsampled** is given by

$$n_2^* = (n_2)\left(\frac{C_0 + C_1 P_1}{C_2 P_1}\right)^{1/2} \qquad (13.4)$$

ILLUSTRATIVE EXAMPLE

For the previous example let us suppose that the cost components are given by

C_0 = $1.00 per questionnaire (initial mailing costs)

C_1 = $10.00 per questionnaire (unit preparation and processing costs)

C_2 = $30.00 per enumeration unit (unit cost of obtaining interview and processing data for nonrespondent eu's)

Then P_1, the observed response rate, is

$$P_1 = \frac{30}{100} = .30$$

and the optimum number to subsample is

$$n_2^* = (70)\left[\frac{1 + (10)(.30)}{(30)(.30)}\right]^{1/2} = (70)\left(\frac{2}{3}\right) \approx 47$$

Thus we should take a subsample of $\frac{2}{3}$, or 47, of the 70 initial nonrespondents.

Determination of Sample Size Needed for a Two-Stage Mail Survey

Suppose we were starting from scratch with the survey of physicians and wish to know how many questionnaires to send out initially. Assuming that 30% of the physicians would respond to the mailing and assuming the cost components used in the previous section, we already know that we should subsample $\frac{2}{3}$ of the initial nonrespondents for intensive effort (i.e., $n_2^*/n_2 = \frac{2}{3}$).

Determination of initial sample size for 100% response

To determine the required number of physicians to sample for initial mailing, we first determine the number n' that would be needed if there were 100% response to the mailing. Since we are using simple random sampling in this case, we use the expression in box 3.4 (for proportion) to obtain n'. Suppose we guess that 80% of all physicians accept patients who cannot pay for their services and that we wish to be virtually certain of estimating this percentage to within 30% of its true value. Then from box 3.4 with $\varepsilon = .30$, $p - .80$, and $N = 300$, we have

$$n' = \frac{9(300)(.8)(.2)}{9(.8)(.2) + (299)(.3)^2(.8)^2} = 23 \text{ physicians}$$

Thus if there were 100% response, we would need a sample of only 23 physicians in order to be virtually certain that the estimated proportion is within 30% of the true proportion.

Determination of sample size considering nonresponse rate

However, we anticipate only a 30% response to the mailed questionnaire, and because of this the estimate is subject to more variability. Hence we need a larger sample size. In fact, the required number n of questionnaires needed can be obtained by multiplying n' (from box 3.4) by a factor that takes nonresponse into consideration. This factor is shown in the formula for n given below:

$$n = (n')\left\{1 + (1 - P_1)\left[\left(\frac{C_2 P_1}{C_0 + C_1 P_1}\right)^{1/2} - 1\right]\right\} \qquad (13.5)$$

Thus for our previous example, from results shown above and earlier, we have

$$\left(\frac{C_2 P_1}{C_0 + C_1 P_1}\right)^{1/2} = \frac{3}{2} \qquad P_1 = .30 \qquad n' = 23$$

and hence

$$n = (23)\left[1 + (.7)\left(\frac{3}{2} - 1\right)\right] = 31.05 \approx 31$$

Thus we would take a simple random sample of 31 physicians for the initial mailing in order to be virtually certain of meeting the specifications set for the estimate.

13.4 WHAT TO DO ABOUT MISSING VALUES: IMPUTATION

One of the most difficult problems confronting investigators who analyze data from surveys is how to deal with missing or clearly erroneous bits of information. In this section we discuss several strategies that can be followed for dealing with such problems. These strategies are collectively referred to as *methods of imputation.*

Irrespective of which sampling method is chosen, the calculation of estimates of population parameters requires that each of possibly multiple items of information be available to the data analyst for each of the sample individuals. Unfortunately, it is rarely the case that a complete set of information is available for each of the study subjects.

To estimate parameters, we need a complete set of data for each subject, which is rarely available

Using a household survey as an example, missing values can occur when no information is obtained concerning any of the members of a household; when information is obtained concerning some but not all of the members of a household; or when specific items of information are not obtained for any member of a household. An erroneous value may arise in several ways. Most often it occurs when an interviewer writes down a value on the interview schedule that is not an accurate representation of the true value of a given individual. For instance, a patient's weight might be 123.5 pounds but the interviewer writes down 1235 instead. Another way for erroneous data to arise is in the process of transferring the data from the data collection instrument to some computer-readable mode such as computer cards or magnetic tape.

Examples of how erroneous or missing information might arise

It is the task of the data analyst to convert the incomplete, unedited data set into one in which every measurement is both present and reasonable. This process is known as **imputation.** This editing function is neither dishonest or unethical. To the contrary, when properly carried out, it allows the data analyst to exercise his or her best judgment by taking maximum advantage of all

In imputation data are edited so that each piece is present and reasonable

relevant information so that the truth is approached as closely as resources allow.

It should be kept in mind that default—or the failure to do anything at all with incomplete data—is a kind of imputation. Therefore, imputation is not only desirable but inevitable as well, and the question is not whether to impute but *how*. The answer depends on the material to be analyzed, the analytical techniques to be used, and the time and resources available. In the following paragraphs we discuss several methods of imputation that are in common use.

Several methods of imputation are in use

The most popular method of dealing with missing or erroneous data is to simply drop all missing or incomplete records from the analysis. We do not, as a rule, advocate this practice for several reasons. First of all, the available sample size may shrink quickly to a small fraction of its original size. Second, if the individuals who were dropped from the analysis are very different from those who remain, the resulting estimates may be highly biased. For this reason no data should ever be discarded without first checking, from any available information, that the individuals whose data are to be dropped do not differ from those whose data will be used. Often this comparison is limited to the few demographic variables that happen to be available for all individuals in the population. Third, if sampling schemes such as PPS cluster sampling are to be employed, the resulting estimates will not be self-weighting unless each of the sample individuals' values are available for analysis. If the imputation strategy is to discard those individuals for whom some or all data are missing, the estimate will no longer be self-weighting. Fourth, in some complex sampling schemes individuals are assigned statistical weights w_i, which may reflect, among other things, their probabilities of selection. If valid estimates are to be produced, it is necessary that $\sum_{i=1}^{n} w_i = N$. Clearly individuals with missing values should not simply be dropped from analyses. At the very least the statistical weights of these individuals should be redistributed among the individuals remaining.

Simply drop all missing or incomplete data

Another popularly employed strategy is simply to create a new category called "unknown" for those individuals on whom there is no data on any particular variable. This technique is best applied in situations in which only one variable is under consideration and there is reason to believe that the set of unavailable measurements does not differ significantly from the set of available measurements.

Create a category "unknown" for missing or incomplete data

Neither of the two methods above involve filling in or substituting one value for another on an individual's data record. The following four methods do, in fact, alter the original appearance of particular data records.

The most commonly used of the methods that alter data involves assigning the mean value $\bar{y}$ of all individuals whose values on a particular variable $\mathcal{Y}$ is present to any individual whose value is missing or erroneous for that variable. In this method the estimate of the population mean for the variable is the same as for those individuals whose data were complete. It replaces the missing

Use the mean value of known data for unknown data

value with an "expected" value that has a relatively high degree of stability. Although easy to do, this method has the unfavorable property that in final tabulations there will be too many observations exactly equal to the mean value, thereby erroneously reducing the standard error.

The disadvantage pointed out in the mean value method has been eliminated by the hot deck and cold deck methods as used, among others, by the U.S. Bureau of the Census.

In the hot deck method the original data file is sorted in such a way that the ordering of subjects corresponds to the structure of the sample design (e.g., individuals from the same clusters might be together in the data file). Cells are established based on the values of selected demographic variables. For each cell a register is set up containing the record of an individual on whom all variables are recorded. In a single pass through the data file each individual's cell is identified, and if the variable of interest for that individual is missing, the value from that cell's register is substituted in place of the missing value. On the other hand, if the individual's record is complete, the complete record is substituted for the one previously serving in the register. In some surveys having much missing data, there may be little change in the registers of certain cells; hence the same values will be imputed repeatedly. To avoid this problem, it is possible to have multiple cases in the registers that are rotated.

The hot deck method; values from a complete data set are substituted for missing data

Another method that has been proposed is similar to the hot deck method except that values from another randomly selected individual in the sample are substituted for those missing from the incomplete record. Even if the random selection occurs within cells similar to those established in the hot deck method, this procedure is not as good as the hot deck method. Since there is often a special ordering among the respondents, by imputing the value of an individual close by in the file, important regional and geographic features may be controlled in the hot deck method. Also, with respect to computational ease the hot deck method is more convenient.

A variation of the hot deck method

In the cold deck procedure cells are identified as in the hot deck procedure, but the cell's registers are composed of records generally compiled in a survey other than the current one. Often this other survey may be a previous one of the same population. There must be at least one case available from the former survey in each of the established cells. When there are multiple records available in a cell, the selection of one for imputation to the current survey is done at random. The cold deck method has the disadvantage that it doesn't use data from the current survey for the purpose of imputation. For this reason a hot deck approach appears to be more appealing.

The cold deck method; values from a complete data set of a previous survey are substituted for missing data

The difficulty with the procedures just described is that when more than two bits of information are missing on the same record, the relationship between the variables must somehow be accounted for in the random generation process. That is, the record of any given individual, which was only partially complete and was later completed during an imputation process, might contain bits of

Disadvantage of some imputation methods

information that are not harmonious. For example, it is possible that imputation of the body weight of a 21-year-old white male would yield a value of 165 pounds. However, if it turns out that this individual was 6′5″ tall, these two bits of information—one real and one imputed—would not be compatible. Fortunately there are imputation strategies available for guarding against this possibility.

When one of a pair of highly related measurements is missing, use the known value of the pair for the missing value

In the situation where one of a pair of highly related measurements—such as the hearing levels of right and left ear, or the visual acuities of right and left eye—is missing, an analyst may elect to fill the gap with the known, correctly recorded measurement. This simple technique is definitely preferred when there is no other information available on an individual that might yield better estimates. Certainly the use of one of a pair of two very highly correlated variables will yield an excellent estimate of the unknown one. This easily applied method is often the best one to use.

Subjective regression; missing data are supplied by an experienced analyst

Another method that is frequently used might best be called "subjective regression." This method is an intuitively deductive process and, as its name implies, relies solely on the analyst's judgment based on strong evidence. For example, if the sex of a sample respondent is the missing item, data recorded on the survey instrument concerning age at menarche would lead the analyst to impute "female." Similarly, an analyst familiar with physical anthropometry could assign a reasonable estimate of height given the presence of other data such as weight, age, sex, and so on.

Objective regression; regression equations are used to fill in missing data

Finally, we discuss a method that may be termed "objective regression." In this method regression equations are generated from either a hot or cold deck based on complete records, with the variable to be imputed serving as the dependent variable. The resulting equation may be of the form.

$$y = a + b_1 x_1 + b_2 x_2 + \cdots + b_k x_k$$

where y is the variable to be imputed for a given individual and $x_1, \ldots, x_k$ are variables known for the individual. The values imputed in this manner may be superior to those derived from the previously described methods since all the relevant information is utilized and allows the imputed value to be harmonious with the rest of the subject's record.

Methods to use when total record of an individual is missing

The methods described to this point are useful when specific items are missing from the records of selected respondents. When the total record is missing, other methods have been proposed.

Substitute responses from a complete record

For example, a possible method of imputation for a sampling unit for which there is no information is to substitute for that unit the responses of another sampling unit for which there is a complete record. This complete record is usually selected from a hot deck. This procedure amounts to increasing the weight of the respondent whose record is duplicated. The difficulty with this method is that the variances of the resulting estimates tend to be larger.

An alternative procedure, which provides smaller variances than are possible with the substitution of another complete record, is to adjust the statistical weights of the respondents so that this group (without the nonrespondents) is representative of the population as a whole. As a rule, this adjustment of weights provides a biased estimate of the population parameters of interest. The amount of bias is an increasing function of the nonresponse rate as well as the difference between responders and nonresponders. Thus if the response rate is high and there is not a great deal of difference between responders and nonresponders, it is likely that the bias will be small. Otherwise, estimates resulting from the redistribution of weights may have considerable bias. Several methods for adjusting statistical weights have been proposed in an attempt to reduce the magnitude of this bias. Among them is a method in which the population is divided into a number of subgroups based on known demographic information, and adjustments for nonresponse take place within each of these subgroups. This approach has been used by many large-scale surveys to impute for missing cases. A description of the procedure used in the Health Examination Survey of the National Center for Health Statistics is given in an NCHS report (6). The approach used by the Current Population Survey of the U.S. Bureau of the Census is documented in a technical report (8).

Adjust the statistical weights of respondents

This method yields biased estimates

As a general rule for any study, a log should be kept documenting all imputation performed on the data file. In addition, it is often advisable to create a new variable that allows for quick retrieval of the exact imputational method used on a given subject.

A detailed discussion of the imputation scheme used in cycle III of the Health Examination Survey of the National Center for Health Statistics is in an NCHS report (5). An excellent review of available imputation methods is given in a paper by David W. Chapman (4). Recently the whole area of imputation has received renewed interest and attention. You may wish to consult the 1978 *Proceedings of the American Statistical Association: Section on Survey Research Methods*, which describes several sessions devoted to the issues of survey imputation, nonresponse, and editing (7).

SUMMARY

In this chapter we discussed problems caused by incomplete data in sample surveys. In particular, we described the effect of nonresponse on estimates obtained from sample surveys of households; we discussed the reasons nonresponse might result; and we suggested several methods for increasing the response rate in such surveys. In one widely used sample design questionnaires are mailed to sample households and then data are obtained on a subsample of the nonrespondents by intensive effort. This sample design, if executed properly, generally results in estimates that are not biased seriously by the nonresponse.

Finally, we discussed the problem of missing items in a data file, and we described several imputation methods that attempt to convert an incomplete data set into a complete one.

EXERCISES

1. In a community containing 200 households, it is desired to conduct a mail survey for purposes of estimating X, the number of persons 18–64 years of age in the community; R_1, the proportion of employed persons among all persons 18–64 years of age; and R_2, the average number of work days lost per employed person per year among employed persons 18–64 years old. From a collection of ten households in a nearby, similar community, the accompanying data were obtained. How large a sample is needed in order to be virtually certain of estimating X to within 20%, R_1 to within 30%, and R_2 to within 25%?

Household	Persons 18–64 Years	Employed Persons 18–64	Work Days Lost in Past Month
a	4	3	1
b	2	1	1
c	3	2	2
d	1	0	0
e	1	1	2
f	0	0	0
g	2	2	3
h	5	4	2
i	0	0	0
j	2	1	2

2. For the data of exercise 1 assume that 20% of the population would not respond to the questionnaire. Assume further that it costs $0.75 per questionnaire for the initial mailing, $5.00 per questionnaire for processing of mailed questionnaires, and $30.00 per interview (cost of obtaining the interview and processing the data) for nonrespondents. Determine the proportion of nonrespondents that should be sampled and the total number of initial questionnaires that should be mailed.

3. Pick a simple random sample of the required number of households, and from the data given in table 13.2, estimate X, R_1, and R_2.

Table 13.2 Data Obtained from Sample Survey

Household	Persons 18–64	Employed Persons 18–64	Work Days Lost in Past Month	Household	Persons 18–64	Employed Persons 18–64	Work Days Lost in Past Month
1	0	0	0	45	3	0	0
2	2	1	1	46	4	0	0
3	*			47	5	1	0
4	*			48	2	2	0
5	1	1	0	49	5	1	0
6	*			50	5	2	3
7	4	1	0	51	4	0	0
8	1	0	0	52	0	0	0
9	4	3	0	53	0	0	0
10	3	3	5	54	0	0	0
11	*			55	3	2	1
12	0	0	0	56	4	1	1
13	2	1	1	57	1	1	1
14	3	0	0	58	0	0	0
15	4	3	6	59	0	0	0
16	*			60	*		
17	2	0	0	61	*		
18	5	3	2	62	*		
19	2	2	1	63	3	3	4
20	1	0	0	64	3	3	1
21	*			65	2	1	2
22	2	2	1	66	2	2	1
23	0	0	0	67	5	0	0
24	2	1	1	68	*		
25	*			69	2	0	0
26	*			70	4	0	0
27	*			71	2	1	1
28	*			72	1	0	0
29	2	0	0	73	*		
30	3	1	1	74	3	2	1
31	4	3	2	75	*		
32	3	3	6	76	*		
33	3	1	1	77	0	0	0
34	5	1	1	78	2	0	0
35	3	2	3	79	*		
36	*			80	1	1	1
37	4	0	0	81	3	1	1
38	2	2	3	82	4	2	1
39	4	1	1	83	5	0	0
40	5	1	1	84	3	0	0
41	5	1	0	85	4	3	1
42	*			86	3	3	1
43	*			87	5	1	0
44	3	3	5	88	*		

Table 13.2 (continued)

Household	Persons 18–64	Employed Persons 18–64	Work Days Lost in Past Month	Household	Persons 18–64	Employed Persons 18–64	Work Days Lost in Past Month
89	*			134	4	3	5
90	1	1	2	135	3	1	2
91	2	2	4	136	4	3	1
92	1	0	0	137	1	1	0
93	*			138	5	4	6
94	2	1	1	139	2	2	3
95	*			140	4	1	0
96	4	2	1	141	2	1	2
97	2	2	1	142	4	1	2
98	4	2	0	143	3	1	0
99	0	0	0	144	*		
100	*			145	*		
101	1	1	2	146	3	3	2
102	5	0	0	147	0	0	0
103	1	0	0	148	3	0	0
104	2	1	1	149	1	1	0
105	*			150	5	4	4
106	4	1	1	151	0	0	0
107	1	1	1	152	5	4	2
108	*			153	1	0	0
109	5	1	2	154	5	5	4
110	3	2	4	155	*		
111	4	2	1	156	2	1	0
112	0	0	0	157	*		
113	*			158	1	0	0
114		2	3	159	4	2	2
115	*			160	4	0	0
116	4	3	3	161	5	2	3
117	4	3	0	162	3	1	1
118	3	2	3	163	3	1	1
119	0	0	0	164	2	1	0
120	0	0	0	165	*		
121	4	3	3	166	2	0	0
122	1	1	0	167	4	2	0
123	0	0	0	168	0	0	0
124	*			169	3	2	3
125	*			170	*		
126	0	0	0	171	0	0	0
127	3	1	0	172	3	1	1
128	5	4	5	173	*		
129	*			174	2	1	1
130	3	1	1	175*			
131	3	1	1	176	*		
132	0	0	0	177	*		
133	4	1	1	178	4	2	2

Table 13.2 *(continued)*

Household	Persons 18–64	Employed Persons 18–64	Work Days Lost in Past Month	Household	Persons 18–64	Employed Persons 18–64	Work Days Lost in Past Month
179	2	1	1	190	*		
180	1	0	0	191	*		
181	4	2	4	192	3	2	0
182	*			193	*		
183	3	1	1	194	*		
184	3	2	0	195	2	2	2
185	2	1	1	196	3	2	3
186	4	3	1	197	*		
187	4	1	1	198	4	3	3
188	*			199	4	2	3
189	3	1	1	200	4	3	3

* Missing information on this household (i.e., nonrespondents). See table 13.3.

Table 13.3   Actual Values for Missing Data in Table 13.2

Household	Persons 18–64	Employed Persons 18–64	Work Days Lost in Past Month	Household	Persons 18–64	Employed Persons 18–64	Work Days Lost in Past Month
3	3	2	2	100	1	0	0
4	3	2	2	105	2	2	1
6	2	1	0	108	1	1	0
11	1	1	1	113	3	3	2
16	2	2	1	115	0	0	0
21	3	2	0	124	2	2	1
25	1	1	0	125	1	1	0
26	2	2	1	129	2	2	2
27	1	1	0	144	1	1	1
28	2	2	2	145	2	2	2
36	1	1	1	155	1	1	1
42	1	1	0	157	2	2	1
43	2	2	1	165	1	1	0
60	3	3	3	170	2	2	2
61	3	2	2	173	2	2	2
62	2	2	1	175	2	2	1
68	1	1	0	176	3	3	2
73	1	1	0	177	2	1	0
75	2	2	2	182	2	2	0
76	1	1	1	188	2	2	2
79	2	2	2	190	3	3	1
88	3	3	1	191	2	1	1
89	1	1	0	193	3	3	1
93	0	0	0	194	3	2	1
95	3	2	0	197	3	2	1

BIBLIOGRAPHY

The following publications discuss some of the issues concerning nonresponse that were presented in this chapter.

1. ERDOS, P. *Professional mail surveys.* New York: McGraw-Hill, 1970.

2. HANSEN, M. H.; HURWITZ, W. N.; and MADOW, W. G. *Sample survey methods and theory.* Vol. 1. New York: Wiley, 1953.

3. National Center for Health Statistics. *A study of the effect of remuneration upon response in the health and nutrition examination survey.* PHS Publication No. 1000, Series 2, No. 67. Washington, DC: U.S. Government Printing Office, 1975.

The following publications discuss methods of imputation for missing values.

4. Chapman, D. W. A survey of nonresponse imputation procedures. *Proceedings of the American Statistical Association: Social Statistics Section* (1976); pp. 245–251.

5. National Center for Health Statistics. *Body weight, stature, and sitting height: White and negro youths 12–17 years, United States.* Vital and Health Statistics, Series 11, No. 126. Washington, DC: U.S. Government Printing Office, 1973.

6. National Center for Health Statistics. *Cycle I of the health examination survey: Sample and response, United States, 1960–1962.* Vital and Health Statistics, Series 11, No. 1, PHS Publication No. 1000. Washington, DC: U.S. Government Printing Office, 1964; p. 6.

7. *Proceedings of the American Statistical Association: Section on Survey Research Methods.* Papers presented at the Annual Meeting of the American Statistical Association, San Diego, CA, August 14–17, 1978.

8. U.S. Bureau of the Census. *The current population survey–a report on methodology.* Technical Paper No. 7. Washington, DC: U.S. Government Printing Office, 1963; p. 53.

14

Constructing Forms and Collecting Data in Sample Surveys

In chapter 1 we mentioned that sample surveys have four major components, namely, sample design, survey measurements, survey operations, and statistical analysis and report writing. Since this book addresses primarily persons functioning as statisticians, we have placed our primary emphasis on statistical methodology relevant to sample surveys, such as sample design and estimation. However, a good sample design will not necessarily result in a good survey if the nonstatistical components are poorly planned and executed. In this chapter we discuss those issues of sample surveys that are basically non-statistical. In particular, we deal with survey measurements and survey operations.

Nonstatistical aspects of sample surveys are considered here

14.1 DESIGNING THE FORM FOR DATA COLLECTION

One of the most important components of a survey design is the set of forms or survey instruments used to collect the data. Form design is considered to be as much an art as a science. However, we feel that it can be organized into a set of operations, which, if followed sequentially, will increase the efficiency of the procedure and result in a product that will do the required job.

Sirken, in a manual for designing forms for use in demographic surveys, has suggested a five-step sequential procedure for designing survey forms (7). Although Sirken's methodology is designed for household surveys, we feel

Form design may be organized into steps

that it is applicable to any type of survey. Sirken's five operations are listed below:

Five steps for designing forms

1. specifying the information to be collected
2. selecting the data collection strategy
3. ordering the questions
4. structuring the questions
5. spacing the questions

We discuss these operations in the paragraphs that follow in the order in which they are listed, which is also the sequence in which they should be performed.

Specifying the Information to Be Collected

The first step in designing the form should be the construction of an inventory of information to be collected. The source of this inventory should be the statement of overall objectives and specific aims of the survey. Let us illustrate this step through an example.

ILLUSTRATIVE EXAMPLE

Let us suppose that in a medium-sized city we are conducting a sample survey having the following aims:

Aims of the survey

1. to estimate the proportion of all persons covered by health insurance
2. to investigate whether the proportion varies according to the age, sex, or race of the household head, according to the family structure of the household, according to the level of family income, and according to the number of persons in the household
3. to estimate, among all persons covered by health insurance, the proportion covered by group (as opposed to individual) insurance policies
4. to estimate the average yearly out-of-pocket premiums paid for health insurance among those households having one or more persons covered by health insurance
5. to estimate the proportion of all persons having hospital visits during the past year, by age and sex

From the five specific aims of the survey stated above, we might abstract the following inventory list of information needed to attain these stated aims:

Information to be collected

1. age and sex of all persons in the household
2. designation of household head
3. relationship of each individual in the household to the household head (e.g., spouse, son, etc.)
4. race of household head

5. income of each individual

6. whether each individual is covered by health insurance and if so whether by individual or group insurance

7. how much each person in the household spends for health insurance

8. whether each individual was hospitalized during the year

Note that each of the eight items on the inventory is needed for the survey to meet the specific aims. For example, the relationship of each household member to the household head must be specified in order for the structure of the household to be characterized (e.g., group of unrelated individuals, parent-child family, etc.). Household structure is one of the variables specified in the second specific aim listed above. In other words, every item in the inventory should have a purpose. The inclusion of irrelevant and unneeded items of information is poor survey practice since it increases the costs of the survey and also increases the burden placed on the respondents.

Selecting the Data Collection Strategy

First of all, we distinguish three basically different methods of collecting data. These are

1. extraction of data from records

2. self-administered questionnaire

3. direct interview (e.g., face-to-face, telephone)

Three methods of collection

The design of data forms depends on which of the three data collection methods listed above is used. In a self-administered questionnaire, for example, the questions must be worded in such a way that every word is understood by the respondent. Thus definitions of words or terms that might be misunderstood by the respondent should be written on the form. In a direct interview, however, this step is less crucial so long as the interviewer tells the respondent the meaning of the question.

Design of forms depends on method of collection

Since the design of the data forms depends to a very large extent on which of the three data collection methods is used, our first step is to decide on which of these three methods to use. In making this decision, we should refer to the inventory constructed earlier of information to be collected, because the data collection method will be determined by the nature of the required information. In the previous example we constructed a list of items needed for our survey. In scanning this list of items, we see that it is unlikely that we can find a set of records that would contain the information listed in the inventory. Clearly some kind of survey of households is required, and so we must choose between a self-administered questionnaire or a direct interview. Although a self-administered questionnaire, possibly sent by mail, would be the less expensive of these two methods, we might feel that the quality of the information on

First step: decide on which method of collection to use

such items as costs and insurance coverage would be better if the data were obtained by direct interview and that this would justify the increased expense.

In our ensuing discussion of data collection strategy, we will discuss issues that are most applicable to direct interview surveys, although many of these issues also apply to surveys conducted by self-administered questionnaire or abstraction of records.

Next step: determine the respondent rule

The next important issue in data collection strategy is that of determining the **respondent rule.** A respondent rule is an algorithm specifying which individuals in an enumeration unit are eligible to serve as respondents. This concept is very important in household surveys conducted by direct interview. A household can be considered as a cluster containing a number of individuals. A respondent rule determines which individuals can give information concerning themselves and concerning other individuals in the household.

For some surveys the respondent rule requires every individual to respond for himself or herself. Other surveys allow the use of **proxy respondents;** that is, an individual can furnish information regarding other individuals in the household. Use of proxy respondents generally results in fewer visits or phone calls and hence in reduction in field costs. On the other hand, the validity of information obtained from proxy respondents might be questionable, at least for certain items. For example, a controversy arose over data reported by the National Center for Health Statistics concerning smoking and disability due to acute illness (2). This report was based on data collected through the Health Interview Survey (HIS), which allows proxy respondents. One critic suggested that women are more likely to be at home than men, and therefore much of the data on both smoking and acute illness in men would be reported by proxy through their wives. He suggested that nonsmoking wives of smoking husbands might tend to exaggerate the acute illnesses of their husbands, which would lead to an overstatement of the association between smoking and disability from acute illness (8). Although NCHS discounted that this had indeed happened (9), the criticism emphasizes the type of pitfalls that can arise from the use of proxy respondents.

If the respondent rule allows the use of proxy respondents, then the data form should indicate which individual supplied the information so that any possible effects of proxy respondents can be investigated later on at the analysis stage.

In the illustrative example of a survey of health insurance coverage, we might allow any person over 18 years of age to respond for any individual in the household.

Ordering the Questions

Group the items of information

Once the inventory of required information is constructed, and the data collection strategy is established, the next step is to group the items of information in some meaningful way and then to order the items within groups. The groups are constructed either on the basis of subject matter or on the basis of some convenient frame of reference.

For example, in our household survey of health insurance coverage, some items pertain to the household whereas others pertain to individuals within the household. In addition, on the basis of subject matter the items can be grouped into demographic items, items on health insurance coverage, and items on hospitalization. Thus we might have the following groupings of the items listed on the inventory: *Ordering the questions for the survey of the previous example*

HOUSEHOLD ITEMS

Age of household head (exact age)

Sex of household head

Race of household head (white, black, or other)

Type of family (group of unrelated individuals, husband-wife nucleus, parent-child nucleus, other)

Total income over all persons in household

Which person is the respondent?

FOR EACH PERSON IN HOUSEHOLD (PERSON ITEMS)

age
sex
relation to head of household } demographic items
annual income

Is individual covered by health insurance?
Is individual covered by group health insurance
or individual policy? } health insurance items
How much in out-of-pocket costs does individual
pay for health insurance?

Hospitalization during past years?} hospitalization item

Structuring the Questions

Once the items of information have been ordered in some meaningful way, the next operation is the actual structuring or wording of the questions to be asked. In structuring each question, we must consider the following issues:

1. Does the question elicit the information that is needed?

2. Would the respondent be willing to answer the question?

3. Would the respondent be able to answer the question (i.e., would he or she have the information or understand the question)?

Issues to consider in structuring questions

*The inventory
can be a checklist
for each question*

If the required information has been listed and ordered as suggested above *before* the structuring and wording of the questions, then the likelihood of missing items of information or of including irrelevant questions is minimized, because we can use the inventory as a checklist for each question. For example, if exact age were required in the inventory, then we would not phrase a question asking for age in 5-year age groups. Rather, we would phrase the question to elicit age as of last birthday or as of nearest birthday, depending on how the characteristic "age" is defined.

*The randomized
response technique
might be considered
for sensitive
questions*

An important issue in structuring the questions is that of *sensitivity*, that is, whether an individual would be willing to answer the question. Some items of information are, of course, more sensitive than others. We could not, for example, easily ask a respondent to provide information about the nature of his or her sexual fantasies or about the number of dollars that he or she cheated the IRS out of on his or her income tax return. One method of asking sensitive questions is the randomized response technique discussed in chapter 8. Assurances of confidentiality will sometimes persuade an unwilling respondent to answer a sensitive question.

Perhaps an equally important issue in the structuring of questions is that of the respondent's ability to provide the information. The respondent may have no knowledge at all of the item being elicited or else may have some but not complete knowledge.

*Telescoping—
shifting events into
or out of the
relevant time
period—may occur*

Another problem, known as *telescoping*, occurs when a respondent shifts an event into or out of the time frame covered by the question. For example, the respondent, when asked about hospitalizations during a particular calendar year, may incorrectly report one that did not take place during that year, or else might not report one that did take place during that year because he or she thought that it occurred during some other time period. One method of dealing with the problem of telescoping is to make the time frame very short.

*Short time periods
may eliminate the
problem of
telescoping*

For example, the Health Interview Survey conducted by the National Center for Health Statistics asks questions about acute illnesses and physician or dental visits that have occurred during the two-week period prior to the date of the interview. On the other hand, more memorable events such as hospitalizations are elicited for a 12-month time frame prior to the interview. Although shortening the time frame decreases the likelihood of telescoping, it also decreases the number of events reported, and this can have an adverse effect on the reliability of the estimates. In other words, we are often caught between the evil of telescoping and that of high standard errors, and we must compromise somewhere between the two.

*Examine published
questionnaires and
use items from
them if applicable*

In the wording of many questions we can make our work easier by examining questionnaires that have already been developed and taking appropriate questions from them. For example, the substantive reports published by the National Center for Health Statistics almost always include in the appendix copies of the relevant portions of the questionnaires. This step can save considerable time and can also result in an improvement in the quality of the form.

Spacing the Questions

Once the wording or structuring of the questions is completed, the last operation in form construction involves the actual appearance of the form. The two most important considerations involved in the layout of the form are the facility with which the interviewer can use the form to elicit information from the respondent and the facility with which the data from the form can be coded and prepared for computer processing. Such matters as the quality of the materials, the kind of typeface used, or the nature of the visual aids given on the form can affect the facility with which the interviewer can use the form. The individual involved in the form construction should consult the data processing staff concerning the layout of the form. Often space can be provided on the form for numerical codes so that a keypuncher can punch data cards from the form itself without the necessity of intermediary coding. Sometimes, however, this is not feasible.

Careful consideration should be given to the physical appearance of the form

An illustration of a form that might be used for the household survey of health insurance coverage and hospitalization is shown in figure 14.1. The layout of the form is such that the interviewer would first ask the respondent to list all persons in the household by name. Then for each individual listed, the interviewer would obtain all the items of information needed for the survey from left to right on the form, beginning with relationship to head of household and ending with hospitalization.

In this section we have outlined some broad strategies in constructing forms for collecting data. More detailed treatment of questionnaire development can be found in the texts by Payne (5) and Oppenheim (4). A detailed treatment of interviewing methodology can be found in an NCHS monograph prepared by Cannell, Marguis, and Laurent (1). This latter publication deals primarily with collection of data on health events and contains an excellent bibliography.

14.2 TESTING THE DATA COLLECTION METHODOLOGY

Once the forms have been designed, the next step is to train the interviewers to collect the data. Ideally, a manual or procedures booklet should be prepared for the interviewers, and one or more training sessions should be held.

The interviewers must now be trained

When the interviewers have been trained on the data collection procedures, the next step is to have a pretest of the data collection process. This step usually entails having the interviewers collect data from a small sample chosen for convenience. The purpose of a pretest is to test the data collection procedures on a dry run. On the basis of the results of the pretest, the data forms and collection procedures might be revised and polished. The size of the sample need not be large for a pretest to provide insight into whether the forms and procedures are adequate.

Next, conduct a pretest

Figure 14.1 Form for Household Survey of Insurance Coverage and Hospitalization

Household Identification ——— Address: ———

What is the name of each person in the household (begin with respondent)?	How is each person related to the head of the household (H.H.)?	Sex	Age at last birthday, in years	Color or race	How much did the person earn in 1978?	Type of health insurance coverage of this individual	How much does this individual pay, out-of-pocket, for health insurance?	Was this individual hospitalized during 1978?
	☐ Head of Household ☐ Spouse of H.H. ☐ Son or daughter of H.H. ☐ Other relative of H.H. ☐ Unrelated	☐ Male ☐ Female	———	☐ White ☐ Negro or Black ☐ Other	$ ———	☐ None ☐ Individual ☐ Group ☐ Both	$ ———	☐ Yes ☐ No
	☐ Head of Household ☐ Spouse of H.H. ☐ Son or daughter of H.H. ☐ Other relative of H.H. ☐ Unrelated	☐ Male ☐ Female	———	☐ White ☐ Negro or Black ☐ Other	$ ———	☐ None ☐ Individual ☐ Group ☐ Both	$ ———	☐ Yes ☐ No
	☐ Head of Household ☐ Spouse of H.H. ☐ Son or daughter of H.H. ☐ Other relative of H.H. ☐ Unrelated	☐ Male ☐ Female	———	☐ White ☐ Negro or Black ☐ Other	$ ———	☐ None ☐ Individual ☐ Group ☐ Both	$ ———	☐ Yes ☐ No
	☐ Head of Household ☐ Spouse of H.H. ☐ Son or daughter of H.H. ☐ Other Relative of H.H. ☐ Unrelated	☐ Male ☐ Female	———	☐ White ☐ Negro or Black ☐ Other	$ ———	☐ None ☐ Individual ☐ Group ☐ Both	$ ———	☐ Yes ☐ No

Sometimes a procedure called a *pilot survey* or *pilot study* is undertaken in addition to a pretest. A pilot survey is generally a full-scale dress rehearsal of the survey. It includes a testing not only of the data collection procedures but of all the components of the survey, from the sampling to the data processing and analysis. A pilot survey is often done on a much larger sample than a pretest. Sometimes a pilot survey may test two or more forms or data collection procedures, and the final procedures used for the survey may depend on the evaluation of the data collected from the pilot study. In addition, the pilot survey may provide estimates necessary for determining the size of sample needed in the actual survey so that final estimates may be made with stated precision.

A pilot study might also be done

14.3 ASSURING THE QUALITY OF THE DATA: QUALITY CONTROL

A sample survey having a good sample design and good data forms can still yield poor data if the execution of the survey is poor. An important part of a survey design is to ensure that the execution of the survey is in accordance with the design. In particular, there should be some formal quality control procedures instituted on both the data collection and data processing components of the survey.

Quality control ensures a good execution of the survey

In very large ongoing data collection systems a subsample of enumeration units is often taken for reinterview (or reabstraction in surveys of records). Data are collected from each enumeration unit in the subsample by experienced personnel, and the data in the subsample are used as a standard against which the performance of each individual doing the initial data collection is evaluated. If the number of discrepancies is large for a particular data collector, that individual may be retrained or subjected to other personnel action. More detailed treatment of the use of reinterview for quality control is given in a manual written by Walt R. Simmons (6). A discussion of quality control procedures used in a survey of hospital records has been published by the National Center for Health Statistics (3).

Reinterviewing can be used for quality control in large ongoing surveys

An important facet of the reinterview subsample is that it pinpoints specific errors on the part of interviewers. This information can then be used to provide feedback to the interviewers so that they do not make the same mistake next time. In smaller surveys, however, there may be no "next time." The entire data collection may cover a very short period of time, such as a day or a week. For such a survey the reinterview subsample may provide information on the dimensions of the interviewer error but would not be of much use in the retraining of interviewers for subsequent data collection in the same survey. For short-term surveys it is advisable that a reinterview subsample be taken and incorporated in the pilot study of the survey and that retraining be done at this stage.

SUMMARY

In this chapter we presented an overview of some of the issues involved in form construction and quality control. We suggested a five-step procedure for designing forms. Finally, we discussed some methods used in quality control, with particular emphasis placed on taking a subsample of the enumeration units initially selected.

BIBLIOGRAPHY

The following publications discuss in more detail the issues presented in this chapter.

1. National Center for Health Statistics. *A summary of studies of interviewing methodology*. Series 2, No. 69, DHEW Publication No. (HRA) 77–1343. Washington, DC: U.S. Government Printing Office, 1977.

2. National Center for Health Statistics. *Cigarette smoking and health characteristics*. Series 10, No. 34, PHS Publication No. 1000. Washington, DC: U.S. Government Printing Office, 1967.

3. National Center for Health Statistics. *Quality control in the hospital discharge survey*. Series 2, No. 68, DHEW Publication No. (HRA) 76–1342. Washington, DC: U.S. Government Printing Office, 1975.

4. OPPENHEIM, A. N. *Questionnaire design and attitude measurement*. New York: Basic Books, 1966.

5. PAYNE, S. L. *The art of asking questions*. Studies in Public Opinion, No. 3. Princeton, NJ: Princeton University Press, 1951.

6. SIMMONS, W. R. *Operational control of sample surveys*. Laboratory for Population Statistics, Manual Series No. 2. Chapel Hill, NC: University of North Carolina, 1972.

7. SIRKEN, M. G. *Designing forms for demographic surveys*. Laboratory for Population Statistics, Manual Series No. 3. Chapel Hill, NC: University of North Carolina, 1972.

8. STERLING, T. D. A review of the claim that excess morbidity and disability can be ascribed to smoking. *Journal of the American Statistical Association* (1971) 66: 251–257.

9. WILSON, R. W. Comment on "Review of claim that excess morbidity and disability can be ascribed to smoking." *Journal of the American Statistical Association* (1973) 68:85–87.

15

Interpretation of Data and Survey Report Writing

Once the sample has been selected and the data collected, edited, and processed, the task remains of analyzing the data and producing a written (or sometimes oral) report that presents appropriate population estimates and interprets the findings of the sample survey. The person responsible for this task should know how to interpret the findings of the survey and to write the report in such a way that is it consistent with the findings.

Once the report of the survey is written, it will often be printed and disseminated. The reader of such a report should be able to evaluate whether the statements made by the author are consistent with the findings of the survey. In order to do this, the reader should be aware of such issues as sample design, estimation procedures, and sampling and measurement errors and should be in a position to evaluate the statements made by the author from the material presented in the body of the report.

Both writers and readers of survey reports should know how to interpret survey data

The objective of this chapter is to discuss the issues that are of importance in interpretation of sample survey data and in statistical report writing. This discussion is addressed to both the writer of survey reports and to the reader of such reports. Much of the material presented here is based on two publications, one from the Bureau of the Census, which addresses the issue of the presentation of sampling and nonsampling errors in statistical reports (1), and the other from the National Center for Health Statistics, which addresses the issue of the kind of statistical statements that are allowable in terms of sampling and measurement errors (7).

15.1 WHAT SHOULD BE INCLUDED IN A SURVEY REPORT

The report consists of the basic text and appendices

A survey report generally consists of a text and one or more appendices. The text often includes a background and introduction section, a methodology section, a results or findings section, a discussion section, and sometimes a summary and conclusion section. The appendices often include definitions of the technical terms used in the survey, detailed tables that present the findings, reproductions of the questionnaires and other materials used in conducting the survey, and detailed discussion of statistical issues such as the sample design, estimation procedures, and survey errors. In the following paragraphs we discuss the types of material that might be presented in each of the major sections of the body of a survey report.

Background and Introduction

Includes survey objectives and rationale

The background and introduction section of the sample survey report should serve to orient the reader concerning such matters as the objectives of the survey, the importance of the subject matter, and a review of the literature on previous relevant work in the subject matter of the survey.

Methodology

The purpose of the methodology section is to provide the reader with information on the methods used in designing the sample, obtaining the data, preparing and processing the data for statistical analysis, and analyzing the data. A good methodology section will discuss all the relevant methodological issues without

This section should not include too much technical detail

going into too much technical detail. Detailed discussion of statistical and other methodological issues should appear in an appendix rather than in the body of the report. Some of the items that should be discussed in general terms in the methodology section (and, if necessary, in more detail in an appendix) are described below.

A precise definition should be given

UNIVERSE OR TARGET POPULATION.   There should be a precise description of what constitutes the universe or target population. This definition is extremely important because it pinpoints the population to which the findings of the survey are extrapolated. The description should include a time reference (e.g., "all persons discharged from short-stay hospitals in the Cleveland standard metropolitan statistical area during the calendar year 1976").

Describe the process and the agency responsible for collection

HOW THE DATA WERE COLLECTED.   There should be an operational description of the data collection process that includes a description of the procedures used for reinterviewing those respondents not at home and other nonrespondents. The agency or organization responsible for the collection of the data should be identified.

SAMPLE DESIGN.   There should be a description of the sampling frame that was used to select the sample. This discussion should include a statement of the extent to which the sampling frame is likely to cover the entire universe or target population as well as a discussion of the sampling units that were used in each stage (e.g., primary sampling units, other clusters, listing units, etc.). There should be a description of the stratification, if any, that was used and the variables on which the strata were formed. The method by which the sample was selected should be described in sufficient detail to provide the reader with information concerning the selection of the sample at each stage of the procedure. There should be a summary of the sample selection, which includes the total number of elementary units selected as well as the total number of sampling units selected at each stage.

Describe the sampling frame and the method of sample selection

SURVEY INSTRUMENTS.   The methodology section should include a description of the materials used to obtain information for the survey. Such materials would include letters of endorsement, covering letters, questionnaires, abstracting forms, and measuring instruments (e.g., sphygnomanometers, written tests, etc.). There also should be a display of these materials in an appendix.

Name and describe materials used

PRETESTS, PILOT SURVEYS, AND OTHER FIELD QUALITY CONTROL PROCEDURES. There should be a description of the pretests or pilot surveys that were performed, including a discussion of changes made as a result of these procedures. In addition, there should be a discussion of the methods used in training interviewers or data abstractors and of quality control procedures used in the field.

DATA PREPARATION AND PROCESSING AND ESTIMATION PROCEDURES.   The methodology section should include a description of the data preparation and processing and the estimation procedures that were used, from the point at which the data were collected to the presentation of the data in tabular form. This description would include a discussion of the methods used in coding, keypunching, encoding (i.e., placing data directly onto magnetic tape), and editing of the computer tapes. There should also be a discussion of the quality control procedures that were used at each stage of the data reduction process. The description of the estimation procedures should include discussion of the weighting that was used at each stage of the estimation as well as other important features of the estimation. Detailed formulas used in the estimation procedures should be included in an appendix.

Include all important features of these procedures

SAMPLING AND NONSAMPLING ERRORS.   In the methodology section there should be a general discussion of the sources of both sampling and nonsampling errors in the estimates. With respect to sampling errors, there should be a discussion of how these errors were estimated and where they are presented. The

Discuss the sources of errors and how they are estimated

actual presentation of the sampling errors is generally best done in the appendix, along with instructions to the user concerning the use of these sampling errors in evaluating the estimates. With respect to the nonsampling errors, the methodology section should discuss the impact of nonresponse on the resulting estimates, the imputation procedures that were used, and the extent of the imputation, as well as the possible effects of response bias and other measurement error on the estimates.

COMPUTATION AND PRESENTATION OF SAMPLING ERRORS.   One of the most difficult tasks in the preparation of a survey report is the computation and presentation of the sampling errors or sampling variances. In the sampling designs discussed in this volume it is generally possible to obtain estimates of the sampling variances from the survey data, although even for some of these relatively simple designs the formulas are quite complex and require a great

This task is often a difficult (and expensive) one

deal of computation. For surveys more complex than those discussed here, it becomes even more difficult (and expensive) to obtain estimates of the sampling variances. Because of the difficulty and expense involved in obtaining estimates of sampling errors, many survey reports include only a very limited presentation and discussion of these errors. In fact, in many survey reports no sampling variances are included, nor is any mention made of the fact that the estimates are subject to sampling as well as nonsampling errors. However, no

But it must be done in order to interpret the findings of the survey

reasonable interpretation of the findings of a survey can be made unless these errors are taken into consideration. Thus it is extremely important that these errors be computed.

Perhaps some idea of the dilemma confronting an individual responsible for writing a survey report can be obtained by considering the following hypothetical example. Suppose that a sample survey includes information on 50 variables and that the findings on each variable are to be presented for two race groups, four age groups, two sex groups, three income groups, and four geographical groups. There are a total of 192 possible subgroups ($2 \times 4 \times 2 \times 3 \times 4$) for which estimates can be presented for each variable and a total of 50×192, or 9600, possible estimates. The presentation of sampling errors for each of these 9600 estimates would add considerably not only to the computation costs of the survey, especially if the formulas for sampling variances are long and complicated, but also to the bulk of the report. On the other hand, these sampling errors are necessary for reasonable interpretations to be made of the data.

Criterion: an estimated standard error for every estimate should be available to reader

A desirable criterion for survey reports is that for every estimate given in the report an estimate of the standard error should be available to the reader. This does not mean that standard errors must be published for every estimate published in the report. The criterion could also be met if the report included material that would provide the reader with the means of computing estimated standard errors for every estimate in the report. For example, estimated standard errors could be given in the form of tables, charts, or similar configurations. Or similar types of estimates could be grouped together and "average" values of standard errors given.

In summary, the reader of a survey report should be able to obtain, either directly or with a small amount of calculation, the estimated standard error for every estimate mentioned in the report. However, it often takes a great deal of thought and imagination on the part of those responsible for the survey report to produce these estimated standard errors without going into prohibitive expense or cluttering the report unnecessarily.

Results or Findings

The results or findings section of a survey report consists of statistical statements about the target population based on the sample estimates. A *statistical statement* is defined as any phrase, clause, sentence, or other grouping of words in which an inference is made from sample estimates to population parameters. Along with tables and graphs, the writer uses these statistical statements to convey the findings of the survey to the readers of the report. It is important that the inferential statements made by the writer be justified by the data. It is also important for the reader of a survey report to be able to evaluate whether or not particular statements in the report are justified. In the next section some methods for evaluating statistical statements will be developed.

This section consists of statistical statements about the target population

Discussion

In this section of the report the analyst discusses the findings that were reported in the previous section. It is this section of the report that gives the analyst the opportunity to discuss the implications of the findings and to relate these findings to those of the previous studies mentioned in the background section of the report. In this section, in contrast to what is done in the results section, the analyst has freedom to extrapolate from the findings of the study.

Implications of the findings are discussed

Summary and Conclusions

In this section the study is summarized and the basic conclusions are listed.

15.2 METHODS OF EVALUATING STATISTICAL STATEMENTS

Much of the discussion that follows is based on the NCHS *Manual on Standards and Procedures for Reviewing Statistical Reports* (7) as well as on earlier publications by Levy and Sirken (4) and Sirken and Levy (6). In these publications statistical statements are classified into various categories and methods are proposed for evaluating each category. Our discussion follows this organization. Alternative strategies for analyzing data from complex surveys have been proposed by Koch, Freeman, and Freeman (3).

Estimates of Population Characteristics

One category of statistical statements is a simple quotation or rounding of an estimate for a population group. For example, the report might state, "Approximately 5% of all hospitalized patients had a length of stay under five days." One method for evaluating the validity of this category of statistical statements is to examine the coefficient of variation of the estimate. If the coefficient of variation is less than a certain amount, then the statement is justified. For example, suppose it is decided to report no survey estimates having a coefficient of variation greater than 25%. If the standard error of the estimated percentage of hospitalized persons with a length of stay under five days is less than 1%, then the estimated coefficient of variation of the estimate is less than 25% (100 × 1%/5%) and the statement is justified. If the coefficient of variation of the estimate is greater than the specified limit (25% in this hypothetical case), the estimate should be considered not reliable enough to be quoted in the survey report. In other words, estimates of population characteristics generally should not be quoted in survey reports unless their reliability meets certain preassigned standards.

Coefficient of variation can be used to evaluate validity

Comparisons of Estimated Population Characteristics with a Constant

A second type of statistical statement frequently found in survey reports is one in which an estimated population characteristic is quoted and compared with a constant. For example, a report might state, "The mean length of stay among patients hospitalized with hip fractures was 17 days, which is less than the standard of 21 days set by the Professional Standards Review Organization for such patients." For this type of statement to be justified not only must the estimate meet standards of reliability but also it should differ significantly from the constant with which it is compared.

The estimate must meet standards of reliability and differ significantly from the constant.

ILLUSTRATIVE EXAMPLE

Suppose that the estimated standard error of the estimated mean length of stay among patients hospitalized with hip fractures is equal to three days. Thus the estimated coefficient of variation of the quoted statistic is 17.6% (100 × 3/17), which is less than the standard of 25% we specified earlier. However, suppose we test the null hypothesis that the mean length of stay is greater than or equal to 21 days against the alternative hypothesis that it is less than 21 days. The usual test statistic z, based on the normal distribution, is given by

$$z = \frac{\bar{x} - 21}{\widehat{SE}(\bar{x})} = \frac{17 - 21}{3} = -1.33$$

where

$$\bar{x} = \text{the estimated mean length of stay} = 17 \text{ days}$$

$$\widehat{SE}(\bar{x}) = \text{the estimated error of } \bar{x} = 3 \text{ days}$$

If we refer the z statistic to tables of the normal distribution (see the Appendix), we obtain a p value of .08, which, if we are using the .05 significance level as a standard, would lead us to conclude that the mean length of stay is not significantly less than 21 days. Hence the statement quoted above does *not* seem to be justified from the data.

Comparison of Two Complementary Groups with Respect to the Level of an Estimated Characteristic

A third type of statistical statement compares two complementary groups of the population with respect to the level of an estimated characteristic. For example, a report might state, "The proportion of white married women 30–39 years of age who admit to having had at least one extramarital sexual relationship was greater among residents of SMSAs (42%) than among non-SMSA residents (25%)." The statement may have been worded, "Among white married women 30–39 years of age, 42% of those residing in SMSAs admit to having had at least one extramarital sexual relationship, as opposed to 25% among those not residing in SMSAs." Although the two statements have different phraseology, the same comparison is implied in both. For this type of statement to be justified by the data, the two estimates quoted in the statement should meet minimum specifications of reliability (e.g., each estimate should have a coefficient of variation less than 25%). In addition, the two estimates should differ from each other statistically when their standardized difference, given by

The estimates must meet standards of reliability and differ from each other statistically

$$z = \frac{\hat{X} - \hat{Y}}{\sqrt{\widehat{\text{Var}}(\hat{X}) + \widehat{\text{Var}}(\hat{Y})}}$$

(where $\hat{X}$ and $\hat{Y}$ are the two quoted statistics) is compared to the cumulative standard normal distribution.

ILLUSTRATIVE EXAMPLE

In the example given above we have

$$\hat{X} = .42 \qquad \widehat{SE}(\hat{X}) = .07$$

$$\hat{Y} = .25 \qquad \widehat{SE}(\hat{Y}) = .04$$

Then

$$\hat{V}(\hat{X}) = \frac{.07}{.42} = .17 \quad \text{and} \quad \hat{V}(\hat{Y}) = \frac{.04}{.25} = .16$$

Thus both estimates meet the preassigned specifications of reliability (less than 25% in this hypothetical example). The standardized difference z between the two estimates is

$$z = \frac{.42 - .25}{\sqrt{(.07)^2 + (.04)^2}} = 2.10$$

Since the p value corresponding to a standardized difference of 2.10 is less than .05, we are justified in concluding that the two population percentages are different, and the statistical statement is justified.

Similar but stronger type of statement

   A type of statement similar to a comparison between two complementary groups with respect to a population characteristic, but somewhat stronger, is one that not only compares the two groups with respect to the variable but also makes a statement concerning the magnitude of the difference between the two groups or the magnitude of the ratio of the levels of the characteristics in the two groups. For example, a report might state, "The percentage of white married women 30–39 years of age living in SMSAs who admit to having had at least one extramarital sexual relationship is 42%, which is approximately 1.7 times as great as the percentage (25%) among white married women in the same age group not living in SMSAs who admit to having had such a relationship." This type of statistical statement gives three estimates (e.g., 42%, 25%, and approximately 1.7), one of which is the ratio of the other two. This statement asserts not only that the level of a characteristic is greater in one group than in another but also that the ratio of the level of the characteristic in one group to that in the other is equal to a quoted value. For this type of statement

Criteria for evaluating the statement

to be justified, (1) the coefficients of variation of all three quoted statistics should be less than the specified standard; (2) the difference between the two groups with respect to their estimated levels of the characteristic should be significant statistically; and (3) the ratio of the levels in the two groups should not be statistically different from the ratio quoted in the statement.

ILLUSTRATIVE EXAMPLE

The statistical statement given above quotes the same two estimates discussed earlier along with their approximate ratio. The method of evaluating this statement is outlined below.

   1. Determine the coefficients of variation.

$$\hat{X} = .42 \qquad \widehat{SE}(\hat{X}) = .07 \qquad \hat{V}(\hat{X}) = \frac{.07}{.42} = .17$$

$$\hat{Y} = .25 \qquad \widehat{SE}(\hat{Y}) = .04 \qquad \hat{V}(\hat{Y}) = \frac{.04}{.25} = .16$$

$$\frac{\hat{X}}{\hat{Y}} = 1.68 \qquad \hat{V}(\hat{X}/\hat{Y}) \approx [\hat{V}^2(\hat{X}) + \hat{V}^2(\hat{Y})]^{1/2} = [(.17)^2 + (.16)^2]^{1/2} \approx .23$$

(The last result is the approximate coefficient of variation of a ratio estimate if the covariance term is ignored.) Since each coefficient of variation is less than 25%, the statement meets the first test of justification.

2. Determine the statistical difference between the two estimates.

$$z = \frac{\hat{X} - \hat{Y}}{\sqrt{\widehat{Var}(\hat{X}) + \widehat{Var}(\hat{Y})}} = 2.10 \qquad \text{so} \qquad p < .05$$

Thus the two estimates differ from each other statistically, and the statement is acceptable from this point of view.

3. Test that the ratio is not significantly different from the rounded value of 1.7 quoted. To do this, we calculate the standardized ratio given by

$$z = \frac{(\hat{X}/\hat{Y}) - R}{\widehat{SE}(\hat{X}/\hat{Y})}$$

where $R = 1.7$, the quoted level of the ratio, and

$$\widehat{SE}(\hat{X}/\hat{Y}) = \left(\frac{\hat{X}}{\hat{Y}}\right)[\hat{V}^2(\hat{X}) + \hat{V}^2(\hat{Y})]^{1/2} = (1.68)(.23) = .388$$

Then

$$z = \frac{1.68 - 1.70}{.388} = .052$$

which is not significantly different from zero. Thus the statement seems to meet all three criteria and appears to be justified.

Comparisons Including Two Groups of a Population That Are Not Complementary

Another type of statistical statement is one that compares two subgroups of the population that are not complementary to each other with respect to the level of a variable. For example, a report might state, "Among seriously injured patients admitted to hospitals having 1000 or more beds, 2.0% were discharged dead, whereas only 1.2% of seriously injured patients admitted to hospitals having fewer than 100 beds were discharged dead." Let us explore the validity of this statement.

Suppose that hospitals were categorized on the basis of number of beds into the five groups given by

under 100 beds

100–249 beds

250–499 beds

500–999 beds

1000 or more beds

Then there are $2\binom{5}{2}$ or 20 pairwise comparisons, taking sign into consideration, that can be made, and the one listed in the statement above, which implies a significant difference, is just one of them.

Use some method of multiple comparisons

This method is based on the Bonferroni inequility

To avoid making too many statements concerning significance, we should use some method of multiple comparisons to evaluate the significance of pairwise differences. One such method, based on the Bonferroni inequality (5), uses the z statistic based on the standardized difference between the two estimates but refers the z statistic to a critical value of the standard normal distribution that gives a probability α of stating that any one of the possible pairwise differences are significant when there are, in reality, no differences among the population parameters. Some of these critical values are given in table 15.1.

Table 15.1   Critical Values for Tests of Hypotheses Based on an Overall Level of $\alpha = .05$

Number of Possible Comparisons, m	*Critical Value, z**	*Number of Possible Comparisons, m*	*Critical Value, z**
1	1.645	16	2.734
2	1.960	17	2.754
3	2.128	18	2.773
4	2.241	19	2.791
5	2.326	20	2.807
6	2.394	21	2.823
7	2.450	22	2.838
8	2.498	23	2.852
9	2.539	24	2.865
10	2.576	25	2.878
11	2.609	26	2.891
12	2.638	27	2.902
13	2.665	28	2.914
14	2.690	29	2.925
15	2.713	30	2.935

The entries in table 15.1 are actually the $[1 - (.05/m)](100)$ percentiles of the standard normal distribution, where $m = 2\binom{k}{2}$ and $k =$ the number of groups. In the example given above $k = 5$, $m = 2\binom{5}{2} = 20$, and $z^* = 2.807$.

In order for this type of statement to be valid, both estimates $\hat{X}$ and $\hat{Y}$ quoted should have coefficients of variation less than or equal to the stated specification and the standardized difference, $z = (\hat{X} - \hat{Y})/\sqrt{\widehat{\mathrm{Var}}(\hat{X}) + \widehat{\mathrm{Var}}(\hat{Y})}$, should be less than the appropriate value of z^* given in table 15.1.   *Criteria for evaluation*

ILLUSTRATIVE EXAMPLE

For the statement cited at the beginning of this section, suppose that the estimated standard error of the first estimate quoted (2.0%) is equal to .3% and that of the second estimate (1.2%) is equal to .1%. Then (expressing everything as proportions) we have

$$\hat{X} = .02 \quad \widehat{\mathrm{SE}}(\hat{X}) = .003 \qquad \hat{Y} = .012 \quad \widehat{\mathrm{SE}}(\hat{Y}) = .001$$

$$k = 5 \qquad m = 2\binom{5}{2} = 20 \qquad z^* = 2.807$$

The coefficients of variation for both $\hat{X}$ and $\hat{Y}$ are less than 25%, so both statistics meet the standards of reliability. The standardized difference z is

$$z = \frac{.02 - .012}{\sqrt{(.003)^2 + (.001)^2}} = 2.53$$

Since $z < z^*$, we cannot conclude that the two groups are different with respect to fatality rates, and we would conclude that the statistical statement is *not justified*.

The use of multiple comparison methods protects us from the results of fishing expeditions in which the report writer examines all possible differences and then reports only those that appear significant, without adjusting for the fishing process.

Statements Involving Monotonic Relationships

Another type of statement quotes a monotonically increasing or decreasing relationship between the level of a variable and a set of ordered subgroups. For example, a report might state, "Among teenage female youths 13–17 years of age, the prevalence of asymptomatic bacteriuria increased consistently with age." For this type of statement to be justified not only should each of the quoted estimates meet the required specifications, but each of the $k - 1$ differences between consecutive subgroups should be significant when subjected to a test based on the Bonferroni inequality.   *Criteria for evaluation*

ILLUSTRATIVE EXAMPLE

Suppose that the statement quoted above is based on the data shown in table 15.2 for women 13–17 years of age. Since there are five subgroups and only ordered differences between consecutive subgroups are considered, there are four possible ordered differences, and each of the standardized differences should be greater than 2.241, the entry in table 15.1 corresponding to $m = 4$. The z statistics for each of the ordered differences are given below.

Table 15.2   Data for Teenage Females and Prevalence of Asymptomatic Bacteriuria

Age Group, i	Estimated Prevalence Per 100 Persons of Asymptomatic Bacteriuria, $\hat{X}_i$	Estimated Standard Error, $\widehat{SE}(\hat{X}_i)$
13	2.3	.2
14	2.8	.3
15	3.4	.3
16	4.0	.4
17	5.6	.5

For age group 13 versus 14:

$$z = \frac{2.8 - 2.3}{\sqrt{(.2)^2 + (.3)^2}} = 1.39$$

For age group 14 versus 15:

$$z = \frac{3.4 - 2.8}{\sqrt{(.3)^2 + (.3)^2}} = 1.41$$

For age group 15 versus 16:

$$z = \frac{4.0 - 3.4}{\sqrt{(.3)^2 + (.4)^2}} = 1.2$$

For age group 16 versus 17:

$$z = \frac{5.6 - 4.0}{\sqrt{(.4)^2 + (.5)^2}} = 2.50$$

Of the four differences tested, only the last one is greater than the required value of 2.241. Thus the statement is not justified.

Statements of Linear Relationships

Although the statement quoted for the previous example is not justified according to the test used to evaluate it, examination of the data indicates intuitively that a linear relationship might exist between age and prevalence of bacteriuria. A somewhat weaker statement than the one quoted above might be justified from the data. For example, consider this statement: "The prevalence of asymptomatic bacteriuria appears to increase with increase in age among teenage female youths." Unlike the previous statement, this statement does not imply a *consistent* monotonic relationship between age and prevalence of bacteriuria.

One way to evaluate this type of statement is to use one of the many nonparametric tests for trend that are available [see Hollander and Wolfe (2)]. Another way of evaluating this type of statement is to determine whether the slope b of the estimated regression line relating the independent variable x (e.g., age) and the dependent variable y (prevalence of asymptomatic bacteriuria) is significantly different from zero. Letting x_i and y_i be the estimated levels of x and y for the ith subgroup, we have the following estimated slope $\hat{b}$ and its estimated standard error $\widehat{SE}(\hat{b})$:

Use a nonparametric test to evaluate this statement

Or use a z statistic based on the estimated slope and its estimated standard error

$$\hat{b} = \frac{\sum\limits_{i=1}^{k} W_i x_i y_i - \left(\sum\limits_{i=1}^{k} W_i x_i\right)\left(\sum\limits_{i=1}^{k} W_i y_i\right) \bigg/ \sum\limits_{i=1}^{k} W_i}{\sum\limits_{i=1}^{k} W_i x_i^2 - \left(\sum\limits_{i=1}^{k} W_i x_i\right)^2 \bigg/ \sum\limits_{i=1}^{k} W_i}$$

where $W_i = 1/\text{Var}(y_i)$;

$$\widehat{SE}(\hat{b}) = \frac{1}{\left[\sum\limits_{i=1}^{k} W_i x_i^2 - \left(\sum\limits_{i=1}^{k} W_i x_i\right)^2 \bigg/ \sum\limits_{i=1}^{k} W_i\right]^{1/2}}$$

If the ratio z, given by

$$z = \frac{\hat{b}}{\widehat{SE}(\hat{b})}$$

is greater than 1.64 (for a statement implying a direct relationship between x and y) or less than -1.64 (for a statement implying an inverse relationship between x and y), then there is evidence of a significant slope, and the statement is justified.

ILLUSTRATIVE EXAMPLE

For the statement given above we have the values of x_i, y_i, and W_i shown in table 15.3.

Table 15.3   Data of Table 15.2 and Calculations of W_i

Group, i	Age, x_i	Estimated Prevalence Per 100 Persons of Asymptomatic Bacteriuria, y_i	W_i
1	13	2.3	$(1/.2)^2 = 25$
2	14	2.8	$(1/.3)^2 = 11.11$
3	15	3.4	$(1/.3)^2 = 11.11$
4	16	4.0	$(1/.4)^2 = 6.25$
5	17	5.6	$(1/.5)^2 = 4$

Using the information in table 15.3, we have the following calculations:

$$\sum_{i=1}^{5} W_i y_i = 173.782 \qquad \sum_{i=1}^{5} W_i x_i = 815.19 \qquad \sum_{i=1}^{5} W_i x_i^2 = 11,658.31$$

$$\sum_{i=1}^{5} W_i y_i^2 = 573.224 \qquad \sum_{i=1}^{5} W_i x_i y_i = 2,530.422 \qquad \sum_{i=1}^{5} W_i = 57.47$$

$$\hat{b} = \frac{2,530.422 - (815.19)(173.782)/57.47}{11,658.31 - (815.19)^2/57.47} = .6872$$

$$\widehat{SE}(\hat{b}) = \frac{1}{[11,658.31 - (815.19)^2/57.47]^{1/2}} = .1025$$

$$z = \frac{.6872}{.1025} = 6.704$$

Thus the estimated slope $\hat{b}$ is significantly different from zero, and the statistical statement is justified.

The statistical statements categorized in the paragraphs above are not meant to constitute an exhaustive list of statistical statements. Rather, they are examples of the type of statistical statements likely to be encountered in a survey report. And the methods chosen to evaluate them are illustrations of how relatively elementary statistical methods, which make use of standard errors of estimates along with normal theory, can help a reader evaluate whether or not particular statistical statements made in a survey report are justified from the data.

15.3 AN ILLUSTRATION OF SURVEY REPORT WRITING

Let us now illustrate with a simple example how we, as analysts writing a sample survey report, might use the methods shown in the previous sections to write the text of the findings.

Before beginning the writing, we should have at hand the necessary estimates and standard errors for each subgroup of interest. Suppose that we are reporting on a sample survey of hospital discharges in a large state and are interested in the distribution of survival (discharged dead or alive) among patients hospitalized for trauma conditions. Suppose further that the data in tables 15.4 and 15.5 are available to us.

Necessary estimates and standard errors must be available before beginning

Table 15.4   Estimated Number of Trauma Discharges in Large Multistate Region for 10-Year Period

Sex	Age Group (years)	Severity of Injury	ESTIMATED NO. OF DISCHARGES (× 1000)			Percentage Discharged Dead
			Alive	Dead	Total	
male	< 45	mild	1990	10	2000	.5
		moderate	1980	20	2000	1.0
		severe	980	20	1000	2.0
	45–64	mild	1986	14	2000	.7
		moderate	2955	45	3000	1.5
		severe	1455	45	1500	3.0
	65+	mild	1485	15	1500	1.0
		moderate	1966	34	2000	1.7
		severe	965	35	1000	3.5
female	< 45	mild	1994	6	2000	.3
		moderate	992	8	1000	.8
		severe	788	12	800	1.5
	45–64	mild	996	4	1000	.4
		moderate	991	9	1000	.9
		severe	980	20	1000	2.0
	65+	mild	1990	10	2000	.5
		moderate	990	10	1000	1.0
		severe	489	11	500	2.2

Table 15.5   Estimated Coefficients of Variation of Estimated Percentages by Estimated Number of Individuals in Base of Percentage

Estimated No. in Base of Percentage (× 1000)	ESTIMATED PERCENTAGE								
	.1	.5	1.0	1.5	2.0	2.5	3.0	3.5	4.0
100	1.00	.45	.31	.26	.22	.20	.18	.17	.15
500	.40	.20	.14	.11	.10	.09	.08	.07	.07
1000	.30	.14	.10	.08	.07	.06	.06	.05	.05
1500	.26	.12	.08	.07	.06	.05	.05	.04	.04
2000	.22	.10	.07	.06	.05	.04	.04	.04	.03
2500	.20	.09	.06	.05	.04	.04	.04	.03	.03
3000	.18	.08	.06	.05	.04	.04	.03	.03	.03
3500	.17	.08	.05	.04	.04	.03	.03	.03	.03

Prepare list of relationships to be studied

As a first step in analyzing data, we should prepare a list of relationships to be examined. This list should be derived from the specific aims of the survey. Suppose, for example, that the survey on which the data in table 15.4 are based has the specific aims as listed below in the form of questions.

1. Is there a relationship between survival and severity of injury, adjusting for the possible effects of such concomitant variables as age and sex?

2. Is there a relationship between survival and age, adjusting for the possible effects of sex and severity of injury?

3. Is there a relationship between survival and sex, adjusting for the possible effects of age and severity of injury?

Draw graph for question 1

In examining the relationship between survival and severity of injury, adjusting for the effect of age and sex, we might first plot survival against severity for each of the six age-sex groups, as indicated in figure 15.1. Since in each of the six age-sex groups the percentage discharged dead increases with increase in severity of injury, we might wish to make a statement such as this:

Statement based on figure 15.1

In both males and females and within each age group, the percentage of persons discharged dead increases consistently with increase in the severity of injury.

This relatively simple statement involves six statements of a monotonically increasing relationship between severity of injury and percentage discharged dead (one for each of the six age-sex groups). For this statement to be justified the relationship should hold in each age-sex group.

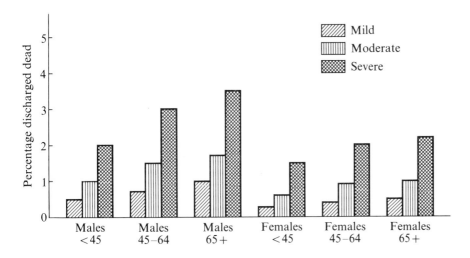

Figure 15.1 Percentage Discharged Dead by Severity of Injury for Males and Females Under 45 Years Old, 45–64 Years Old, and 65 Years Old and Over

Let us now examine the data for males under 45 years of age. The relevant data extracted from tables 15.4 and 15.5 are shown in table 15.6. The standard errors are obtained by first finding the coefficient of variation from table 15.5 and then multiplying the coefficient of variation by the estimated percentage. For example, for males under 45 having mild injuries, the estimated percentage discharged dead, .5%, is based on an estimated 2000 discharges. From table 15.5 we see that this corresponds to a coefficient of variation of .10. On multiplying the estimated percentage discharged dead (.5) by its coefficient of variation (.10), we obtain a standard error of .05.

After obtaining the standard errors, we then test the significance of the differences in the percentage discharged dead between mildly and moderately

Examine relationship in each age-sex group

Table 15.6   Data for Males Under 45

Injury Severity	Estimated Percentage Discharged Dead	Approximate Coefficient of Variation of Estimate	Approximate Standard Error of Estimate
mild	.5	.10	.05
moderate	1.0	.07	.07
severe	2.0	.07	.14

injured persons and between moderately and severely injured persons. These comparisons are shown below.

Mild versus moderate:

$$z = \frac{1.0 - 0.5}{\sqrt{(.05)^2 + (.07)^2}} = 5.81$$

Moderate versus severe:

$$z = \frac{2.0 - 1.0}{\sqrt{(.07)^2 + (.14)^2}} = 6.39$$

Using an overall level of significance set at .05, our critical value of z^* from table 15.1 (with $m = 2$ possible comparisons) is 1.96. Since both the standardized differences shown above exceed 1.96, the statement is justified for males under 45 years of age.

Similar analysis on the five other subgroups would show that all the standardized differences exceed 1.96. Thus the statement quoted above is justified. Hence we infer from the data that there is a relationship between survival and severity within each age and sex group.

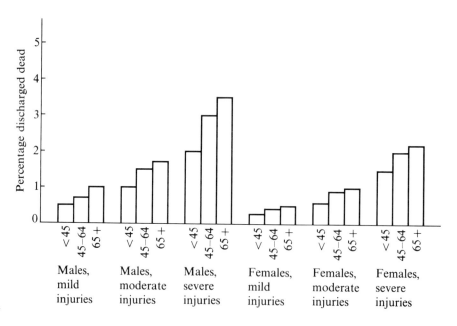

Figure 15.2   Percentage Discharged Dead by Age for Males and Females at Each Level of Severity

The second specific aim suggests that we examine the relationship between survival and age, taking into consideration possible effects of sex and severity of injury. A first step might be to plot survival against age for males and females at level of severity (figure 15.2). Examination of figure 15.2 shows that in each of the six sex-severity groups the percentage discharged dead shows a consistent increase with age. Thus we may wish to make a statement such as the following:

Draw graph for question 2

Statement based figure 15.2

> The percentage discharged dead increases consistently with increase in age, and this relationship holds in males as well as in females and in mildly and moderately injured patients as well as in severely injured patients

However, when the appropriate statistical tests are performed, the *z* scores shown in table 15.7 are obtained.

Examine each subgroup

Table 15.7 *z* Scores for Subgroups Shown in Figure 15.2

	z SCORES	
Sex and Level of Severity	*Age Group < 45 vs. Age Group 45–64*	*Age Group 45–64 vs. Age Group 65 +*
mildly injured males	2.52	2.97
moderately injured males	4.87	1.65
severely injured males	4.87	2.17
mildly injured females	1.16	1.18
moderately injured females	.74	.71
severely injured females	2.54	.78

From the table we see that among males five of the six *z* scores are above the required value of 1.96. However, among females only one of the six *z* scores is above 1.96. On the basis of these *z* scores we might be safer in restricting our statement to males.

For females, if we compute the estimated slope $\hat{b}$ and estimated standard error of $\hat{b}$, we obtain the results shown in table 15.8. Since each of the estimated

Table 15.8 *z* Scores for Females Based on $\hat{b}$ and $\widehat{\text{SE}}(\hat{b})$

Group	*Estimated Slope,* $\hat{b}$	$\widehat{\text{SE}}(\hat{b})$	$z = \hat{b}/\widehat{\text{SE}}(\hat{b})$
mildly injured females	.015	.0015	10.0
moderately injured females	.0037	.0010	3.41
severely injured females	.0150	.0047	3.19

slopes is significantly different from 0, as determined from table 15.1, we are justified in making the following statement concerning females:

> Among mildly, moderately, and severely injured females, there is evidence of an increase in the percentage discharged dead with increase in age.

The complete statement might then read as follows:

Revised statement based on evaluations

> Among mildly, moderately, and severely injured males, the percentage discharged dead increases consistently with increase in age. Among females, whether mildly, moderately, or severely injured, there is evidence of an increase in percentage discharged dead with increase in age

Note that the statement for females is somewhat weaker than the statement for males.

As the discussion above shows, care should be taken by the analyst in making statistical statements. Clearly, a great deal of thought and analysis should go into the writing of a survey report, and sufficient time should be allocated for the data analysis and report writing.

SUMMARY

In this chapter we discussed statistical report writing. In particular, we discussed what should be included as the major components of a statistical report: the background and introduction, the methodology, the results or findings, the discussion, and the summary and conclusions. In addition, we discussed the types of statistical statements commonly found in statistical reports, and we presented methods for evaluating the inferences made in statistical statements.

BIBLIOGRAPHY

The following publications discuss in greater detail the issues raised in this chapter concerning statistical report writing and the evaluation of statistical statements.

1. GONZALEZ, M.; OGUS, J.; SHAPIRO, G.; and TEPPING, B. Standards for discussion and presentation of errors in survey and census data. *Journal of the American Statistical Association* (1975) 70: 1–23.

2. HOLLANDER, M., and WOLFE, D. A. *Nonparametric statistical methods.* New York: Wiley 1973.

3. KOCH, G. G.; FREEMAN, D. H.; and FREEMAN, J. L. Strategies in the multivariate analysis of data from complex surveys. *International Statistical Review* (1975) 43: 59–78.

4. LEVY, P. S., and SIRKEN, M. G. Quality control of statistical reports. *Proceedings of the American Statistical Association: Social Statistics Section* (1972); pp. 356–359.

5. MILLER, R. G. *Simultaneous statistical inference.* New York: McGraw-Hill, 1966.

6. SIRKEN, M. G., and LEVY, P. S. Multiplicity estimation of proportions based on ratios of random variables. *Journal of the American Statistical Association* (1974) 69: 68–73.

7. SIRKEN, M. G.; SHIMIZU, I.; FRENCH, D.; and BROCK, D. *Manual on standards and procedures for reviewing statistical reports.* National Center for Health Statistics, DHEW (unpublished).

Appendix

Table A1   Random Number Table

Line/Col.	(1)	(2)	(3)	(4)	(5)	(6)	(7)	(8)	(9)	(10)	(11)	(12)	(13)	(14)
1	10480	15011	01536	02011	81647	91646	69179	14194	62590	36207	20969	99570	91291	90700
2	22368	46573	25595	85393	30995	89198	27982	53402	93965	34095	52666	19174	39615	99505
3	24130	48390	22527	97265	76393	64809	15179	24830	49340	32081	30680	19655	63348	58629
4	42167	93093	06243	61680	07856	16376	39440	53537	71341	57004	00849	74917	97758	16379
5	37570	39975	81837	16656	06121	91782	60468	81305	49684	60072	14110	06927	01263	54613
6	77921	06907	11008	42751	27756	53498	18602	70659	90655	15053	21916	81825	44394	42880
7	99562	72905	56420	69994	98872	31016	71194	18738	44013	48840	63213	21069	10634	12952
8	96301	91977	05463	07972	18876	20922	94595	56869	69014	60045	18425	84903	42508	32307
9	89579	14342	63661	10281	17453	18103	57740	84378	25331	12568	58678	44947	05585	56941
10	85475	36857	53342	53988	53060	59533	38867	62300	08158	17983	16439	11458	18593	64952
11	28918	69578	88231	33276	70997	79936	56865	05859	90106	31595	01547	85590	91610	78188
12	63553	40961	48235	03427	49626	69445	18663	72695	52180	20847	12234	90511	33703	90322
13	09429	93969	52636	92737	88974	33488	36320	17617	30015	08272	84115	27156	30613	74952
14	10365	61129	87529	85689	48237	52267	67689	93394	01511	26358	85104	20285	29975	89868
15	07119	97336	71048	08178	77233	13916	47564	81056	97735	85977	29372	74461	28551	90707
16	51085	12765	51821	51259	77452	16308	60756	92144	49442	53900	70960	63990	75601	40719
17	02368	21382	52404	60268	89368	19885	55322	44819	01188	65255	64835	44919	05944	55157
18	01011	54092	33362	94904	31273	04146	18594	29852	71685	85030	51132	01915	92747	64951
19	52162	53916	46369	58586	23216	14513	83149	98736	23495	64350	94738	17752	35156	35749
20	07056	97628	33787	09998	42698	06691	76988	13602	51851	45104	88916	19509	25625	58104
21	48663	91245	85828	14346	09172	30163	90229	04734	59193	22178	30421	61666	99904	32812
22	54164	58492	22421	74103	47070	25306	76468	26384	58151	06646	21524	15227	96909	44592
23	32639	32363	05597	24200	13363	38005	94342	28728	35806	06912	17012	64161	18296	22851
24	29334	27001	87637	87308	58731	00256	45834	15398	46557	41135	10307	07684	36188	18510
25	02488	33062	28834	07351	19731	92420	60952	61280	50001	67658	32586	86679	50720	94953
26	81525	72295	04839	96423	24878	82651	66566	14778	76797	14780	13300	87074	79666	95725
27	29676	20591	68086	26432	46901	20849	89768	81536	86645	12659	92259	57102	80428	25280
28	00742	57392	39064	66432	84673	40027	32832	61362	98947	96067	64760	64584	96096	98253
29	05366	04213	25669	26422	44407	44048	37937	63904	45766	66134	75470	66520	34693	90449
30	91921	26418	64117	94305	26766	25940	39972	22209	71500	64568	91402	42416	07844	69618
31	00582	04711	87917	77341	42206	35126	74087	99547	81817	42607	43808	76655	62028	76630
32	00725	69884	62797	56170	86324	88072	76222	36086	84637	93161	76038	65855	77919	88006
33	69011	65795	95876	55293	18988	27354	26575	08625	40801	59920	29841	80150	12777	48501
34	25976	57948	29888	88604	67917	48708	18912	82271	65424	69774	33611	54262	85963	03547
35	09763	83473	73577	12908	30883	18317	28290	35797	05998	41688	34952	37888	38917	88050

Table A.1 (*continued*)

Line/Col.	(1)	(2)	(3)	(4)	(5)	(6)	(7)	(8)	(9)	(10)	(11)	(12)	(13)	(14)
36	91567	42595	27958	30134	04024	86385	29880	99730	55536	84855	29088	09250	79656	73211
37	17955	56349	90999	49127	20044	59931	06115	20542	18059	02008	73708	83517	36103	42791
38	46503	18584	18845	49618	02304	51038	20655	58727	28168	15475	56942	53389	20562	87338
39	92157	89634	94824	78171	84610	82834	09922	25417	44137	48413	25555	21246	35509	20468
40	14577	62765	35605	81263	39667	47358	56873	56307	61607	49518	89656	20103	77490	18062
41	98427	07523	33362	64270	01638	92477	66969	98420	04880	45585	46565	04102	46880	45709
42	34914	63976	88720	82765	34476	17032	87589	40836	32427	70002	70663	88863	77775	69348
43	70060	28277	39475	46473	23219	53416	94970	25832	69975	94884	19661	72828	00102	66794
44	53976	54914	06990	67245	68350	82948	11398	42878	80287	88267	47363	46634	06541	97809
45	76072	29515	40980	07391	58745	25774	22987	80059	39911	96189	41151	14222	60697	59583
46	90725	52210	83974	29992	65831	38857	50490	83765	55657	14361	31720	57375	56228	41546
47	64364	67412	33339	31926	14883	24413	59744	92351	97473	89286	35931	04110	23726	51900
48	08962	00358	31662	25388	61642	34072	81249	35648	56891	69352	48373	45578	78547	81788
49	95012	68379	93526	70765	10592	04542	76463	54328	02349	17247	28865	14777	62730	92277
50	15664	10493	20492	38301	91132	21999	59516	81652	27195	48223	46751	22923	32261	85653
51	16408	81899	04153	53381	79401	21438	83035	92350	36693	31238	59649	91754	72772	02338
52	18629	81953	05520	91962	04739	13092	97662	24822	94730	06496	35090	04822	86774	98289
53	73115	35101	47498	87637	99016	71060	88824	71013	18735	20286	23153	72924	35165	43040
54	57491	16703	23167	49323	45021	33132	12544	41035	80780	45393	44812	12515	98931	91202
55	30405	83946	23792	14422	15059	45799	22716	19792	09983	74353	68668	30429	70735	25499
56	16631	35006	85900	98275	32388	52390	16815	69293	82732	38480	73817	32523	41961	44437
57	96773	20206	42559	78985	05300	22164	24369	54224	35083	19687	11052	91491	60383	19746
58	38935	64202	14349	82674	66523	44133	00697	35552	35970	19124	63318	29686	03387	59846
59	31624	76384	17403	53363	44167	64486	64758	75366	76554	31601	12614	33072	60332	92325
60	78919	19474	23632	27889	47914	02584	37680	20801	72152	39339	34806	08930	85001	87820
61	03931	33309	57047	74211	63445	17361	62825	39908	05607	91284	68833	25570	38818	46920
62	74426	33278	43972	10119	89917	15665	52872	73823	73144	88662	88970	74492	51805	99378
63	09066	00903	20795	95452	92648	45454	69552	88815	16553	51125	79375	97596	16296	66092
64	42238	12426	87025	14267	20979	04508	64535	31355	86064	29472	47689	05974	52468	16834
65	16153	08002	26504	41744	81959	65642	74240	56302	00033	67107	77510	70625	28725	34191
66	21457	40742	29820	96783	29400	21840	15035	34537	33310	06116	95240	15957	16572	06004
67	21581	57802	02050	89728	17937	37621	47075	42080	97403	48626	68995	43805	33386	21597
68	55612	78095	83197	33732	05810	24813	86902	60397	16489	03264	88525	42786	05269	92532
69	44657	66999	99324	51281	84463	60563	79312	93454	68876	25471	93911	25650	12682	73572
70	91340	84979	46949	81973	37949	61023	43997	15263	80644	43942	89203	71795	99533	50501

71	91227	21199	31935	27022	84067	05462	35216	14486	29891	68607	41867	14951	91696	85065
72	50001	38140	66321	19924	72163	09538	12151	06878	91903	18749	34405	56087	82790	70925
73	65390	05224	72958	28609	81406	39147	25549	48542	42627	45233	57202	94617	23772	07896
74	27504	96131	83944	41575	10573	03619	64482	73923	36152	05184	94142	25299	84387	34925
75	37169	94851	39117	89632	00959	16487	65536	49071	39782	17095	02330	74301	00275	48280
76	11508	70225	51111	38351	19444	66499	71945	05422	13442	78675	84031	66938	93654	59894
77	37449	30362	06694	54690	04052	53115	62757	95348	78662	11163	81651	50245	34971	52924
78	46515	70331	85922	38329	57015	15765	97161	17869	45349	61796	66345	81073	49106	79860
79	30986	81223	42416	58353	21532	30502	32305	86482	05174	07901	54339	58861	74818	46942
80	63798	64995	46583	09785	44160	78128	83991	42865	92520	83531	80377	35909	81250	54238
81	82486	84846	99254	67632	43218	50076	21361	64816	51202	88124	41870	52689	51275	83556
82	21885	32906	92431	09060	64297	51674	64126	62570	26123	05155	59194	52799	28225	85762
83	60336	98782	07408	53458	13564	59089	26445	29789	85205	41001	12535	12133	14645	23541
84	43937	46891	24010	25560	86355	33941	25786	54990	71899	15475	95434	98227	21824	19535
85	97656	63175	89303	16275	07100	92063	21942	18611	47348	20203	18534	03862	78095	50136
86	03299	01221	05418	38982	55758	92237	26759	86367	21216	98442	08303	56613	91511	75928
87	79626	06486	03574	17668	07785	76020	79924	25651	83325	88428	85076	72811	22717	50585
88	85636	68335	47539	03129	65651	11977	02510	26113	99447	68645	34327	15152	55230	93448
89	18039	14367	61337	06177	12143	46609	32989	74014	64708	00533	35398	58408	13261	47908
90	08362	15656	60627	36478	65648	16764	53412	09013	07832	41574	17639	82163	60859	75567
91	79556	29068	04142	16268	15387	12856	66227	38358	22478	73373	88732	09443	82558	05250
92	92608	82674	27072	32534	17075	27698	98204	63863	11951	34648	88022	56148	34925	57031
93	23982	25835	40055	67006	12293	02753	14827	23235	35071	99704	37543	11601	35503	85171
94	09915	96306	05908	97901	28395	14186	00821	80703	70426	75647	76310	88717	37890	40129
95	59037	33300	26695	62247	69927	76123	50842	43834	86654	70959	79725	93872	28117	19233
96	42488	78077	69882	61657	34136	79180	97526	43092	04098	73571	80799	76536	71255	64239
97	46764	86273	63003	93017	31204	36692	40202	35275	57306	55543	53203	18098	47625	88684
98	03237	45430	55417	63282	90816	17349	88298	90183	36600	78406	06216	95787	42579	90730
99	86591	81482	52667	61582	14972	90053	89534	76036	49199	43716	97548	04379	46370	28672
100	38534	01715	94964	87288	65680	43772	39560	12918	80537	62738	19636	51132	25739	56947

Abridged from *Handbook of Tables for Probability and Statistics*, Second Edition, edited by William H. Beyer (Cleveland: The Chemical Rubber Company 1968.) Reproduced by permission of the publishers, The Chemical Rubber Company.

Table A2   Normal Curve Areas

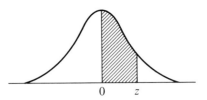

z	.00	.01	.02	.03	.04	.05	.06	.07	.08	.09
0.0	.0000	.0040	.0080	.0120	.0160	.0199	.0239	.0279	.0319	.0359
0.1	.0398	.0438	.0478	.0517	.0557	.0596	.0636	.0675	.0714	.0753
0.2	.0793	.0832	.0871	.0910	.0948	.0987	.1026	.1064	.1103	.1141
0.3	.1179	.1217	.1255	.1293	.1331	.1368	.1406	.1443	.1480	.1517
0.4	.1554	.1591	.1628	.1664	.1700	.1736	.1772	.1808	.1844	.1879
0.5	.1915	.1950	.1985	.2019	.2054	.2088	.2123	.2157	.2190	.2224
0.6	.2257	.2291	.2324	.2357	.2389	.2422	.2454	.2486	.2517	.2549
0.7	.2580	.2611	.2642	.2673	.2704	.2734	.2764	.2794	.2823	.2852
0.8	.2881	.2910	.2939	.2967	.2995	.3023	.3051	.3078	.3106	.3133
0.9	.3159	.3186	.3212	.3238	.3264	.3289	.3315	.3340	.3365	.3389
1.0	.3413	.3438	.3461	.3485	.3508	.3531	.3554	.3577	.3599	.3621
1.1	.3643	.3665	.3686	.3708	.3729	.3749	.3770	.3790	.3810	.3830
1.2	.3849	.3869	.3888	.3907	.3925	.3944	.3962	.3980	.3997	.4015
1.3	.4032	.4049	.4066	.4082	.4099	.4115	.4131	.4147	.4162	.4177
1.4	.4192	.4207	.4222	.4236	.4251	.4265	.4279	.4292	.4306	.4319
1.5	.4332	.4345	.4357	.4370	.4382	.4394	.4406	.4418	.4429	.4441
1.6	.4452	.4463	.4474	.4484	.4495	.4505	.4515	.4525	.4534	.4545
1.7	.4554	.4564	.4573	.4582	.4591	.4599	.4608	.4616	.4625	.4633
1.8	.4641	.4649	.4656	.4664	.4671	.4678	.4686	.4693	.4699	.4706
1.9	.4713	.4719	.4726	.4732	.4738	.4744	.4750	.4756	.4761	.4767
2.0	.4772	.4778	.4783	.4788	.4793	.4798	.4803	.4808	.4812	.4817
2.1	.4821	.4826	.4830	.4834	.4838	.4842	.4846	.4850	.4854	.4857
2.2	.4861	.4864	.4868	.4871	.4875	.4878	.4881	.4884	.4887	.4890
2.3	.4893	.4896	.4898	.4901	.4904	.4906	.4909	.4911	.4913	.4916
2.4	.4918	.4920	.4922	.4925	.4927	.4929	.4931	.4932	.4934	.4936
2.5	.4938	.4940	.4941	.4943	.4945	.4946	.4948	.4949	.4951	.4952
2.6	.4953	.4955	.4956	.4957	.4959	.4960	.4961	.4962	.4963	.4964
2.7	.4965	.4966	.4967	.4968	.4969	.4970	.4971	.4972	.4973	.4974
2.8	.4974	.4975	.4976	.4977	.4977	.4978	.4979	.4979	.4980	.4981
2.9	.4981	.4982	.4982	.4982	.4984	.4984	.4985	.4985	.4986	.4986
3.0	.4987	.4987	.4987	.4988	.4988	.4989	.4989	.4989	.4990	.4990

Abridged from Table I of *Statistical Tables and Formulas* by A. Hald (New York: John Wiley & Sons, Inc., 1952). Reproduced by permission of A. Hald and the publishers, John Wiley & Sons, Inc.

Answers to Exercises

CHAPTER 2

1. (a) $\bar{X} = 370$; $\sigma_x = 277.20$; $\sigma_x^2 = 76,840$

   (b) 10 possible samples

   (d) $E(\bar{x}) = 370$

   (e) $\text{Var}(\bar{x}) = 28,815$; $\text{SE}(\bar{x}) = 169.7498$

   (f) 5 possible samples

   (g) $E(\bar{x}) = 370$; $\text{Var}(\bar{x}) = 4802.5$

3. (c) 15 possible samples

   (d) $E(r) = .537$; $R = .529$

   (e) $\text{Var}(r) - .02775$

CHAPTER 3

2. $2.073746998 \times 10^{14}$

3. $p_y = .275$; $.137 \leq P_y \leq .413$

4. $N = 1200$; $n = 40$; $y = 12$; $y' = 360$; $z = 8$; $\hat{\sigma}_z = .49$; $\widehat{\text{SE}}(z/y) = .139$; $.40 \leq P \leq .94$

5. $p_y = .30$; $.16 \leq P_y \leq .44$

6. (a) $p_y = .275$; $n = 3276$

   (b) $n = 84$

7. $n = 216$

8. (a)

Random Number	No. of Visits
06	0
08	0
14	4
22	0
17	7
03	1

$\bar{x} = 2$; $s_x^2 = 8.4$

   (b) $.30 \leq \bar{X} \leq 3.70$

   (c) $0 \leq X \leq 100.54$

   (d) $0 \leq P_y \leq .87$

CHAPTER 4

1. (a) $n = 40$; $p_y = .05$

   (b) $0 \leq P_y \leq .106$

   (c) $E(p_y) = .0333$; $\text{Var}(p_y) = .000139$; $\widehat{\text{Var}}(p_y) = .000812$

   (d) $P_y = .0333$; $\text{Var}(p_y) = .00054$

313

2. (a) $n = 24$; $p_y = 0$

(b) We cannot construct a confidence interval.

(c) $E(p_y) = .0333$; $\text{Var}(p_y) = .000278$

(d) $\text{Var}(p_y) = .001082$

3. (a) $p_y = .04167$; $\widehat{\text{Var}}(p_y) = .001389$; $0 \le P_y \le .115$

(b) $\widehat{\text{Var}}(p_y) = .001389$ (repeated systematic);
$\text{Var}(p_{sys}) = .000278$ (systematic 1 in 5)

4. $N = 162$; $m = 6$; $n = 18$; for P_y:
$.0889 \le P_y \le .4668$; for X: $706.41 \le X \le 183.59$

5. (a) $\bar{x} = 2.33$; $s^2 = 4.0$; $1.383 \le \bar{X} \le 3.277$

CHAPTER 6

1. (b) Proportional allocation:

Stratum	n_h
1	20
2	33
3	7
4	40
	100

(c) Optimum allocation (based on income):

Stratum	n_h
1	33
2	33
3	7
4	27
	100

(d) Optimum allocation (based on age):

Stratum	n_h
1	24
2	39
3	5
4	32
	100

(f) $\sigma_{bx}^2 - 11.05$; $\sigma_{wx}^2 = 10.2$; $\sigma_x^2 = 21.25$

2. (a)

Stratum	n_h
high	28
medium	6
low	6
	40

(b) $\bar{x}_{str} = 80.4$

(c) $\widehat{\text{Var}}(\bar{x}_{str}) = 3.82$; $76.57 \le \bar{X} \le 84.23$

(d) $\widehat{\text{Var}}(\bar{x}) = 3.72$; $76.62 \le \bar{X} \le 84.18$

3. Costs: screening, $5; interviewing, $25; total amount available, $5000. For stratum 1: total cost = $11.25; for stratum 2: total cost = $8.75; for stratum 3: total cost = $7.50. $n_1 = 140.11$; $n_2 = 317.74$; $n_3 = 85.80$; total sample size = 542

4. (a) $\bar{x} = 80.4$; $s^2 = 153.94$; $\widehat{\text{Var}}(\bar{x}) = 3.72$;
$77.23 \le \bar{X} \le 83.57$

(b) $\bar{x}_{pstr} = 79.825$; $\widehat{\text{Var}}(\bar{x}_{pstr}) = 4.00$;
90% confidence interval: $76.535 \le \bar{X} \le 83.115$

CHAPTER 7

1. (a) $24.131 \le \bar{X} \le 30.851$

(b) $r = 7.376$; $\widehat{\text{SE}}(r) = .522$; $6.353 \le R \le 8.399$

(c) $r = 1256$; $\widehat{\text{SE}}(r) - .007662$; $.1106 \le R \le .1406$

(d) $x'' = 19,914.07$; $\widehat{\text{SE}}(x'') = 1409.4$;
$17,151.65 \le X \le 22,676.49$

(e) $r = .1437$. For income less than $200 per week:
$n = 12$; $\widehat{\text{SE}}(r) = .0155$; $.1133 \le R \le .1741$. For income greater than $200 per week: $n = 21$;
$\widehat{\text{SE}}(r) = .00854$; $.102 \le R \le .135$

CHAPTER 10

1. $x'_{clu} = 280$; $\hat{\sigma}_{1x} = 3.16$; $\widehat{\text{SE}}(x'_{clu}) = 52.8$;
$176.47 \le X \le 383.53$; $r_{clu} = .019$;
$\hat{\sigma}_{1y} = 57.81$; $\widehat{\text{SE}}(\bar{x}_{clu}) = 1.76$; $\widehat{\text{SE}}(\bar{y}_{clu}) = 32.21$;
$\widehat{\text{SE}}(r_{clu}) = .0023$; $.0144 \le R \le .0236$

2. (a) $n = 654.7$

(c) $m = 33$

3. (b) $x'_{clu} = 7293$; $\bar{x}_{clu} = 221$; $\hat{\sigma}_{1x} = 143.94$;
$\widehat{\text{SE}}(x'_{clu}) = 1273.46$; $4797.02 \le X \le 9788.98$

(c) $y'_{clu} = 99$; $\bar{y}_{clu} = 3$; $\hat{\sigma}_{1y} = 2.63$;
$\widehat{SE}(y'_{clu}) = 23.27$; $53.40 \le Y \le 144.61$

(d) $r_{clu} = .0136$; $\widehat{SE}(\bar{y}_{clu}) = .7051$;
$\widehat{SE}(\bar{x}_{clu}) = 38.59$; $\widehat{SE}(r_{clu}) = .0033$;
$.0071 \le R \le .0201$

4. (a) $\bar{x}_{clu} = 221$; $\bar{y}_{clu} = 353$; $r_{clu} = .6261$;
$Y = 7217$; $x''_{clu} = 4518.29$; $\hat{\sigma}_{1y} = 214.32$;
$\widehat{SE}(\bar{y}_{clu}) = 57.46$; $\widehat{SE}(r_{clu}) = .025$;
$4160.59 \le X \le 4875.99$

(b) $r_{clu} = .0085$; $x''_{clu} = 61.34$; $\hat{\sigma}_{1x} = 2.63$;
$\bar{x}_{clu} = 3$; $\widehat{SE}(\bar{x}_{clu}) = .7051$; $\hat{\sigma}_{1y} = 214.32$;
$\bar{y}_{clu} = 353$; $\widehat{SE}(\bar{y}_{clu}) = 57.46$; $\widehat{SE}(r_{clu}) = .002$;
$32.35 \le X \le 90.33$

CHAPTER 11

2. $x'_{clu} = 700$; $\bar{x}_{clu} = 23.33$; $\widehat{SE}(x'_{clu}) = 136.4$;
$432.65 \le X \le 967.35$

3. $r_{clu} = .0189$; $x'_{clu} = 700$; $\bar{x}_{clu} = 23.3$; $y'_{clu} = 36,975$;
$\bar{y}_{clu} = 1232.5$; $\widehat{SE}(\bar{x}_{clu}) = 4.547$; $\widehat{SE}(\bar{y}_{clu}) = 83.150$;
$\widehat{SE}(r_{clu}) = .0024$; $.0142 \le R \le .0236$

4. $m = 280$

5. (a) $x'_{clu} = 13,420$; $\bar{x}_{clu} = 1342$; $\widehat{SE}(x'_{clu}) = 2513.3$;
$8,493.93 \le X \le 18,346.07$

(b) $y'_{clu} = 70$; $\bar{y}_{clu} = 7$; $\widehat{SE}(y'_{clu}) = 34.61$;
$14 \le Y \le 137.836$

(c) $\bar{x}_{clu} = 1342$; $\widehat{SE}(\bar{x}_{clu}) = 251.33$;
$849.4 \le \bar{X} \le 1834.6$; $\bar{y}_{clu} = 7$;
$\widehat{SE}(\bar{y}_{clu}) = 3.461$; $.22 \le \bar{Y} \le 13.78$

(d) $\bar{\bar{x}}_{clu} = 223.67$; $\widehat{SE}(\bar{\bar{x}}_{clu}) = 41.89$;
$141.57 \le \bar{\bar{X}} \le 305.77$; $\bar{\bar{y}}_{clu} = 1.17$;
$\widehat{SE}(\bar{\bar{y}}_{clu}) = .5269$; $.04 \le \bar{\bar{Y}} \le 2.30$

(e) $r_{clu} = .005$; $\widehat{SE}(r_{clu}) = .0016$;
$.0018 \le R \le .0082$

6. (a) $x'_{clu} = 14,685$; $\hat{\sigma}_{1x} = 1057.9$; $\widehat{SE}(x'_{clu}) = 7052.7$;
$2,937 \le X \le 28,508.23$

(b) $y'_{clu} = 100$; $\hat{\sigma}_{1y} = 6.708$; $\widehat{SE}(y'_{clu}) = 44.72$;
$20 \le Y \le 187.65$

(c) $\bar{x}_{clu} = 1468.5$; $\widehat{SE}(\bar{x}_{clu}) = 705.27$;
$86.18 \le \bar{X} \le 2850.8$; $\bar{y}_{clu} = 10$;
$\widehat{SE}(\bar{y}_{clu}) = 4.472$; $1.23 \le \bar{Y} \le 18.77$

(d) $\bar{\bar{x}}_{clu} = 244.75$; $\widehat{SE}(\bar{\bar{x}}_{clu}) = 117.545$;
$14.36 \le \bar{\bar{X}} \le 475.14$; $\bar{\bar{y}}_{clu} = 1.67$;
$\widehat{SE}(\bar{\bar{y}}_{clu}) = .7453$; $.21 \le \bar{\bar{Y}} \le 3.13$

(e) $r_{clu} = .0068$; $\widehat{SE}(\bar{y}_{clu}) = 4.472$; $\bar{y}_{clu} = 10$;
$\widehat{SE}(\bar{x}_{clu}) = 705.27$; $\bar{x}_{clu} = 1468.5$;
$\widehat{SE}(r_{clu}) = .0002$; $.0064 \le R \le .0072$

7. $\sigma_{1x}^2 = 277,768.4$; $\sigma_x^2 = 9343.43$; $\delta_x = .791$

8. $\bar{n} = 1$

CHAPTER 12

1. $M = 25$; $N = 22,965$

Random Number Selected	Health Center
10480	8
22368	25
9429	8
10365	8
7119	8

2. take $\bar{n} = 2$ from clusters of size $\bar{N} = 9$

3. $M = 37$; $N = 49$; $\sigma_{1y}^2 = 25.69$; $\bar{Y} = 7.135$;
$\bar{\bar{Y}} = 5.388$; $m = 28$

4. $\bar{x}_{clu} = 5.62$; $\bar{y}_{clu} = 77.2$; $\widehat{SE}(r_{clu}) = .0054$;
$.06 \le R \le .08$

Index

Boldface numerals indicate the pages on which a term or concept is defined.